*Abét · Prenzlau · Richter*

# Prenatal Diagnosis of Foetal Malformations and Diseases

*Teaching Atlas of Amniofoetography*

*by Lothar Abét,*

*Peter Prenzlau and*

*Johannes Richter*

*with technical assistance*

*contributed by*

*Rainer Bollmann,*

*Horst Schilling and*

*Wolfram Natho*

*Akademie-Verlag Berlin*

# Prenatal Diagnosis of Foetal Malformations and Diseases

*Teaching Atlas of Amniofoetography*

*with 88 Figures and 3 Tables*

Team of authors:
Doz. Dr. sc. med. *Lothar Abét*, specialist in radiology, gynaecology and obstetrics, senior physician at the Institute of Radiological Diagnosis (Director: Prof. Dr. sc. med. *M. Lüning*), School of Medicine (Charité), Humboldt-Universität zu Berlin – Head of the Division of Ultrasonic Diagnosis

Doz. Dr. sc. med. *Peter Prenzlau*, specialist in gynaecology and obstetrics, senior physician at the Department of Gynaecology and Obstetrics (Director: Prof. Dr. med. habil. *H. Bayer*), School of Medicine (Charité), Humboldt-Universität zu Berlin

Dr. sc. med. *Johannes Richter*, specialist in radiology, medical superintendant

Translated into English by *W. Ghantus*, Berlin

**Front cover:** Normal foetogram.
**Back cover:** Normal foetogram.

ISBN 3-05-500611-9

Erschienen im Akademie-Verlag Berlin,
Leipziger Straße 3–4, O-1086 Berlin

Printed in Germany
Satz und Druck: Druckhaus Köthen GmbH, O-4370 Köthen
Lektor: Karl Abel
Gestaltung: Sirko Wahsner
LSV 2145
Bestellnummer: 763 920 7 (9173)

# Contents

## Prefatory note

Tempestuous progress of sonographic facilities for prenatal detection of foetal malformations and diseases has necessarily resulted in substantial decline in the use of amniofoetography. Yet, substantial decline does not mean abandonment at all or fall into oblivion. Amniofoetography is used at present and will certainly continue to be used with benefit in the foreseeable future to cope with dubious findings of ultrasound diagnosis and, perhaps, also to support "secured" diagnoses which may lead to decisions with serious implications for mother and child. It has been particularly this aspect of rare indications that has encouraged the authors to respond to the demand for a competent illustrated account of important findings so far obtained from that method. This is actually a compendium of equal interest for the experienced and unexperienced, carrying substantial information on efficacy, limits, and indications of amniofoctography together with a strategic programme for its use within the complex network of diagnostic tools.

This "Atlas of Amniofoetography" by Abet, Prenzlau, and Richter, to which contributions were made by several specialists of the Department of Gynaecology and Obstetrics and the Institute of Radiological Diagnosis at Charité, is a product of genuine interdisciplinary teamwork. Born out of practice, it has been designed for use in practice. Modern obstetrics is no longer thinkable without amniofoetography, since the latter has become interconnected with ultrasound diagnosis as well as with other modern complementary methods, such as chorionic biopsy, foetoscopy, and also genetic investigations. Viewed from the position of the obstetrician, this Atlas is likely to open up access to an area that is not free from doubt and that is somewhat burdened with moral-ethic and legal problems. The authors, therefore, have taken a courageous step. May their courage be accompanied by real success, and may this be reflected in widespread dissemination of this book among the widest possible circles of practitioners to the benefit of mother and child.

*H. Bayer*
*M. Lüning*

## Preface

X-ray diagnosis, primarily in conjunction with amniofoetography, used to be the only way for prenatal detection of foetal malformations, before the ultrasound era had begun to make its way into obstetrics. When ultrasound had been, finally, introduced to obstetric diagnosis, a suspicion of monstrous malformation in the early days was still considered as some sort of an accidental sideline finding which had to be confirmed and cleared up by complementary amniofoetography. Ultrasound and X-ray techniques and hardware have ever since undergone tempestuous development. The treasure of experience in X-ray diagnosis which had become accumulated in the course of time and now provided a lead proved to be helpful in interpreting ultrasonic findings, while, on the other hand, growing resolution power of ultrasound equipment together with growing experience of examiners enabled continuously improving interpretation of radiographs. Charité, too, has seen increasing cooperation between the Department of Gynaecology and Obstetrics and the Institute of Radiological Diagnosis, and this proved to be conductive to parallel progress of amniofoetography and ultrasonic diagnosis. The authors have performed 361 amniofoetographies within ten years, from 1976 to 1988, some of them being accompanied by invasive methods for complementary foetal examination. This relatively low figure produces evidence to the stringent criteria used on indication.

The author's efforts for prenatal diagnosis led to the establishment of an interdisciplinary team, in 1985. That team was set up for the explicit purpose of perinatal diagnosis and therapy of foetal malformations and diseases. This means that children involved in prenatal diagnosis, in the first place, will be postnatally looked after in long-term programmes. Included in the team are obstetricians, radiologists, neonatologists, paediatric surgeons, neurosurgeons, geneticists, cardiologists, biochemists, and paediatric pathologists. All of them are affiliated to institutes and departments in one and the same compound, which is an invaluable advantage. We are fully satisfied that the growing demands on perinatal medicine as well as on persistent reduction of perinatal mortality and morbidity can be met only by an approach of such complex nature.

Notwithstanding the advent of sonography for highly subtle diagnosis, amniofoetography has retained its position in the authors' spectrum of diagnostic approaches. Similar developments are assumed to take place at numerous medical centres, and interest in amniofoetography has been strongly expressed at meetings and postgraduate courses, which, together with repeated encouragement, has prompted the authors to communicate their own experience in the form of this Atlas. It will, hopefully, help to provide inspiration to other colleagues also interested in the subject and to cut short for them the long road of collecting experience which is certainly quite tedious due to relatively infrequent indications for amniofoetography.

*L. Abét*
*P. Prenzlau*
*J. Richter*

# 1.

## Historic account

Tempestuous progress of radiological diagnosis has been affected, last but not least, by obstetrics and related medical problems. While radiographs of pregnancy conditions had been used for diagnosis even in the past, the advent of new positive contrast media opened up the possibility of direct representation of the embryonic cavity and the entire foetus. *Menees* et al. (1930) as well as *Kerr* and *McKay* (1933) were the first to report introduction of water-soluble contrast media into the amniotic cavity. This was the birth hour of **"amniography"**, that is indirect representation of the foetus in the mother's body by contrasting of amniotic fluid. Other examiners (*Erbslöh*, 1941/42, 1942a, b, c; *Utzuki* and *Hashidzume*, 1941) injected fat-soluble contrast media which dissolved in the fatty vernix caseosa of the foetus and thus enabled its direct representation. That approach has ever since been called **"foetography"**. Use of both methods and their combination, **"amniofoetography" (AFG)**, has been reported time and again throughout all subsequent decades (*Queenan* and *Gadow*, 1970; *Da Cunha* et al., 1974; *Rubino* and *Messana*, 1974, 1976; *Ang* et al., 1975; *Vincenzoni* et al., 1975; *Hesseldahl* et al., 1980; *Fernhoff* et al., 1980; *Christensen* et al., 1982). The development taken by AFG certainly cannot be called spectacular, but it has been spreading all over the globe, as may be seen from countless publications in different languages.

More details on the development of AFG as well as on its value, indications, methods, symptomatology, and risks, some of them illustrated and supplemented with lists of cases and references, have been published by *Fochem* (1967), *Noonan* (1974), *Halle* et al. (1977), *Leitsmann* et al. (1980), *Skovbo* and *Smith-Jensen* (1981) as well as by *Balsam* and *Weiss* (1981). *Krause* (1983) made reference to most recent experience and correctly emphasized the important position of AFG in modern obstetric diagnosis.

The requirements of AFG in terms of hardware and methodology are just as low as the molestation inflicted on the patient, while the informative potential is really great owing to relatively easy interpretation. Nevertheless, AFG has so far failed to make a decisive breakthrough. This probably may be attributable to unsubstantiated fear of clearly increased risk which has assumed nearly mystic dimensions. Amniocentesis, part of and prerequisite for AFG, is performed much more often despite comparable risk. Radiation load is the only additional risk, but this has never impeded medically necessary developments.

Attitudes towards AFG throughout the decades of its existence had been characterised by the development of alternative or complementary diagnostic methods. The beginnings were rather determined by scientific interest, in the first place. Substantial insights have been gained thanks to AFG. *Erhardt* (1937) found that the foetus is continuously drinking amniotic fluid, a condition of diagnostic implications. Reifferscheid and *Schliemann* (1939) in a publication, two years later, reported that the foetus because of intra-uterine respiratory movements took up amniotic fluid also into the bronchopulmonary tract. The same phenomenon was recorded by *Szendi* (1940) from a foetus, eight weeks of age. *McLain* (1963) on the basis of 75 amniograms, taken in the 20th through 40th weeks of pregnancy, observed steady increase in motility of the gastro-intestinal tract in the course of foetal development.

The field of indications has become quite narrow now, but it used to be much wider before. *Möbius* (1967) in a comprehensive survey listed the following indications for amniofoetography:

I. Proceeding from the uterus –
(a) Assessment of uterus wall during pregnancy or birth to look for malformations or myoma not detectable by soft tissue radiation techniques;
(b) Scientific observation of uterus contractions in various phases during pregnancy and at childbirth;
II. Proceeding from the child –
(c) Sexing;
(d) Scientific observation of embryonic movement;
(e) Retardation of childbirth;
(f) Hydrops foetus universalis;
(g) Malformations in embryonic soft tissue;
III. Proceeding from embryonic accessories –
(h) Localisation of placenta;
(i) Retention of umbilical cord.

Ultrasonic diagnosis in obstetrics, diagnostic amniocentesis, determination from serum and amniotic fluid of alpha-foetoproteins, and genetic cytology are some of the new diagnostic methods which have actually eliminated earlier situations in differential diagnosis, such as suspicion of hydatide mole,

# 2.

dubious intrauterine embryonic death, foetal maturity rating, retardation of childbirth, malpresentation of foetus, placental localisation, resistance of uterine scar following caesarean section etc., in that these situations are no longer a subject for AFG. The same is true for preparations for intrafoetal intraperitoneal transfusion in cases of rhesus incompatibility. Owing to the advanced technical standards of sonography and high skills of experienced examiners AFG can be abandoned even in a great number of cases with findings supporting suspicion of malformations. It appears to be paradoxical that modern obstetric ultrasonic diagnosis and alpha-foetoprotein determination have resulted in qualitatively more exacting demands on AFG (*Halle* et al., 1977; *Leitsmann* et al., 1980; *Balsam* and *Weiss*, 1981; *Zanke*, 1983). Persistent advance towards diagnosis of relatively obscure syndromes of malformation together with an upswing in therapeutic possibilities in the context of neonatology and paediatric surgery have given AFG an established position in the process of antenatal diagnosis.

## Methods for prenatal diagnosis of malformations

Generations of obstetricians have been preoccupied with the desire and quest for early detection of foetal maldevelopment, before parturition. Ignorance about the genesis of maldevelopment and helplessness in prenatal diagnosis have inflicted untold suffering on countless patients and their families. Decisive change has been brought about only by introduction of modern diagnostic and therapeutic methods to the search for congenital malformations and intra-uterine diseases. While in the past members of families with hereditary chromosomal abnormalities or metabolic diseases had to be discouraged from full-term pregnancy, these families today can enjoy the cheerful experience of birth of a healthy child, owing to the achievement of prenatal diagnosis.

However, should a foetal disease be realised by prenatal diagnosis, the obstetrician will not find himself confronted with the problem all of a sudden in the delivery room. The patient can be guided beforehand. Treatment of a viable child can be prepared. Precautions can be taken to cope with complications to be expected at childbirth. Pregnancy may be prematurely terminated in case of need. Finally, briefing and education of parents can be initiated in good time. Delivery as such can be performed and controlled with due consideration of the infant's disease. Termination of pregnancy, of course, will be the approach to non-viable malformations. Time and place of delivery can be planned in advance to have all specialists and adequate equipment available for postnatal immediate action. The prognosis of malformed children and of those with intrauterine diseases can be favourably influenced by early diagnosis and by interdisciplinary cooperation between gynaecologists, neonatologists, paediatric surgeons, neurosurgeons, geneticists, and radiologists.

In the diagnosis of malformations, a decisive role is played, no doubt, by sonography. Ultrasonic diagnosis has not only revolutionised prenatal diagnosis, but it has become a predominant discipline in its own right in perinatal medicine.

### 2.1. Ultrasonic diagnosis

Thirty years have passed ever since *Ian Donald* has performed a pioneer action in publishing his first results, 1958, after having worked on ultrasound for gynaecological diagnosis since 1955. At the beginning, the procedure received little attention and was sceptionally appraised even by the inventor, but in the meantime it has become an established method and has been accepted worldwide thanks to intensive cooperation between medical practitioners, on the one hand, and engineers, on the other. The underlying working principle is simple; it is based on echo tracking along the interface in between tissues which differ by acoustic impedance. The procedure is non-invasive and is harmless to mother and foetus and is, consequently, reproducible as often as necessary. Transition took place in a historically short period of time from the A-scan of minor informative power to the two-dimensional B-scan and from compound scanner to high-resolution real-time instruments.

The spectrum of prenatally detectable malformations has enormously grown owing to the introduction of modern hardware. More than 200 foetopathological conditions are sonographically detectable today. Possible differentiation of intrafoetal structures has opened up a brandnew dimension in prenatal diagnosis. Accurate knowledge of foetal sonographic anatomy is a prerequisite for proper use of the method. Major anatomic deviations, such as anencephalus, hydrocephalus, and hydrops, would not cause problems in diagnosis, whereas minor sono-anatomic abnormalities will be grasped only by an experienced examiner. A multi-step programme for sonographic monitoring of pregnant women has been devised, with the view to enhancing diagnostic accuracy and is described in greater detail in Chapter 9 (Diagnostic strategy ...). Probands giving rise to suspicion of foetal malformation or exhibiting indicative signs will be transferred to a larger centre for detailed diagnosis.

Roughly 70 measurable parameters and indices are being used at present to rule out or confirm foetal malformation, including assessment of intracerebral, intrathoracic, and intra-abdominal structures, epiphyseal spacing, eye distance, mandibular length, undeveloped fingers, facial profile, vertebral column etc. Parameters for purely morphological determination are increasingly supplemented in importance with functional diagnosis, that is monitoring of foetal functions, such as sleeping-waking rhythm, motility behaviour, thoracic excursions, and swallowing movements.



### 2.2. Amniocentesis

Ever since foetal cells have been successfully cultured and alpha-foetoproteins determined from amniotic fluid (*Steele* et al., 1966), amniocentesis has proved to be a standard method properly applicable to prenatal diagnosis of genetic defects and has been used worldwide. It is also used for diagnosis of infections and for measurement of numerous laboratory parameters.

### 2.3. Foetoscopy

Access to the pregnant uterus had become possible through amniocentesis, and this paved the road for the invention of a high-sensitivity endoscope by which the foetus could be watched. Intra-uterine inspection of the foetus was the purpose of the exercise to rule out or identify foetal malformations which had escaped common diagnostic methods before or had not been reliably identifiable. Malformations of vertebral column, extremities, and face (schistasis) were of particular interest.

Foetoscopy, introduced twelve years ago, is being used as a routine procedure by a number of medical centres. The instrument is transabdominally introduced into the embryonic cavity under ultrasonic control, with the patient being in local anaesthesia. Bores are provided next to the lenses to insert cannulae and biopsy forceps. The risk of abortion associated to this method is not higher than that resulting from amniocentesis, provided that the method is used by experienced examiners at appropriate centres. Foetoscopy and sonography today are competing each other. Ultrasound instruments have become available, in the meantime, to handle most of the problems of interest. Emphasis, consequently, has been shifted to collection of foetal blood and biopsy of foetal tissue. Foetal blood is aspirated from umbilical cord vessels at the placental insertion. Blood testing is undertaken, for example, for diagnosis of haemoglobin or coagulation disorders, metabolic shortcomings or immune defects. Diagnosis of foetal myopathies, metabolic diseases, and dermatoses would required collection of foetal tissue from skin, liver, and muscles. Punch biopsy of intrafoetal solid growths can be helpful in tumour identification.

# 3.

## 2.4. Chorion biopsy

Conceptionalised as early as in 1968 (*Mohr*), the method was adopted in China and the USSR in the mid-seventies and has been practised, in the meantime, by several teams. Chorion biopsy is an enrichment to prenatal diagnosis and has substantially reduced the time one had to wait for the result of cytogenetic investigation. Possible access to chorionic tissue has enables its sampling as of the eighth week of pregnancy, with appropriate instruments being transcervically or transabdominally introduced under ultrasonic control and without anaesthesia. Sexing, chromosomal analysis, haemoglobin disorders or leucodystrophy are some of the indications for chorion biopsy. The method, used in DNA technology, will help to open up new areas.

## Methods of amniofoetography

AFG is comparable to amniocentesis but is supplemented with intra-amniotic application of water-soluble and fat-soluble contrast media to produce a general image of the abdominal cavity at pre-selected p.i. (post injectionem) junctures. The following aspects can be covered by numerous methodological and technological variants which have been introduced, ever since the invention of the tecnique:

- Type and quantity of contrast media administered;
- Point of injection;
- Mode of diagnostic radiography and exposure data;
- Time of diagnostic radiography and steps of documentation;
- Other conditions of diagnostic radiography, such as radiation shielding, instruments, etc.

Numerous studies have been conducted, in the meantime, into possible complications and risks of both amniocentesis and amniofoetography. These together with many case reports have been conductive to several methodological conclusions. Certain diagnostic procedures have been adopted in the wake of the advent of more modern diagnostic methods, such as ultrasound, alpha-foetoprotein determination, and cytogenetic tests. Today, the risk associated with the investigation has been reduced to an acceptable level owing to stringent criteria for indication, thorough preparatory examinations of the patient concerned, clinical, sonographic, and in terms of laboratory chemistry, performance of the diagnostic procedure by most modern rules of asepsis and antisepsis, and most up-to-date standards of the X-ray process. Risk and effort must be justifiable by the relevance of the diagnostic question to which an answer is sought.

Amniocentesis is performed in a non-placental area under strict observance of aseptic conditions, with the proband in local anaesthesia. Part of the amniotic fluid may be slowly drained off in case of polyhydramnion, but at least an amount equivalent to the quantity of contrast medium applied. Correct intraamniotic position is ensured by sonographic control of puncture, a demand which is compulsory today. Then, something between 40 ml and 80 ml of a water-soluble contrast medium, for example, Visotrast 290®, and between 3 ml and 6 ml of Lipiodol UF® are consecutively injected through a

# 4.

cannula, depending on the sonographically estimated quantity of amniotic fluid and the age of the foetus. Thirty minutes are allowed to pass from injection, before the first general radiograph is made of the abdominal cavity, following withdrawal of the cannula. The amniograph depicts the foetus as a recess in the contrasted amniotic fluid. Amniotic fluid with high levels of contrast medium will accumulate after short time in the foetal intestine. The fat-soluble contrast medium, distributed in the form of large drops at the beginning, will then become dissolved in the foetal skin coating, the vernix caseosa. A foetograph is then obtained from the second general radiograph of the abdominal cavity made within 18 and 24 hours from injection of contrast medium. The foetus may be seen completely depicted by contrast, with even the smallest details of the foetal surface being visible. No native radiograph is required under the conditions of the highly advanced sonography, and even amniography may become superfluous, for example, in a case in which the examiner's interest is restricted to a very specific, delimited question.

Optimum conditions in terms of X-ray technology and equipment are absolutely essential. High-performance generators, highly sensitive X-ray film, first-class exposure mechanisms, highly accurate positioning (prone!), and optimum focussing are prerequisites of crucial importance to high-quality images for adequate assessment. Padding of the pregnant woman's thorax and lateral buttressing of the abdominal region may be required to handle very large abdominal surfaces (twins or strongly pronounced polyhydramnion). High-kV radiation, as required for native radiography (U = 100 kV) is not mandatory in this case. Image contrast might be too low for proper evaluation, and for absence of any benefit the risk may prove to be unnecessary. Good contrast may be ensured by voltage levels about 70 kV with sufficiently short exposures, provided that first-class hardware be used.



## Diagnostic potential of amniofoetography

Amniography may be used in isolation as of the 16th week of pregnancy. Celes in the central nervous system and other regions are visualised as recesses in amniotic fluid with contrast medium. Should no optimum sagittal-plane image of the foetus be provided by a general radiograph, target fluoroscopy will be possible, using an image amplifier television chain and image amplifier photography.

Amniography also can be helpful in detecting malformations of the uterus and provide information indicative of a uterus tumour.

Water-soluble contrast medium normally is eliminated from amniotic fluid, 24 hours after amniocentesis. If an amniographic effect without detectable foetal malformation is still visible from a radiograph made at that juncture, in comparison to the radiograph 30 minutes after injection, impairment of amniotic fluid absorption can be assumed as the cause of polyhydramnion.

If two radiographs are made in an interval of 24 hours, the foetus will be usually found to be in a clearly different position on the second radiograph. No such positional change would be indicative of oligohydramnion, and motility disorder can be assumed, for example, in case of a neural tube defect.

The foetal stomach and the beginning part of the small intestine will be clearly recordable from the radiograph 30 minutes from injection due to drinking by the foetus of amniotic fluid with contrast medium. Sections of the small intestine with residual contrast and the entire colon up to the rectal ampulla will be usually visualised after 24 hours. The contrast medium tends to stay bonded to the meconium for many weeks up to childbirth, as has been confirmed by post-AFG radiographs of newborns. Earlier non-detectability of contrast medium in the colon by post-AFG X-ray is indicative, with high probability, of past or present hypoxia of the foetus, which may have caused discharge of meconium.

Water-soluble contrast medium is not only accumulated in meconium but is also eliminated via foetal membranes by maternal circulation. A maternal excretory urogram has quite often been recordable from a radiograph made 24 hours after injection of contrast medium.

Insufficient formation of vernix caseosa due to retardation of foetal maturity must be assumed in cases of poor Lipiodol marking of foetal skin by amniofoetography as of the 28th calculated week of pregnancy.

This information regarding the kinetics of contrast media is relating to the combination used by the authors, Visotrast 290® (VEB Fahlberg List, Magdeburg, GDR) and Lipiodol UF® (Byk-Gulden, Konstanz, FRG). Other contrast media, used in the past and at present, may exhibit deviating behaviours in time (strontium-iodide, potassium iodide, sodium iodide, Abrodil, Perabrodil, Uroselectan, Uroselectan B, Immetol, pyelophanine, Skiodan, Neo-Skiodan, Umbrenal, Umbrathor, Lithiumbral, Tetragnost, moliodole, Thorotrast, Cholumbral, Hypopaque, Pantopaque, Lipiodol UF alone).

Contrast formation of the foetal gastro-intestinal tract may enable a number of diagnostic conclusions which are summarised in Table 1.

**Table 1**
**Diagnostic information potentially obtainable from AFG contrast formation of gastro-intestinal tract**

**Displacement**
- caudal direction in case of hepatomegaly
- ventral direction in cases of urinary congestion kidneys, renal cysts, and megaloureter
- crancial or dorsal direction in cases of enlarged urinary bladder, ovarian and urachus cysts
- ahead of abdominal wall in cases of omphalocele and gastroschisis
- into thorax in case of (left-side) defect of diaphragm (left congenital diaphragmatic hernia)

**Absence of contrast formation**
- in cases of stenosis/atresia of gastro-intestinal tract and stenosis due to volvulus or pancreas anulare
- dysphagia caused from central nervous system
- severe disease of foetus
- intra-uterine foetal death.

**Retarded passage and inhomogeneous contrast formation**
- in cases of intra-uterine infections
- peritonitis, usually concomitant with bulged abdomen due to ascites
- hypothyreosis of foetus, with struma
- neural tube defect.

**Megacolon, Dolicocolon**
**Conjoined twins**
- for assessment of gastro-intestinal situation in cases of partitional malformations, such as thoracopagus.

While the skeletal system can be examined and properly assessed without AFG, discernibility of abnormalities is often facilitated by the foetographyc effect of Lipiodol UF. Conditions which would call for particular attention, in this context, are given in Table 2.

**Table 2**
**Malformations of skeletal system detectable by AFG**

Osteogenesis imperfecta (types I–IV)
Hypophosphatasia
Dysplasia (thanatophoric disease, achondrogenesis, achondroplasia, diastrophic disease etc.)
Cranial dysmorphia
Macrocephalus
Insufficient calcification of skull cap in cases of internal hydrocephalus, without enlargement of biparietal head diameter
Microcephalus
Anencephalus
Aplasia
Dysmelia
Polydactyly
Abnormalities of ribs
Defects of skull cap
Dysplasia and other malformations of vertebral bodies
Dysraphism of vertebral column
Gibbus of vertebral column
Caudal regression
Intra-uterine foetal death.

Additional diagnostic conclusions may be derived from Lipiodol labelling of the foetal surface and are summarised in Table 3.

**Table 3**
**Diagnostic information recordable from labelling of soft tissue surface in conjunction with AFG**

Assessment of foetal proportions; foetal hydrops; facial profile; lowered insertion of ears; neural tube celes; spinal schisis; nape region; thoracic deformation; clubfoot; clubhand; sex; intrauterine foetal death; defects of abdominal wall (omphalocele, gastroschisis); abdominal protrusion (ascites, abnormalities of urinary tract, ovarian cyst, hepatomegaly); assessment of multiple pregnancy (mon-/diamniotes, extent of bond between conjoined twins).

Combination of AFG with more thorough but invasive diagnostic approaches can prove useful to cope with problems of differential diagnosis in conjunction with sonography. For example, intrathoracic, intra-abdominal or retroperitoneal cystic growths may be punctured and visualised by means of contrast medium (*Prenzlau* and *Abét*, 1983). Intra-uterine ventriculography with intracranial pressure measurement will be practicable, as well. However, such procedures will not be taken into consideration unless intra-uterine therapy or premature termination of pregnancy are under discussion.

# 5.

## Diagnostic problems of amniofoetography

A more or less substantive role is played by adequate dosage of contrast medium, which is of particular relevance to the oily contrast component rather than to water-soluble contrast media. Too much Lipiodol UF, not completely bonded to the vernix caseosa, may cause diagnostically confusing superimpositions, primarily in the region of the foetal spine. The following Lipiodol UF doses are recommended for application in different phases of pregnancy:

| | |
|---|---|
| 24th to 28th weeks | 3 ml |
| 28th to 30th weeks | 4 ml |
| 30th to 32nd weeks | 5 ml |
| 33rd week and beyond | 6 ml |

Errors in foetal assessment may be caused by osseous structures of the maternal skeleton, so that particular attention ought to be given to this potential source of error.

Extremity bones which are not accurately imaged in film parallelism may appear to be shortened or deformed, another source of malinterpretation. An extremital malformation, on the other hand, may be misinterpreted as lack of film parallelism in bone position. Yet, correct assessment is usually possible, if skeleton together with proportions between head, trunk, and extremities are imaged in totality. Target-oriented fluoroscopy or even better targeted sonographic examination can be used for verification in cases of doubt.

In cases of oligohydramnion or anhydramnion, clubhand or clubfoot positions may be misrepresented by constrained positions of the foetus.

Time-adjusted passage of contrast media through the gastrointestinal tract may entail atresia due to frequent combination with surrounding fistulation. Yet, absence of contrast formation in the gastro-intestinal tract does not necessarily mean presence of atresia (cf. Table 1).

With diamniotes, water-soluble contrast medium may diffuse through foetal membranes, so that even in a case in which only one embryonic cavity had been punctured, contrast formation may be visible in the gastro-intestinal tract of the second foetus in a radiograph taken after 24 hours. Yet, misinterpretation as a monoamniote can be prevented by Lipiodol labelling of only one foetus or by contrast medium recess of one embryonic cavity in the amniogram. Diagnostic mistakes and associated problems of interpretation may result also from erroneous placing of contrast medium, such as Lipiodol UF in an omphalocele. Situations of that kind may be avoided by ultrasonically controlled amniocentesis.

Presence of pronounced polyhydramnion may occasionally prevent image quality good enough for adequate diagnosis. Amniofoetographic information may become impossible at all, if an image is getting additionally blurred by foetal movements. The examiner confronted with such a situation will have to decide, if AFG should not better be repeated, following relief of the polyhydramnion. Inadequate image quality may result also from adiposity. In such cases, dubious sonographic findings, such as internal hydrocephalus, may be possibly cleared up by computed tomography.

# 6.

## Relevance of amniofoetography in our days

Basically, all the diagnostic information described in Chapter 4 as being obtainable from AFG can be attained, as well, by sonography. However, those taking a self-critical approach to their own use of prenatal sonographic diagnosis will certainly come across, up to our days, some points and reasoning in favour of AFG.

1. About 200 sonographically detectable intra-uterine malformations and diseases of the foetus are known at present. True, the questions of interest to the transferring doctor and the experience of the examiner are factors which limit the range of pathological findings that may be subject of search, but plenty of possible constellations of findings may be left hardly determinable even after a one-hour check or repetitive examinations. The authors have been intensively dealing for years with sonographic prenatal diagnosis under optimum hardware conditions, and yet, on childbirth they have been frequently taken by surprise at malformations or at least signs of syndromes actually detetable but not detected before delivery.

2. There is a subjective element of bias that must not be underestimated: Examiners detecting a dubious or pathological pattern may become fixed to it, and other deviations which might change the findings escape attention (for example, a genetically determined syndrome).

3. Prenatal diagnosis of malformations and search for foetal diseases will not make any sense unless conclusions are drawn from it. Possible conclusions are

(a) full-term completion of pregnancy under regular ultrasonic monitoring;

(b) premature termination of pregnancy at a juncture considered optimal, followed by postnatal care for the newborn;

(c) intra-uterine palliative therapy up to childbirth on term; and

(d) premature termination of pregnancy in case of malformations that would be incompatible with decent postnatal life.

It seems to be at least questionable to accept the idea of making far-reaching decisions, such as those associated with Items (c) and (d) solely dependent on one single diagnostic method, since erroneous judgement is always a possibility. Double confirmation of findings or at least complementary information, therefore, is a legitimate demand. No doubt, there are unambiguous findings which do not require any additional diagnosis (e.g. anencephalus).

4. An examination may be burdened with technical problems which may even conceal actually present pathological conditions and make them escape sonographic detection. Unfavourable child presentation and oligohydramnion would be of relevance, in that context.

It is because of the above experience that in the authors' team AFG has continued to be part of the repertoire of prenatal diagnosis. AFG is an approach complementary to sonography. It may confirm sonographic findings or invalidate them or may be helpful in arriving at a different interpretation. AFG may reveal additional pathological findings or uncover suspicious elements for more targeted sonography. Both methods strengthen each other and, at the same time, are likely to contribute to steadily growing accuracy of diagnostic information. Indications for AFG are on a declining trend, as experience is growing in prenatal sonographic detection of malformations and other diseases of the foetus and as a widening range of laboratory-chemical and genetic parameters has become available. Nevertheless, AFG can prove to be quite a promising method for people beginning to specialise in this subject. In the authors' environment, sonography and AFG have developed in interaction.

# 7.

## Indications for amniofoetography

No additional diagnosis would be necessary for decision-making on premature termination of pregnancy, once safe sonographic evidence has been produced to a non-viable malformation. Anencephalus, Potter's sequence, strongly pronounced and rapidly progressing non-immunological hydrops fetus universalis, progressing hydrocephalus with the cerebral cranium below 10 mm in thickness and in combination with neural tube defect as well as paraplegiform symptoms are some examples, in this context. The lethal variant of osteogenesis imperfecta (type II), too, is likely to exhibit sonographic findings which are so typical that additional radiography would not be necessary. Yet, the examiner will be hardly capable of safely identifying such condition unless he or she had seen it before. The less experienced examiner should resort to AFG as an additional aid. On the other hand, the more bland manifestations of osteogenesis with no major intra-uterine skeletal deformations would be more reliably identifiable by AFG, on account of inadequate skeletal calcification. Sonography and AFG are complementary in an ideal way also for all other suspicious signs of skeletal malformation.

All sonographically detected malformations of major relevance to preservation of the child's life, associated with a question for the acceptable risk to the child during parturition, should be made subject to more complex diagnosis. Counselling of parents could then be more professional, and the defect and resulting ailment could be more reliably prognosticated. Date of birth, obstetric management, and postnatal care, consequently, could be optimally adjusted to each other.

Occasionally, sonographic differentiation may be difficult between hydronephrosis and renal cystic dysplasia or between hydroureter and enlargement of intestinal convolution, though it may be of crucial importance to decision-making, especially with bilateral findings. Here, AFG might be helpful, perhaps in combination with puncture and instillation of contrast medium into the cystic cavity. Cystic formations in the thoracic region may be indicative of cystic malformations of lungs or intestinal loops along with defect of the diaphragm (left diaphragmatic hernia). However, non-enlarged loops of the small intestine in the thorax may just as well escape the examiner's attention, if they become superimposed by a rib shadow. In such cases, intestinal motility of the pregnant woman can be stimulated to sonographic visibility by application of medicaments, and AFG, through intestinal contrast build-up, can be helpful in clearing up the situation.

AFG would be indicated, as well, in all cases of unambiguous deviation of amniotic fluid quantity-polyhydramnion and oligohydramnion, if no pathological findings had been revealed by ultrasonic examination.

It is well known that sonographic assessment of a foetus is impeded in a condition of oligohydramnion. This can be compensated by fill-up of the amniotic cavity and use of AFG.

AFG may be also helpful in clearing up a genetic risk, repetitive on account of an unfavourable case history but with no sonographically detectable pathological findings, provided that the type of possible malformation is detectable by amniofoetography.

A dense coronal scalp may occasionally generate the sonographic impression of scalp edema hydrops of the galea. This can be safely cleared up by AFG.

Sonography and AFG, finally, support each other in adequate assessment of type and extent of fusion of conjoined twins, with sonography being applicable to heart and liver and AFG to intestines and body surface.

# 8.

## Radiation load and complications of amniofoetography

Possible complications of AFG cannot be properly explained unless attention is simultaneously given to possible complications associated with amniocentesis. There have been scores of literature reports on amniocentesis and studies based on high numbers of examinations. All of them are, more or less, general accounts (*Gautray* et al., 1980; *Klein*, et al., 1981; *Verjaal* et al., 1981; *Nolan*, et al., 1981; *Mikusova* et al., 1982; *Porecco* et al., 1982; *Gillberg* et al., 1982; *Galle* and *Meis*, 1982; *Cruiskshank* et al., 1983; *Finegan* et al., 1984; *Sant-Cassia* et al., 1984; *Crane* and *Kopta*, 1984; *Hinst* and *Stengl*, 1985).

The number of amniocenteses quoted in the majority of these publications is rarely below 7,000. Therefore, the experience reported in them can be considered representative. Particular conclusiveness may be claimed for the results obtained by *Leschot* et al. and published in 1985. By targeted use of ultrasonic diagnosis in conjunction with amniocentesis, they succeeded in reducing their rate of foetal deaths or abortions from originally 1.8 per cent (27 in 1,500 amniocenteses **without** sonography) to 0.5 per cent (seven in 1,500 amniocenteses **with** sonography). In other words, this has been the most substantial complication, and here is the approach to minimising the risk.

*Ron* et al. (1982) recorded clearly higher rates of abortion along with blood-tinged amniotic fluid samples, as compared to 1.7 per cent in their control group. For example, maternal contamination was recorded from 152 in 706 amniocenteses (rate of abortion being 6.6 per cent), while 28 were foetally contaminated (rate of abortion amounting to 14.3 per cent). *Palle* et al. (1983) recorded higher abortion risk also for twin gravidities (six and 17 per cent). *Shapiro* et al. (1983) reported five unexplained immediate foetal deaths among 7,254 amniocenteses at four centres in the USA. *Bremme* et al. (1984) found that in cases of damaged gravidity amniocentesis, through foetal adrenal stress, would possibly result in spontaneous abortion. *Stock* (1982) reported another foetal death in the wake of amniocentesis, probably due to head injury.

Those more general accounts are accompanied by a great number of publications on individual cases or more specific complications. A contribution of basic importance to more understanding of the pathogenetic mechanisms undelying complications was made by *Finegan* (1984) when he investigated amniocentesis in the second trimester of pregnancy and related it to the formation, properties, and importance of amniotic fluid. He was particularly interested in the role played by loss of amniotic fluid in the course of amniocentesis and consequences of such loss which he studied in animal experiments and in man. Such loss was thought to be relevant primarily to respiratory disorders and orthopaedic malformations (*Finegan*, 1984; *Wald* et al., 1983; *Moessinger* et al., 1983).

The following amniocentesis-related risks should be mentioned, as well, for the sake of completeness:
(a) Persistent loss of amniotic fluid and its possible negative consequences for body weight and lung development (*Alumina* et al., 1981; *Simpson* et al., 1981; *Hislop* et al., 1984);
(b) Foeto-maternal bleeding due to injury of vessels and its increasing effect on alpha-foetoprotein values (*Dallaire* et al., 1980; *Lele* et al., 1982; *Portman* et al., 1982; *Memuti* et al., 1980, 1983; *Thomsen* et al., 1983; *Selpuveda* et al., 1984; *Lenke* et al., 1985); *Goldmann* and *Peleg* (1980) reported about the rare complication of massive maternal retroperitoneal bleeding;
(c) Injury of foetal membranes (*Yeast* et al., 1984), foetal soft tissues (*Broome* et al., 1976; *Raimer* and *Raimer*, 1984; *Bruce* et al., 1984), eye (*Merin* and *Beyth*, 1980), brain due to formation of porencephalic cysts (*Youroukos* et al., 1980; *Schinzel*, 1981), and thorax with subsequent lung prolapse (*Prenzlau* et al., 1986);
(d) Injury and strangulation of the umbilical cord (*Moessinger* et al., 1983; *Zakut* et al., 1984);
(e) Disorders of cardiac functionality (*Neldam* and *Pedersen*, 1980; *Sadovsky* et al., 1981; *Spinapolice* et al., 1983; *Haberstroh* et al., 1983);
(f) Accidental rhesus iso-immunisation as a consequence of foeto-maternal blood transfusion (*Queenan*, 1966; *Schneider*, 1972; *Schmidt* et al., 1980; *Hill* et al., 1980; *Hensleigh* and *Cann*, 1981; *Golbus* et al., 1982; *Grant* et al., 1983; *Tabsh* et al., 1984);
(g) Infection in the wake of amniocentesis (*Wurster* et al., 1982; *Delaplane* et al., 1983; *Elliot*, 1984);
(h) Amniotic fluid embolism (*Hasaart* and *Essed*, 1983);
(i) Extramembranous pregnancy, following amniocentesis (*Vago* and *Charkin*, 1980);

(j) Intestinal atresia as a consequence of amniocentesis (*Therkelsen* and *Rehder*, 1981).

In other publications, reference was made to pericardial tamponade, eye traumata, pneumothorax, and spleen injuries (*Holzgreve* and *Hansmann*, 1984; *Roberts* et al., 1983; *Schlensker* et al., 1984; *Weise* and *Gabriel*, 1984).

AFG goes along with additional risk factors caused by radiation load and application of contrast medium. However, a major contribution to an elucidation of radiation exposure of the general public should not be expected from AFG, given the low number of examinations so far conducted. Yet, while AFG does not add substantially to radiation exposure, in general, its relevance to the individual pregnant woman must not be neglected. The mother-child combination is actually exposed to a twofold risk, since two indivudals are involved. And taken the age of both of them, both somatic and genetic risks ought to be taken into serious consideration. Most recent estimates of organ doses affecting maternal ovaries are likely to support the assumption that they are exposed to 1.2 mGy in antero-posterior radiography of the lumbovertebral column and to 1.3 mGy in antero-posterior radiography of the pelvis (*Angerstein* et al., 1986). The entire body is exposed to 0.6 mGy. For the foetus, it should be the very first whole-body exposure, and its dose level might be assumed to be somewhere between 0.6 and 1.3 mGy. Foetal gonadal exposure should be rated somewhat lower. The radiation risk implied in AFG is certainly related to the stochastic nature of radiation action. This is duly observed in practice by confirmed rare use of the method as a result of most stringent indication criteria as well as by scrupulous compliance with radiation shielding and image quality standards and rules in the production of the radiographs proper. Targeted fluoroscopy of the foetus is permissible only as an exception, when highly specific questions have to be answered. One foetogram rather than two should be made, whenever clinically justifiable. In 1977, the point was made in a report of the National Council on Radiation Protection and Measurement (NCRP) that the risk of foetal malformations as a result of radiography in pregnancy, using radiation doses of 0.05 Gy and below, was negligible when compared to other risk sources. *Balsam* and *Weiss* (1981) postulated a foetal dose of less than 0.01 Gy for AFG. According to them, the risk of oncogenesis was higher than that of teratogenesis in response to AFG in the "mid trimester". They failed to detect any malignoma in 1,000 children who had been exposed to "irradiation" at foetal stage in a pelvimetry programme. The risk associated with irradiation should be matched against the risk that might emanate from omission or delay of an examination (*Neumeister*, 1982).

Other complications may result from application of contrast medium, with an accident due to hypersensitivity to contrast medium being the most common risk factor, though no reports have so far come to the authors' knowledge.

There has been repeated reference in the literature, on the other hand, to possible development of foetal transitory hypothyreosis caused by administration of iodine in the contrast medium (*Rodesch* et al., 1976; *Becroft* et al., 1980; *Stubbe* et al., 1980; *Miething* et al., 1981; *Oide* et al., 1983,; *Storm*, 1986; *Muti* et al. 1986). Yet, no hard evidence has so far been produced to a relationship. The authors, on account of their own sonographic studies, are rather inclined to seeing a relationship the other way round. Children with postnatal hypothyreosis had prenatally exhibited struma colli, prior to AFG. "Dipsophobia" thus induced had caused polyhydramnion, and the latter had then provided the indication for AFG.

Mechanical injuries caused by intrafoetal injection of contrast medium have been described, as well (*Grech* and *Spitz*, 1977). There is also a hypothetic danger of fat embolism, for example, if fat-soluble contrast medium is allowed to enter into the maternal or foetal circulation, say, when celes or cysts are punctured. Both types of accidents, however, are avoidable by sonographic control of the puncturing procedure.

Too much Lipiodol UF (20 ml and more) may possibly cause meconium ileus. However, this complication has so far been described only in connection with an intra-uterine exchange transfusion, ad ileus conditions have become known also in situations in which no contrast medium was involved at all. Hence, no causative relationship can be safely claimed to exist between oily contrast medium and ileus.

# 9.

## Diagnostic strategy for prenatal detection and differentiation of foetal malformations and diseases

It is undisputed today that sonography will not come to its full potential effectiveness unless it is applied to all pregnant women. Ultrasonographic diagnosis, therefore, must not be left to individual discretion or accidental circumstances. General and systematic integration of the method with the general pregnancy care system has to be demanded. Possible solutions and programmes have been published by several authors and teams, with the view to adapting the entire spectrum of prenatal sonographic diagnosis to the requirements of practice. The following insights have been gained from an analysis of comprehensive material handled at the Department of Gynaecology and Obstetrics of Humboldt-Universität zu Berlin (*Bayer*, 1981):

(a) Three routine ultrasonic examinations in the course of a normal pregnancy have proved to be sufficient for 64.8 per cent of all pregnant women. (Postnatal check-up of this group revealed that not a single ultrasonically recordable foetal finding had been overlooked in the patients concerned.)

(b) The majority of all abnormal findings, requiring follow-up and repetitive sonography, has been detected up to the 28th week of pregnancy. Thereafter, abnormal findings were present merely in 3.8 per cent of all cases. The purpose of the exercise, to detect and identify the largest possible number of foetal maldevelopments at the earliest possible juncture, can be accomplished only by means of a stage-wise programme on the basis of high-continuity sonographic control throughout pregnancy.

A strategy has been devised to meet that demand, and it can be put into practice by due consideration of international experience as well as of national and regional peculiarities of education and equipment. This model must be such that the requirement of highly skilled prenatal diagnosis are fully met. It has to provide realistic guidelines to examiners and must be in line with their professional competence. It ought to cover the full range of aspects, from basic check-up at primary level to highly specialised diagnosis. Quality criteria should be stipulated for sonographic equipment used at all levels, and a code of practice should be formulated for purpose-oriented diagnosis of malformations.

Included in the multi-stage programme are ultrasonic investigations at basic level (Stage I), specialised investigations (Stage II), and highly specialised diagnosis, including follow-up attention to established malformations and research (Stage III).

**Ultrasonic investigation at basic level (Stage I)**

Ultrasonic investigations at basic level are used in sonographic monitoring and supervision of all pregnant women. Pregnancy development and progress are monitored in correlation with established parameters of foetal development. Probands are screened for signs of foetal maldevelopment or malformation. Pathological or dubious pregnancies are sorted out. The following recommendations are made for chronological action:

The first check should be made between the 14th and 16th weeks of pregnancy for the following purposes –

- Determination of gestational age;
- To establish intact condition of pregnancy;
- Detection or exclusion of multigravidity;
- Detection or exclusion of pathological findings.

The second investigation should be made between the 20th and 24th weeks of pregnancy for the following purposes –

- Check on somatic development of foetus;
- Assessment of foetal organs;
- Identification or exclusion of developmental disorders or malformations of foetus.

The third investigation should be made between the 28th and 32nd weeks of pregnancy for the following purposes –

- Check on somatic development of foetus (retardation);
- Differentiated organ diagnosis;
- Identification or exclusion of developmental disorders or malformations of foetus;
- Placental diagnosis.

The following more specific recommendations are given for ultrasonic investigation at basic level, against the background of latest knowledge and with reference to the authors' own results:

(a) Attention should be given to general indicators of malformations.

(b) A defined sequence should be adopted for examinations, for example, as follows –
Head, longitudinal section of trunk with body contour, cranial-to-caudal cross-section of trunk with spepwise analysis of foetal organs, extremities.

(c) Compulsory foetometry: measurement of biparietal head diameter, largest trunk diameter in cross-section, and length of femoral diaphysis; determination, if possible, of head circumference at fronto-occipital plane; determination of largest ab-

dominal diameter in cross-section; determination of quotient of biparietal head diameter to length of femoral diaphysis to secure data on gestational age.
(d) Optional foetometry: Determination from foetal body regions of biometric parameters conspicuous in structural assessment.
(e) Particular attention may be given to certain points of predilection for higher incidence of foetal malformations.

**Specialised ultrasonic diagnosis (Stage II)**
At this level, emphasis is laid on more specialised and differentiated diagnosis of foetal malformations. Stage II investigations should be linked to or supervised by a somewhat larger centre with facilities for adequate immediate prepartum hospitalisation. Examinations will be continued by interdisciplinary teams. All necessary biophysical (external cardiotocography) and biochemical facilities for supervision should be available for assessment of short-term foetal changes of relevance to foetal life. Pregnant women will have to be transferred to Stage II for problematic individual, familial, and obstetric histories and in case of pathological pregnancy, that is following suspicious diagnosis from Stage I screening. Particular attention will have to be given to pregnant women who fall into high-risk or target groups, including probands with records of frequent delayed abortions, premature childbirths, obstetric retardation, metabolic disorders, rhesus conflict, teratogenic exposures, and multigravidity.

Transfer to Stage II should be accompanied by transfer to that stage of all other pregnancy services under the given National Health Scheme for reasons of higher effectiveness. Checks should be continued from now on by examiners of longstanding experience in sonographic diagnosis, that is doctors who are highly familiar with normal and pathological sonographic anatomy and who are skilled in measuring foetal parameters (biometry) as well as in assessing embryonic and foetal mobility. Sonographic diagnosis is highly time-consuming and takes 30 minutes on average. Repetitive attempts are required in cases in which adequate visualisation of a region of interest is not possible at the first strike.

Sonographic equipment should meet the growing demands. A twosystem scanner should be available (real-time with linear and sector scans). Recording (video) should be desirable of characteristic structures and functional aspects.



**Highly specialised ultrasonic diagnosis (Stage III)**
Stage III is used in differential diagnosis for elucidation and possible treatment of cases filtered out from Stages I and II and not safely defined. Its function is that of a "problem solver" (*Hansmann*, 1981). It is also used in research for persistent scientifically founded integration of ultrasonographic diagnostics with the system of gestational monitoring. Organisation of interdisciplinary cooperation and counselling for highly specialised and, if so required, invasive early therapy, timing of termination of pregnancy, adequate postnatal care of the newborn or discontinuation of pregnancy for infaust prognosis of the child are the major purposes at that stage. Maximum diagnostic dependability is desirable at that level of highly specialised medical attention. Examinations require much time, competent personnel, and expensive hardware.

Individual experience of all specialists involved in Stage III is absolutely imperative. This should be consolidated by systematic referral to such centres of rare pathological cases. The following conditions should be called for, in that context:
1. Availability of highly effective sonographic apparatus, including Doppler scanner;
2. Longstanding experience of examiner;
3. High time commitment to individual check-up;
4. Masterhood in use of invasive diagnostic techniques, including amniocentesis, foetoscopy, and intrafoetal puncture;
5. Acquisition of techniques of minor surgical interventions;
6. Consideration of complementary biochemical, biophysical, and image-generating parameters, including alpha-foetoprotein, maturity diagnosis, external cardiotocography, foetal mobility analysis, amniofoetography, computed tomography, and magnetic resonance;
7. Close cooperation with centre of human genetics, neonatologists, paediatric surgeons, neurosurgeons, cardiologists, and paediatric pathologists.

# 10.

## Case histories

Case 1

**Patient B.K./76,** 28 years, first gravidity.
**Clinical findings:** 33rd week of pregnancy; polyhydramnion.
**Ultrasonic findings:** Polyhydramnion known from 28th week of pregnancy; no foetal malformations detectable.
**Indication for AFG:** Polyhydramnion.
**AFG findings** (Fig. 1: plain abdominal scan prior to

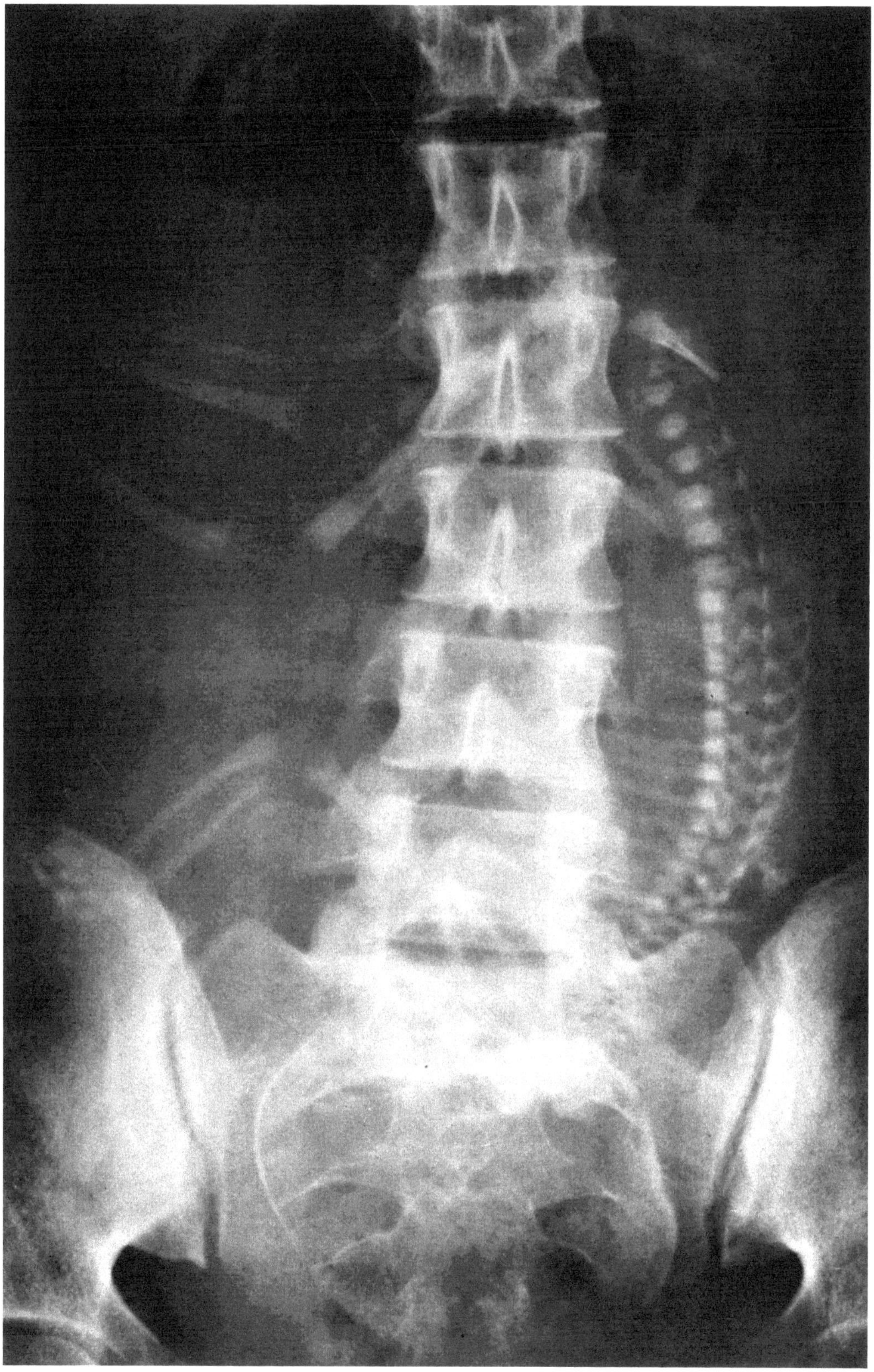

Fig. 1

**Case 1** amniocentesis; Fig. 2: amniogram 30 minutes hours from injection; Fig. 3: foetogram 20 hours from injection): No sign indicative of skeletal malformation was only information obtained from plain abdominal scan; amniogram (Fig. 2) and foetogram (Fig. 3) enabled assessment of soft tissue, gastro-intestinal passage of contrast medium as well

Fig. 2

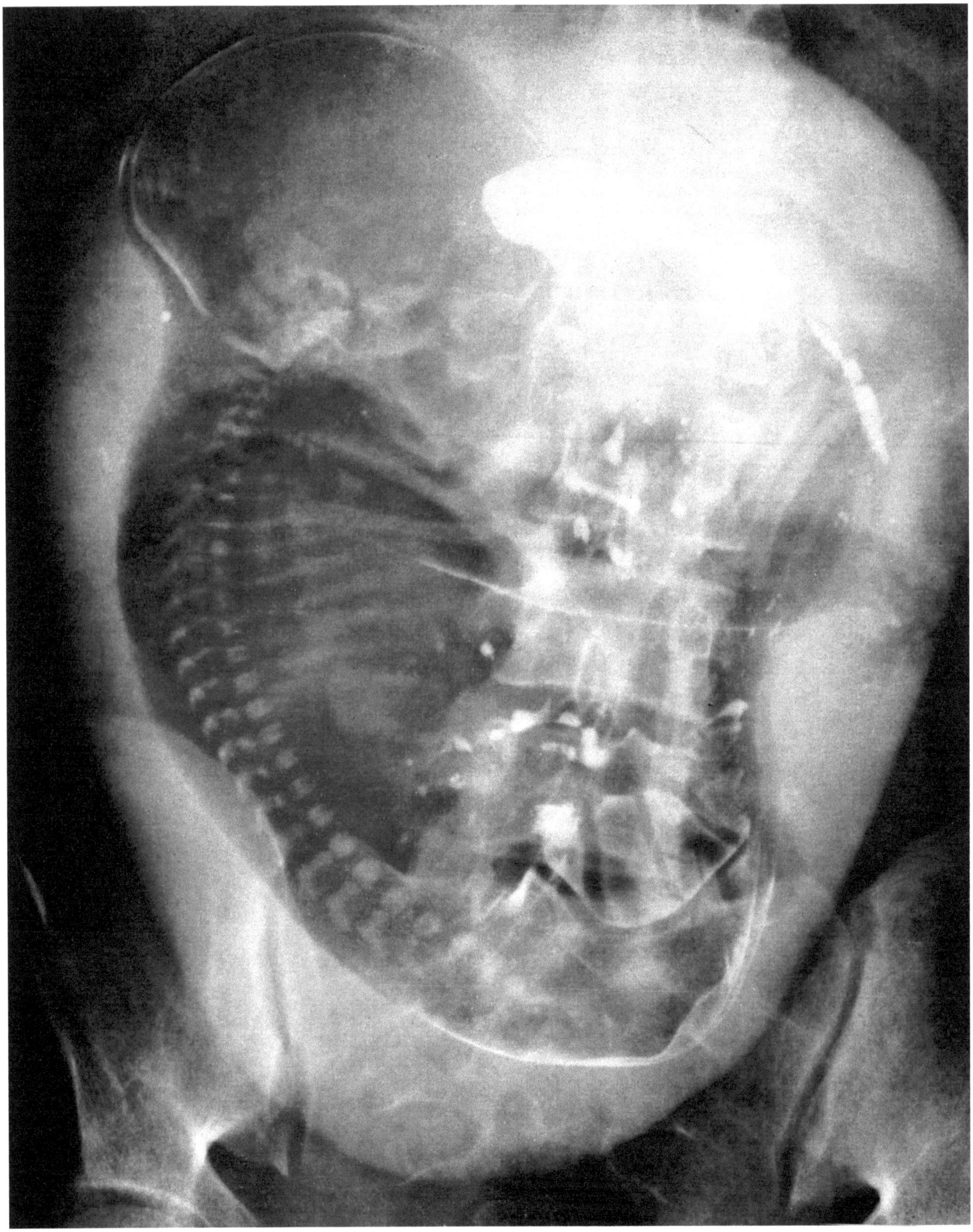

as assessment of vitality of foetus due to change of positions and also sexing (male foetus).
**Prenatal summary diagnosis:** No pathological findings.

**Clinical course:** Spontaneous labour in 34th week of pregnancy; clinically intact child, 1,830 g, 43 cm. ◁

Case 1

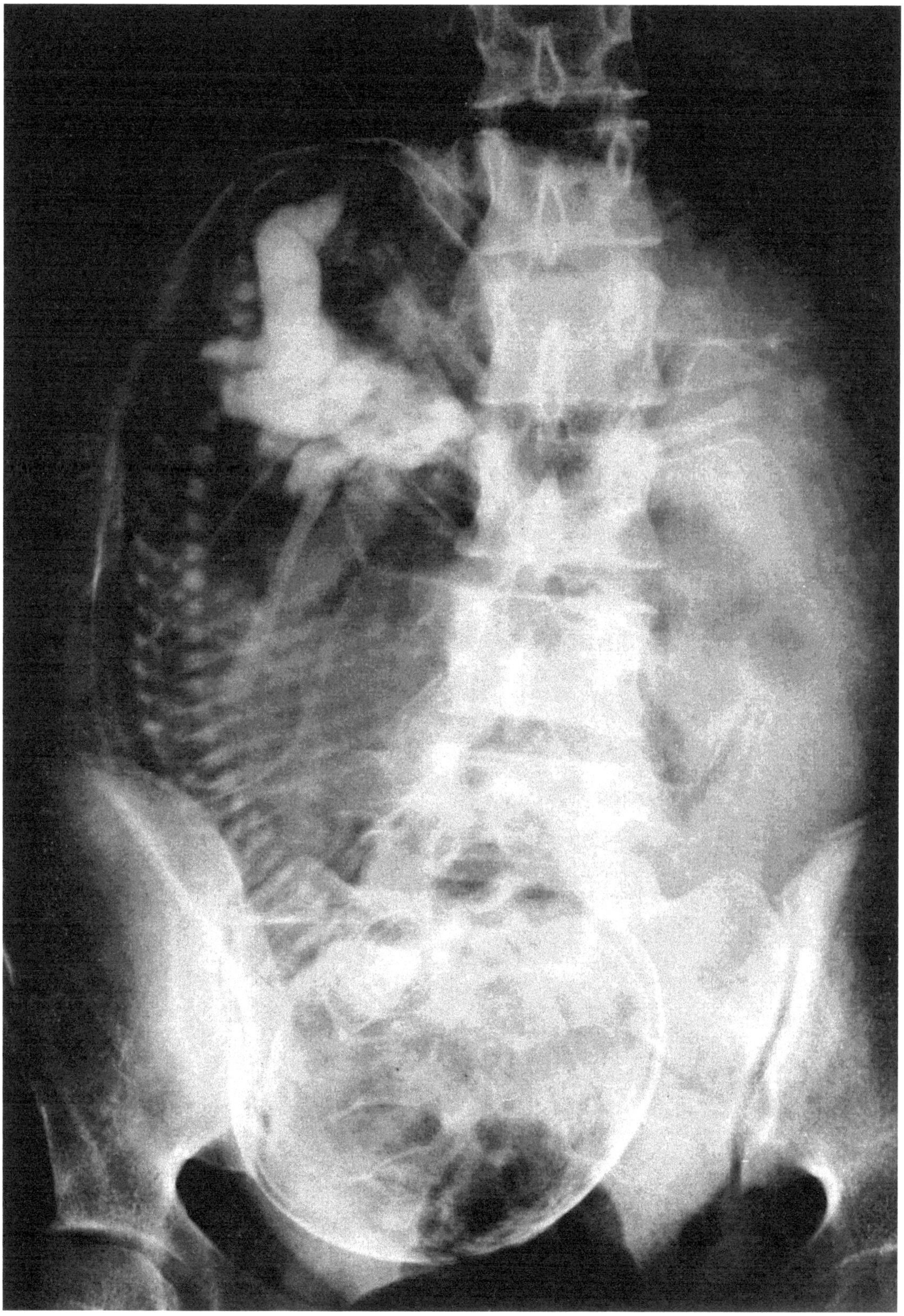

Fig. 3

**Case 2** **Patient F.S./78,** 39 years, sixth gravidity, five parturitions.
**Record:** Two live-born children; death few hours post-partum for multiple malformations; two stillbirths; one live-born child with omphalocele and cleft palate.

**Clinical findings:** 36th week of pregnancy; no contributory findings.
**Ultrasonic findings:** No signs indicative of malformations.

Fig. 4a

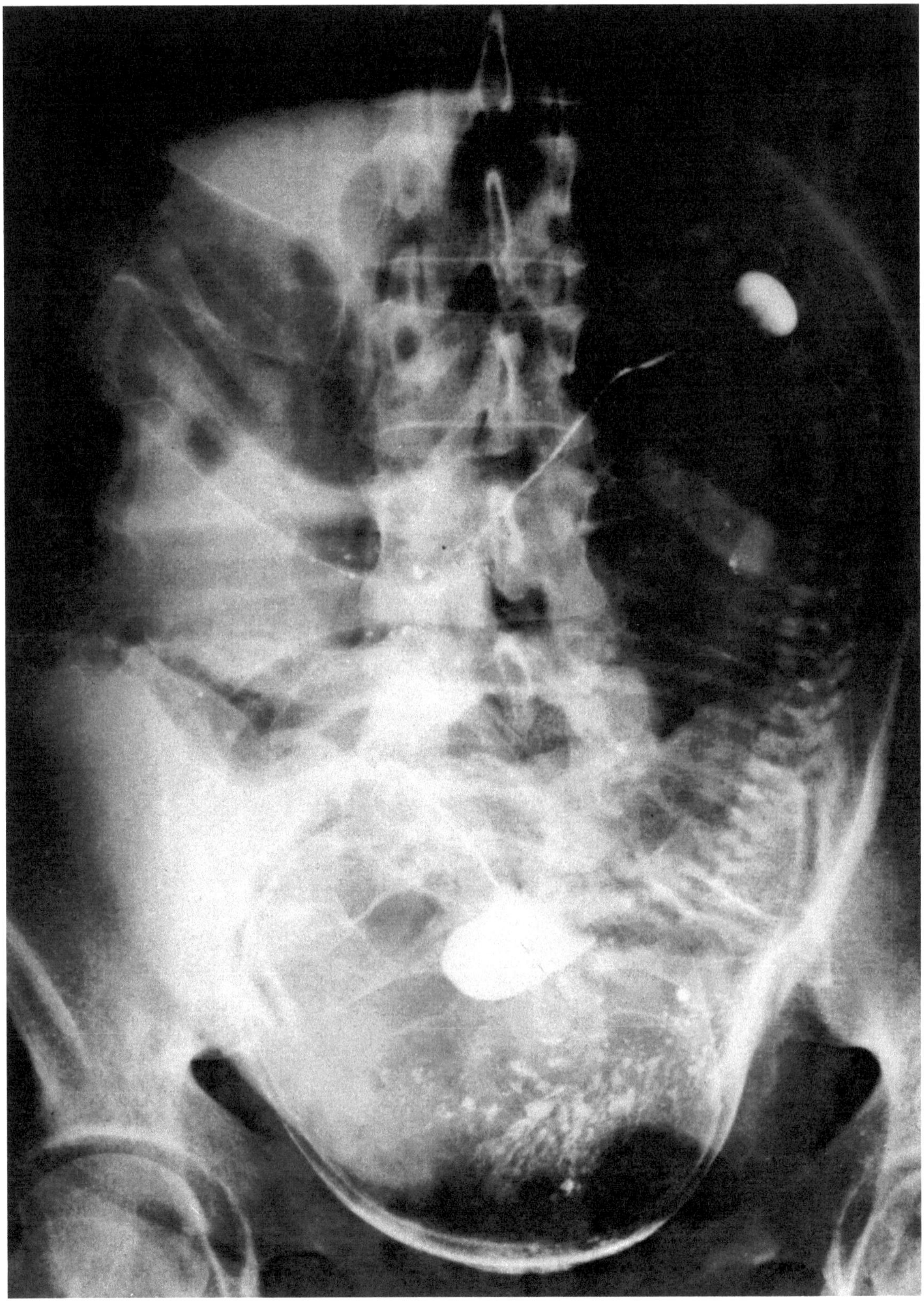

Indication for AFG: Infavourable record.
**AFG findings** (Fig. 4a: amniogram 60 minutes from injection; Fig. 4b: foetogram 20 hours from injection): Male foetus; cephalic presentation; no malformation detectable.
**Clinical course:** Spontaneous labour in 38th week of pregnancy; 3,240 g, 52 cm, clinically intact. ◁

Case 2

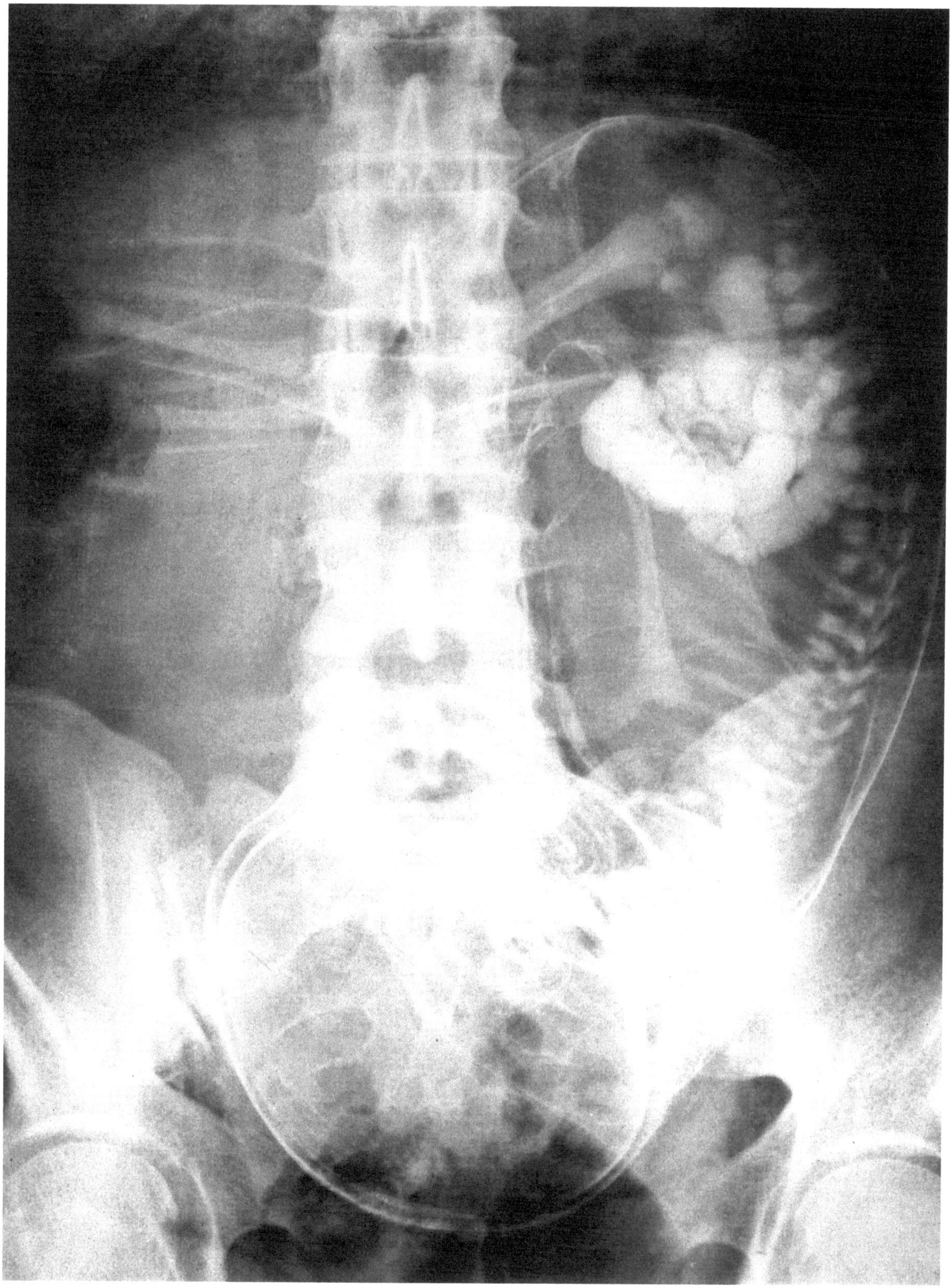

Fig. 4b

**Case 3** **Patient K.M./83,** 29 years, second gravidity, one parturition.
**Record:** One clinically intact child.
**Clinical findings:** 33rd week of pregnancy; polyhydramnion.
**Ultrasonic findings** (Fig. 5a): Polyhydramnion; no detectable malformation.
**Indication for AFG:** Polyhydramnion; to rule out malformations.
**AFG findings** (Fig. 5b: foetogram 24 hours from injection):

Fig. 5a

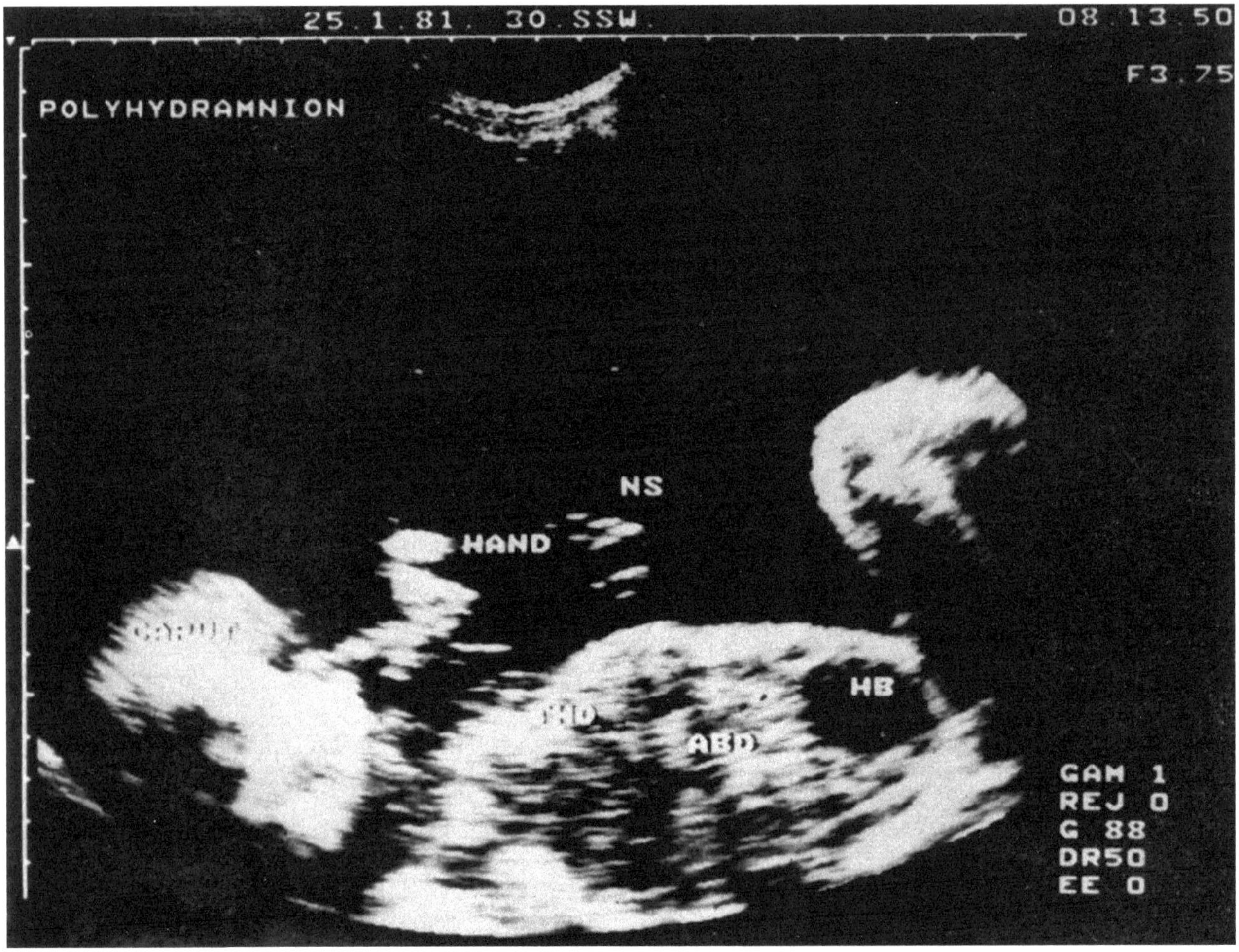

Male foetus; cephalic presentation; projection-dependent limitation of spine assessment; time-adequate gastro-intestinal passage of contrast medium up to rectal ampulla.
**Prenatal summary diagnosis:** No detection of foetal malformations.
**Clinical course:** Spontaneous labour in 35th week of pregnancy; 2,840 g, 51 cm; clinically intact newborn. ◁



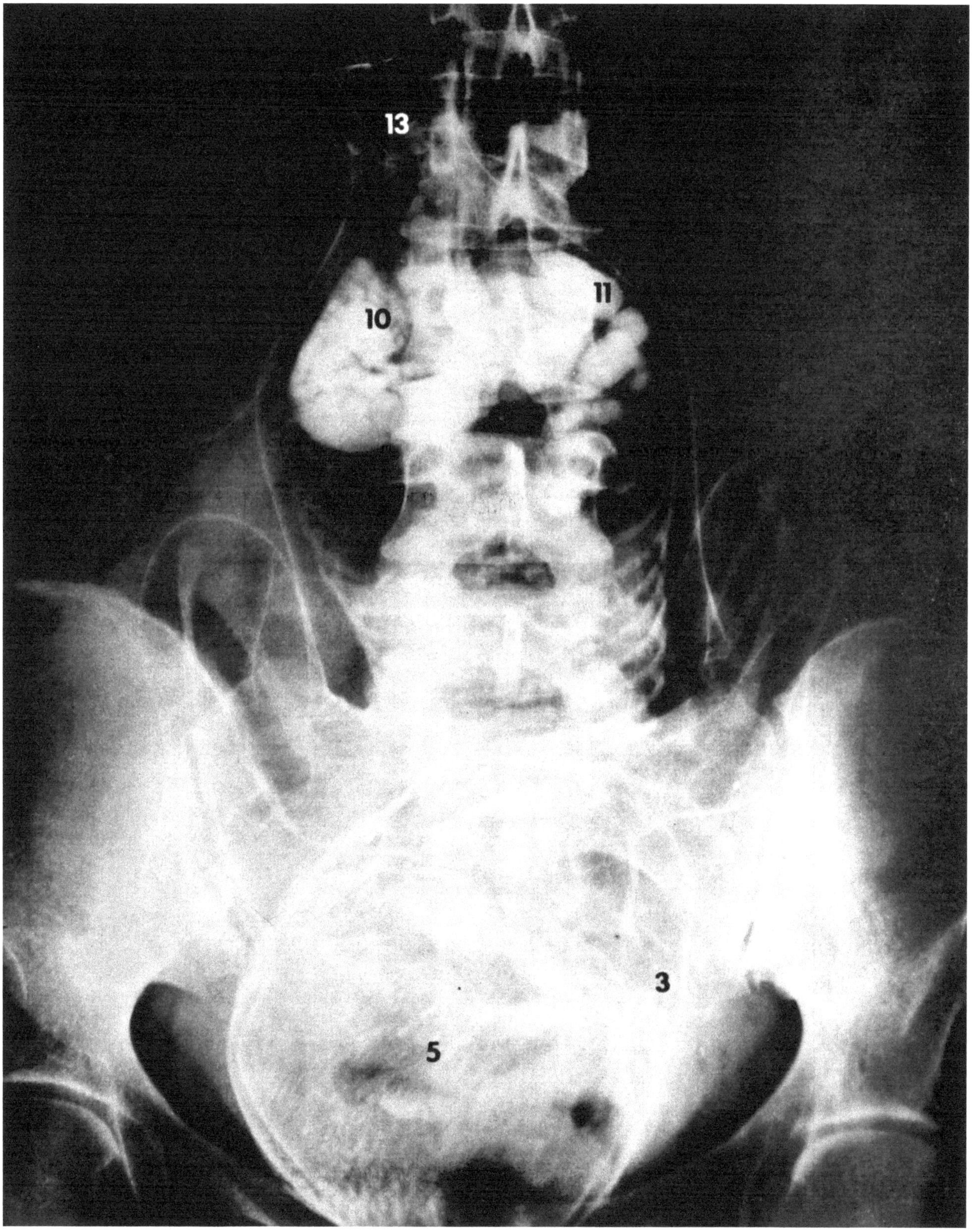


Fig. 5 b

**Case 4** **Patient F.H./78,** 24 years, fourth gravidity, no parturition. **Record:** Three abortions (in third, fourth, and sixth month). **Clinical findings:** 32nd week of pregnancy; no contributory findings.

**Ultrasonic findings** (Fig. 6a, b): No clue to malformation. Amniotic band (arrows).
**Indication for AFG:** Infavourable record.
**AFG findings** (Fig. 6c: amniogram 30 minutes from injec-

Fig. 6a

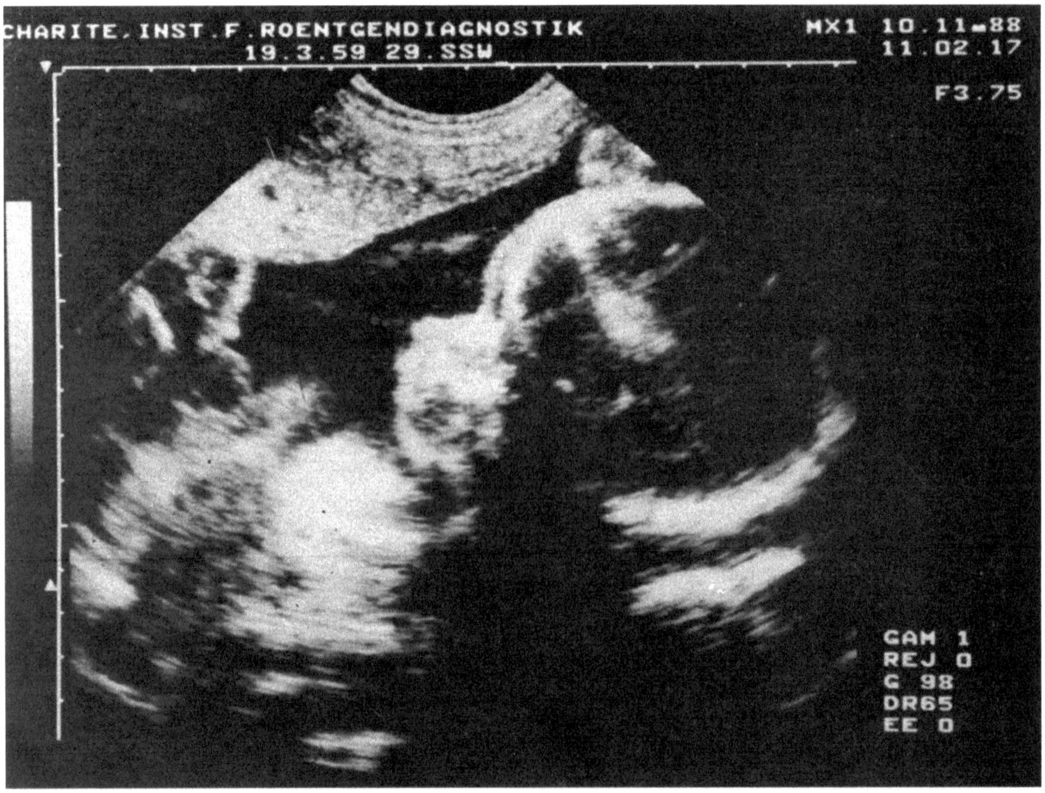


Fig. 6b

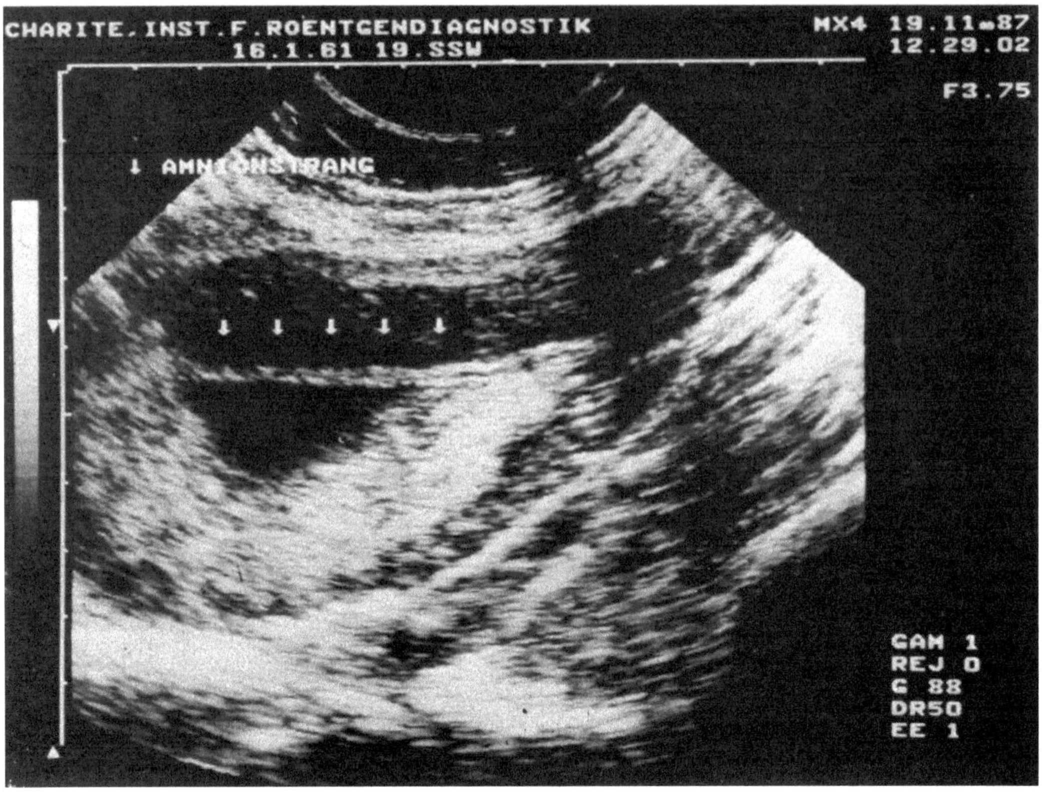

tion): Visualisation of uterus subseptus; foetus in breech presentation; sex not safely determinable; foetal head located in left cornu of uterus; lower extremities in right cornu; free Lipiodol UF in cranial region; no clue to malformation.

**Prenatal summary diagnosis:** Uterus subseptus.
**Clinical course:** Spontaneous labour in 36th week of pregnancy; clinically intact girl. ◁

Case 4

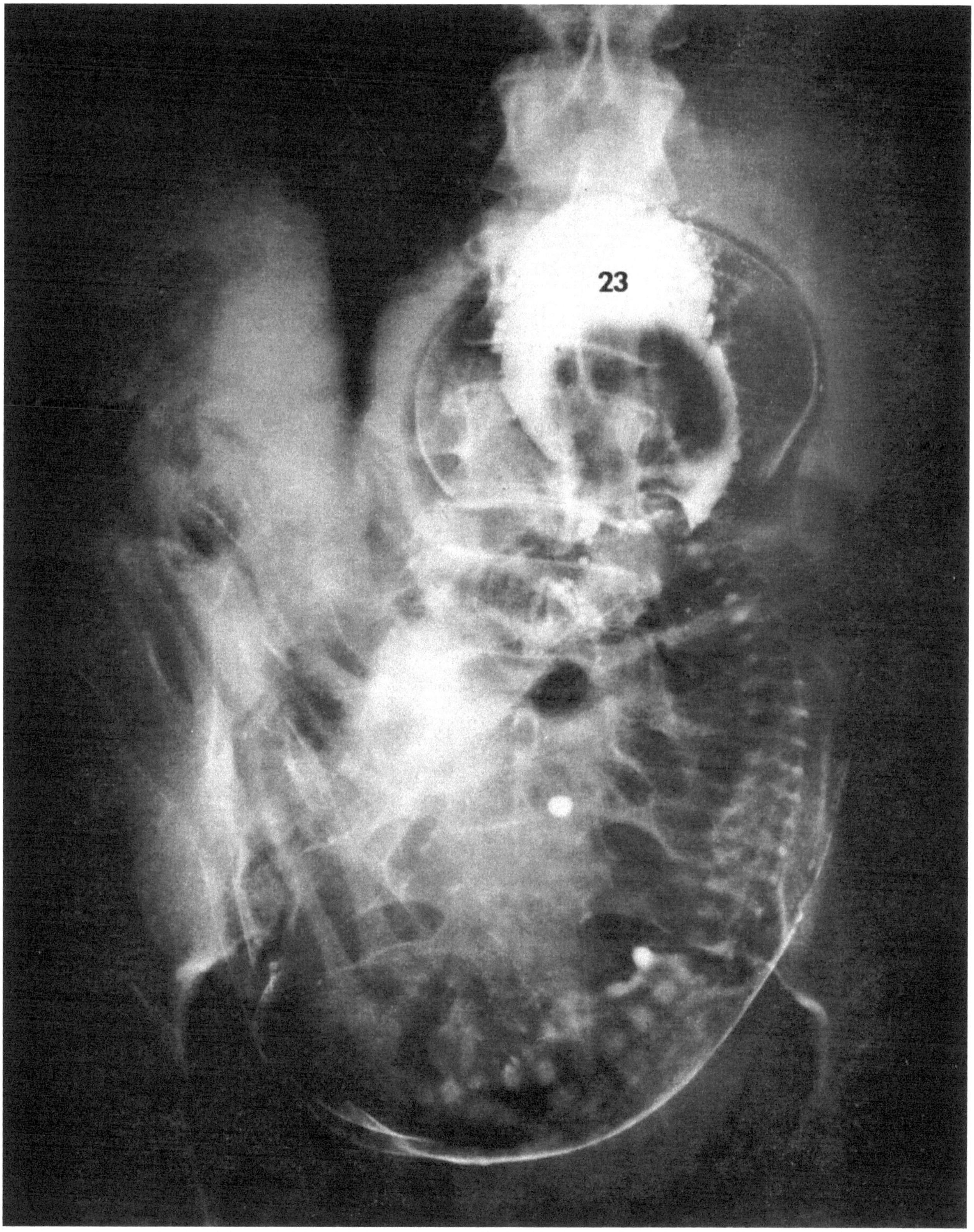


Fig 6c

**Case 5** **Patient H.H./86,** 21 years, fourth gravidity, no parturition.
**Record:** Three abortions in third, fourth, and fifth months.
**Clinical findings:** 26th week of pregnancy; oligohydramnion.
**Ultrasonic findings:** Dubious placental findings; large lacunae (chorangioma?); forced posture of foetus.
**Indication for AFG:** To clear up ultrasonic findings; in-favourable record; search for malformations.
**AFG findings** (Fig. 7a: amniogram 30 minutes from injection; Fig. 7b: foetogram 20 hours from injection): Fluoroscopy shows uterus bicornis and, in the meantime, accumulation of free Lipiodol in left cornu of uterus; foetus visualised in forced posture as recess in amniotic fluid with

Fig. 7a

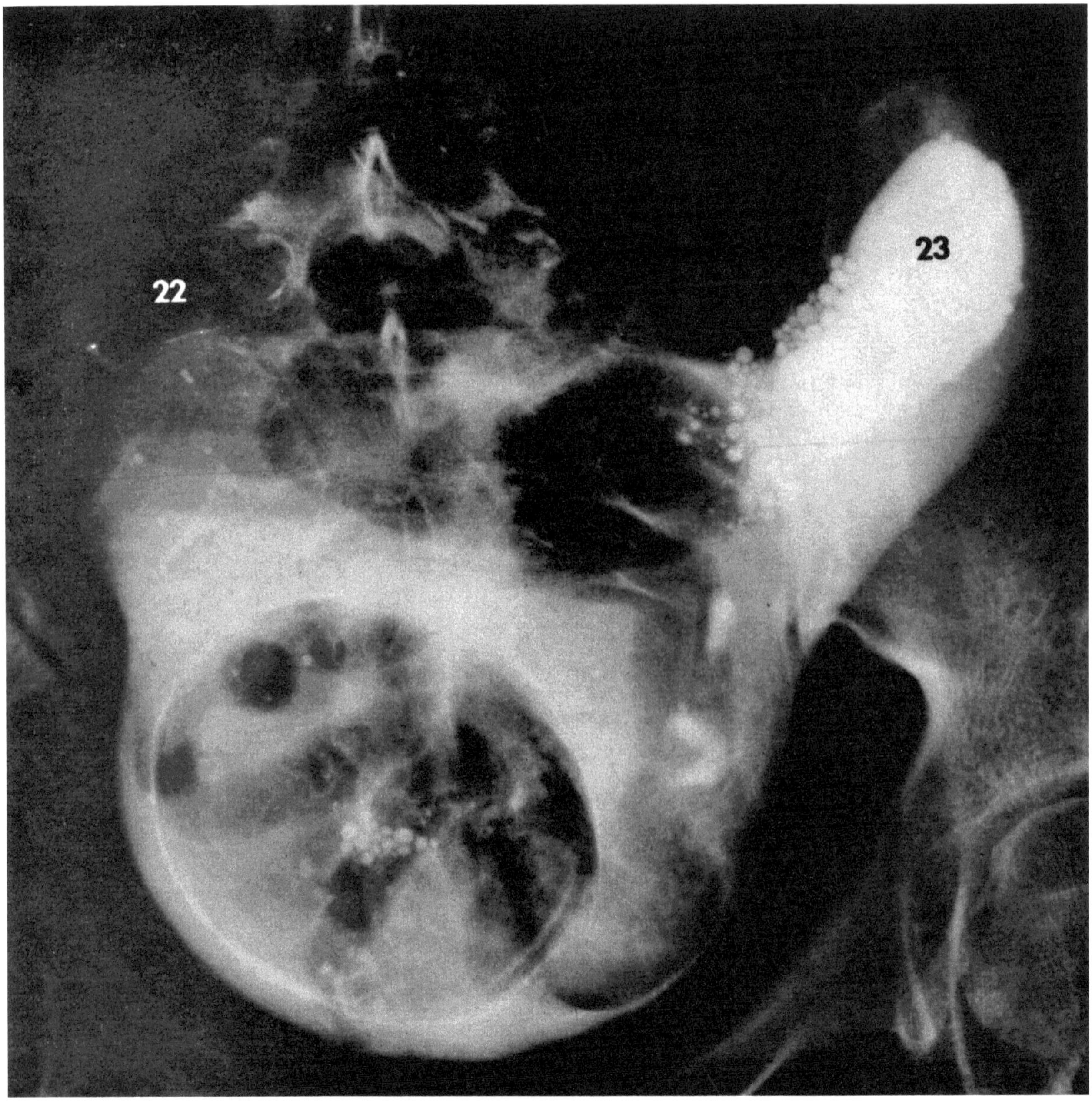

contrast medium. Cephalic presentation; oligohydramnion; contrast medium detectable in small intestine; no additional information of substantial value due to superimposition by maternal skeleton and presence of free Lipiodol UF; maternal excretory urogram.
**Prenatal summary diagnosis:** Bicornuate uterus; no foetal malformation detectable.
**Clinical course:** Spontaneous labour in 30th week of pregnancy; 750 g; no malformation; premature partial placental detachment; no signs of chorangioma; death of newborn eight weeks from birth. ◁

Case 5

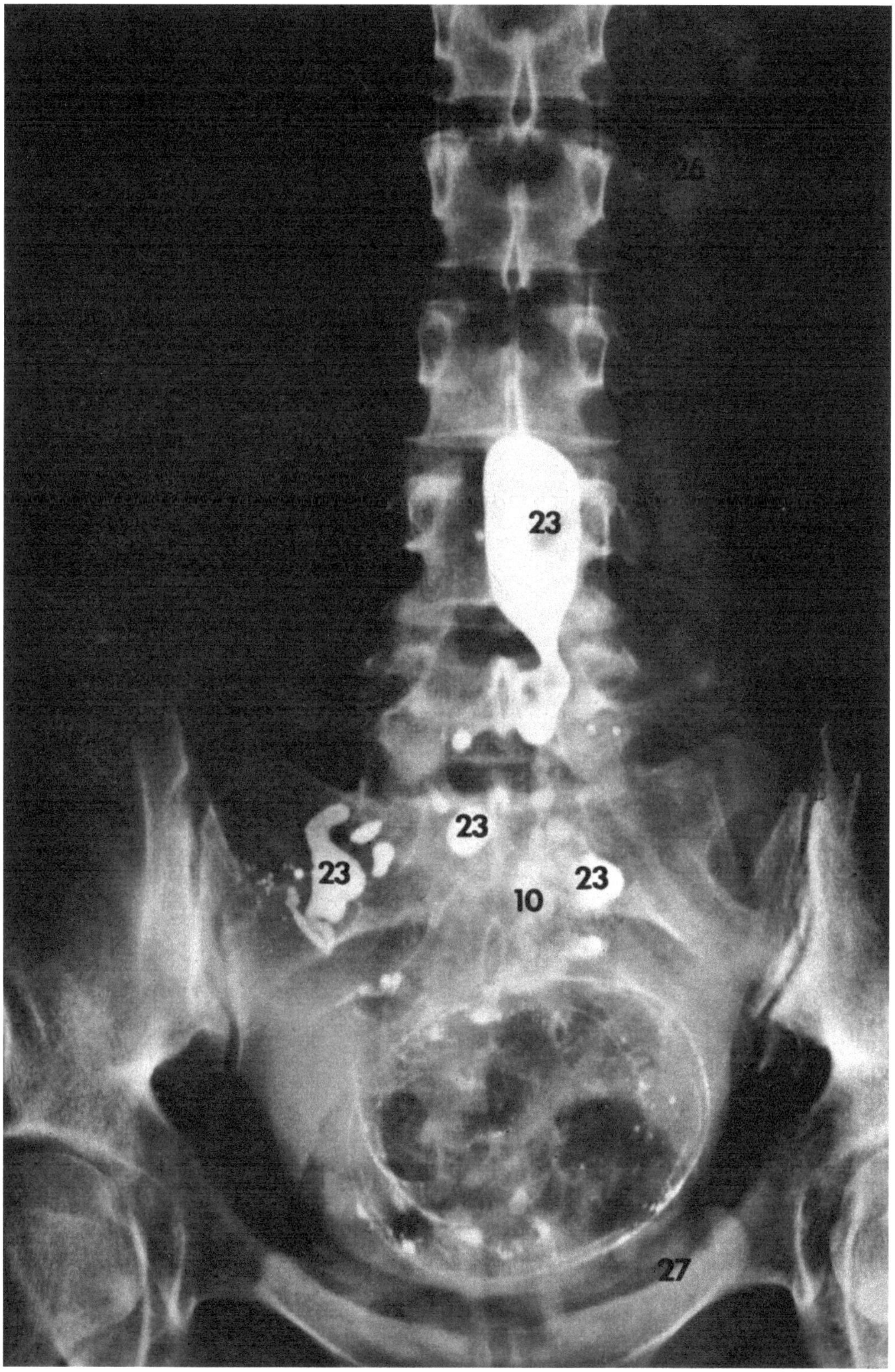


Fig. 7b

**Case 6** **Patient P.S./86,** 19 years, first gravidity.
**Clinical findings:** 35th week of pregnancy; no contributory findings.
**Ultrasonic findings** (Fig. 8a, b): Inhomogeneous echo structure with irregular surface of entire skeleton; extremities are shortened and curved.
**Indication for AFG:** Verification of ultrasonic findings.
**AFG findings** (Fig. 9: foetogram 24 hours from injection):

Fig. 8a

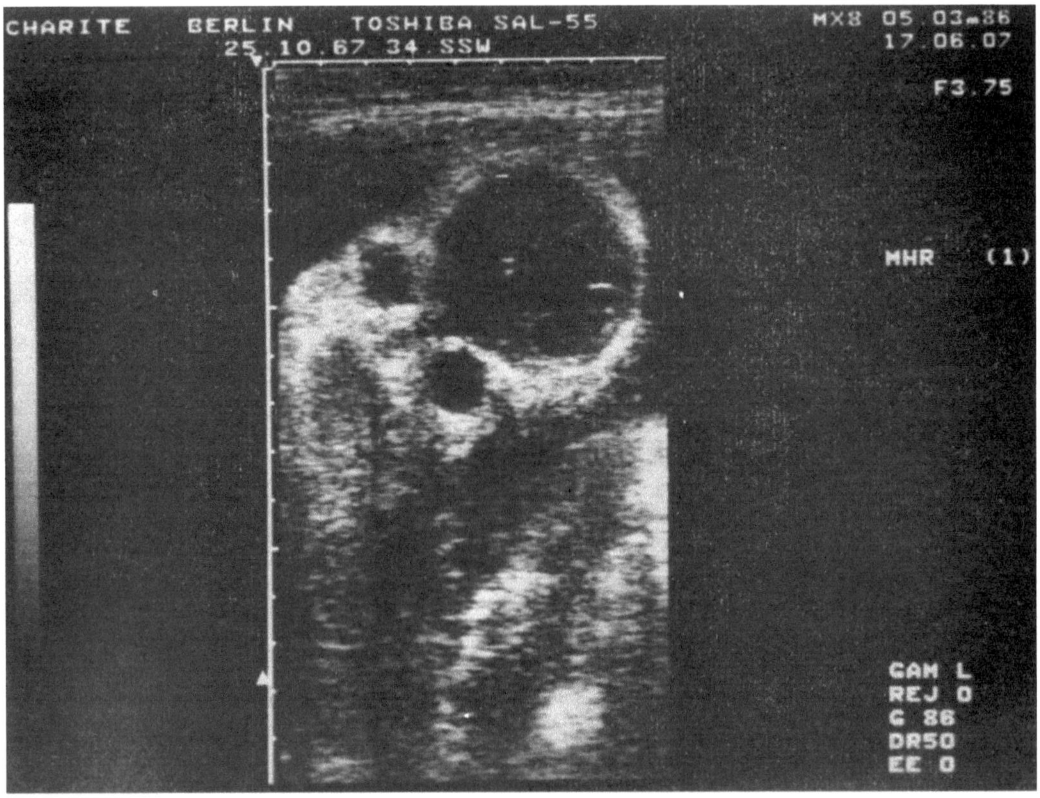


Fig. 8b

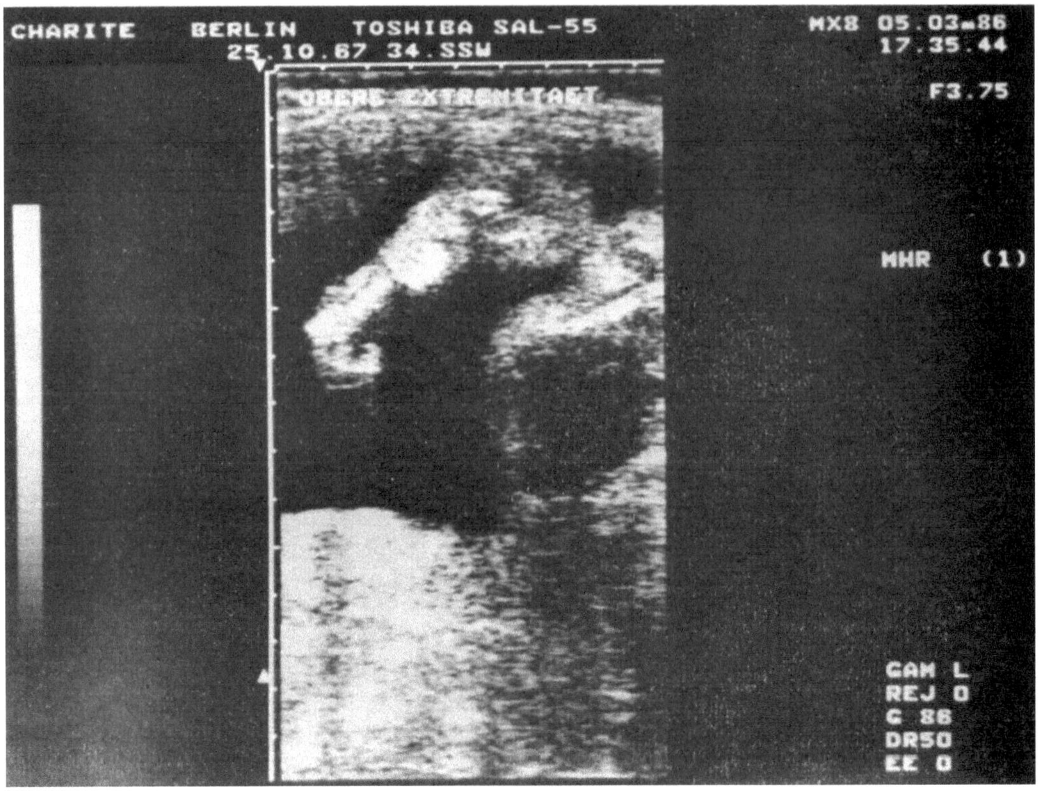

Female foetus; cephalic presentation; skeletal visibility limited to shortened, ungainly ribs, flattened vertebral bodies of cuneiform deformation, and vague contours of pelvic girdle; only marking of soft tissue of shortened, ungainly extremities, no calcification of skull cap; normal gastro-intestinal passage of contrast medium up to rectal ampulla; projection to cheek shows accumulation of free Lipiodol. **Prenatal summary diagnosis:** Osteogenesis imperfecta con-

Case 6

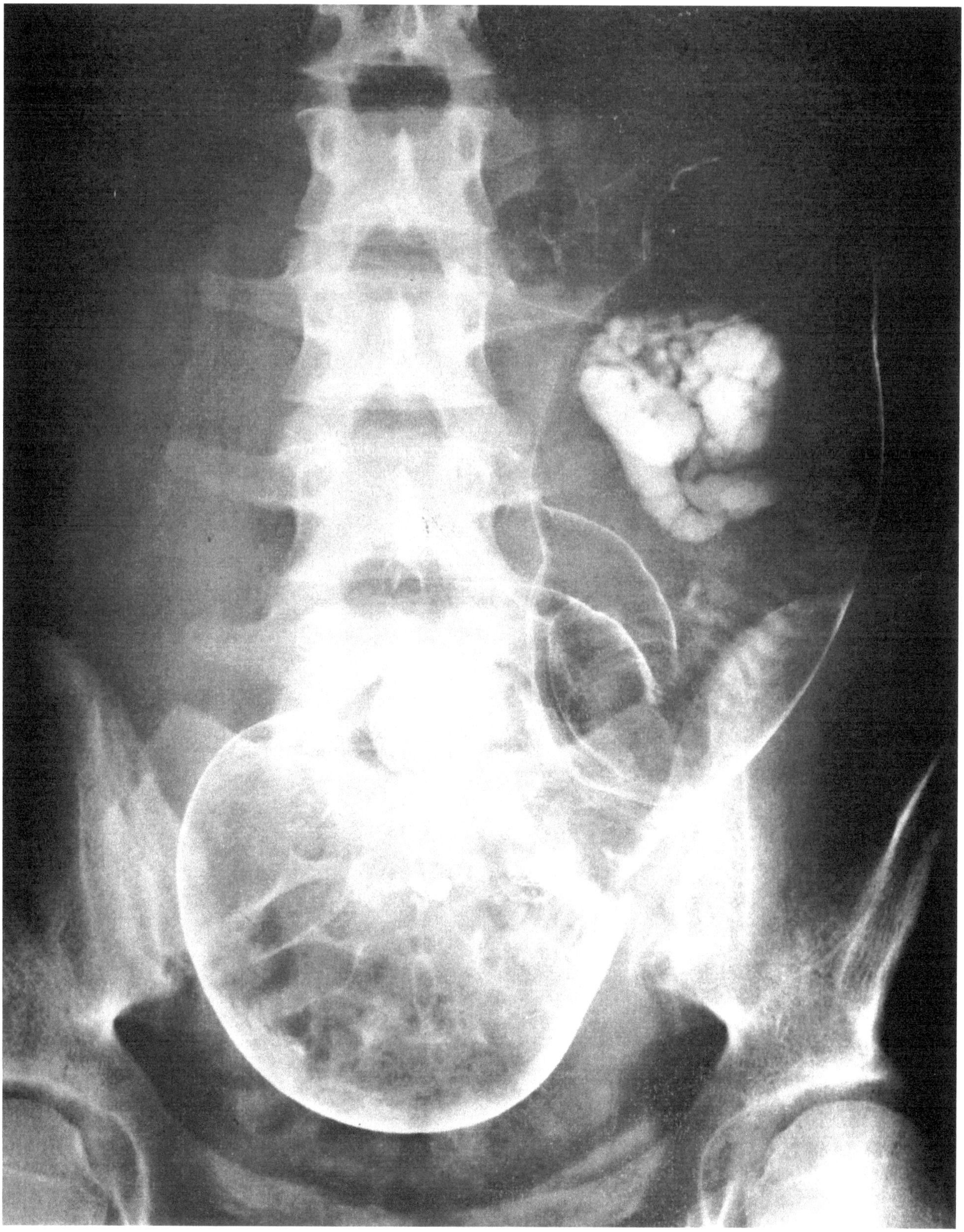

Fig. 9

Case 6 genita, type II (lethal variant Vrolik disease).
**Clinical course:** Termination of pregnancy in 35th week; intrapartum death; 1,140 g, 33 cm.
**Radiogram** (Fig. 10) and **post-mortem findings:** Confirmation of prenatal diagnosis; severest deformation and vesicular distension of costal and tubular bones with thickening of structures typical of multiple intra-uterine fractures. ◁

Fig. 10

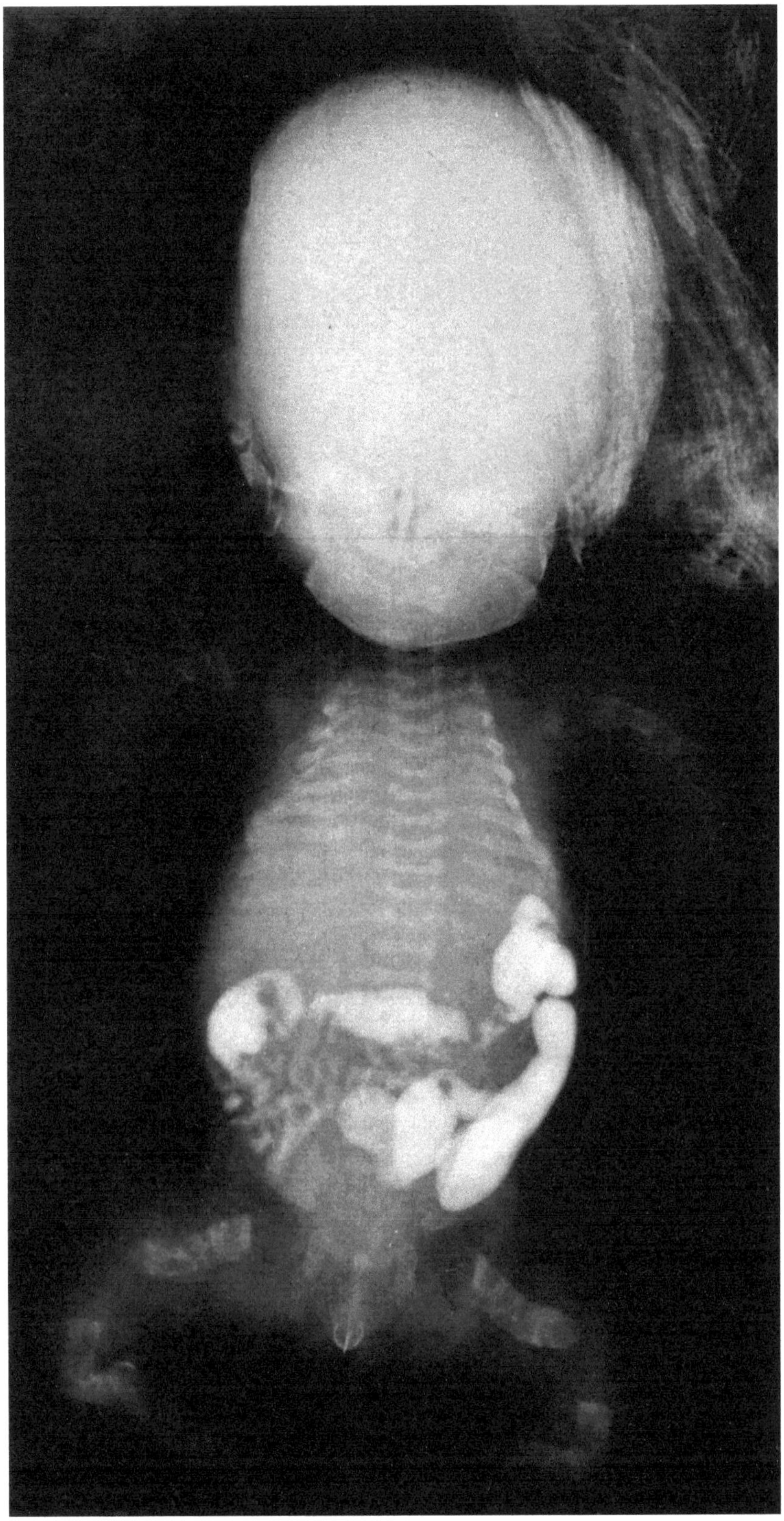

**Patient T.A./78,** 35 years, second gravidity, one parturition.
**Record:** One clinically intact child.
**Clinical findings:** 34th week of pregnancy; polyhydramnion.
**Ultrasonic findings:** No prenatal ultrasonic diagnosis.
Fig. 11 a, b (another patient): Typical ultrasonic aspect of thanatophoric dysplasia.

**Indication for AFG:** Polyhydramnion.
**AFG findings** (Fig. 11 c: foetogram 23 hours from injection): Sex of foetus not determinable; breech presentation; macrocephalus (A); protrusion of forehead; incomplete calcification of skull cap; disproportionality between trunk and extremities; shortened and ungainly extremities (B); shortened

**Case 7**

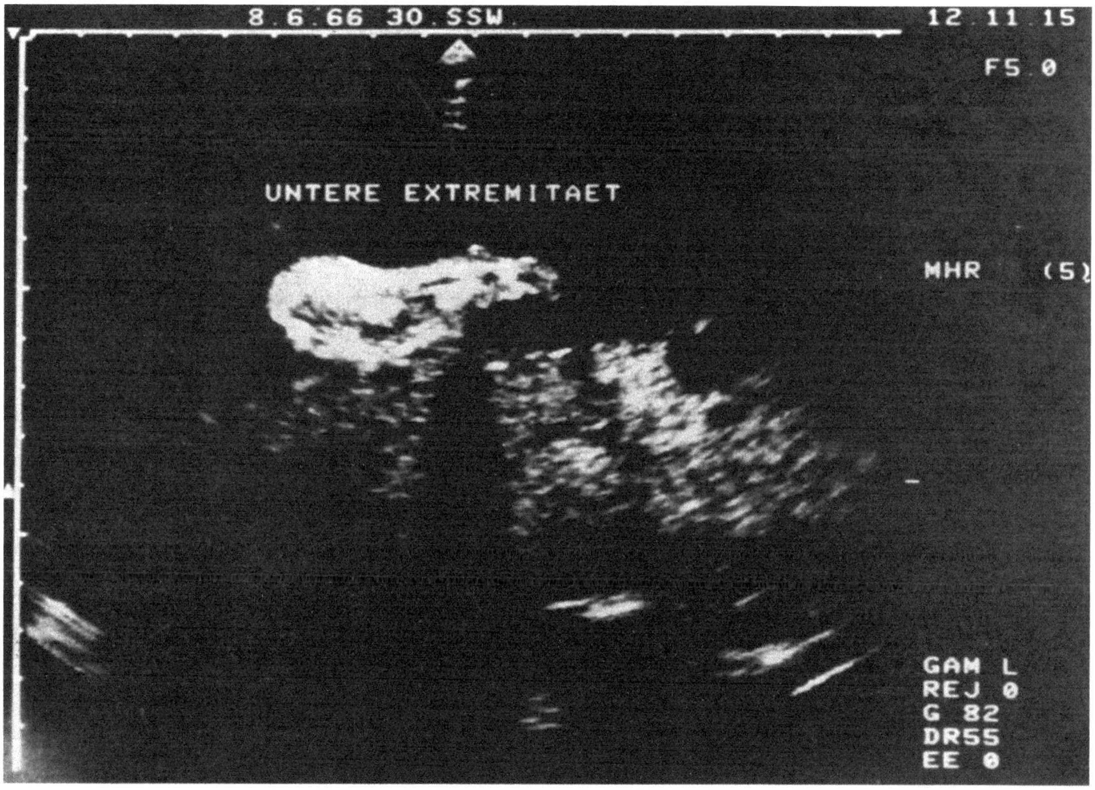


Fig. 11 a

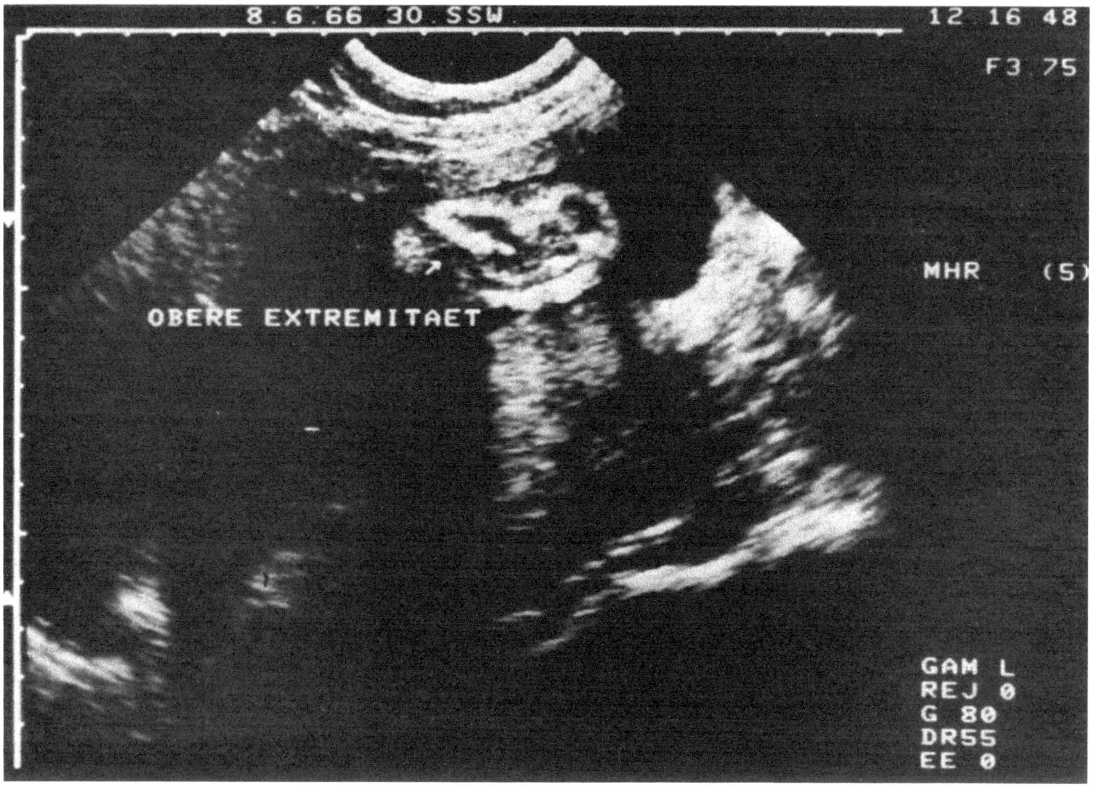


Fig. 11 b

Case 7 ribs; no safe assessment of vertebral column; protrusion of abdominal region; regular gastro-intestinal passage of contrast medium.
**Prenatal summary diagnosis:** Hydrocephalus; skeletal dysplasia.
**Clinical course:** Spontaneous labour in 35th week of pregnancy, following premature rupture of the amnion; female foetus; cranioclasty; 2,000 g, 43 cm.
**Post-mortem findings:** Internal hydrocephalus; achondroplasia; ventricular septal defect, 4 cm in diameter; dilatation of urinary bladder. ◁

Fig. 11 c

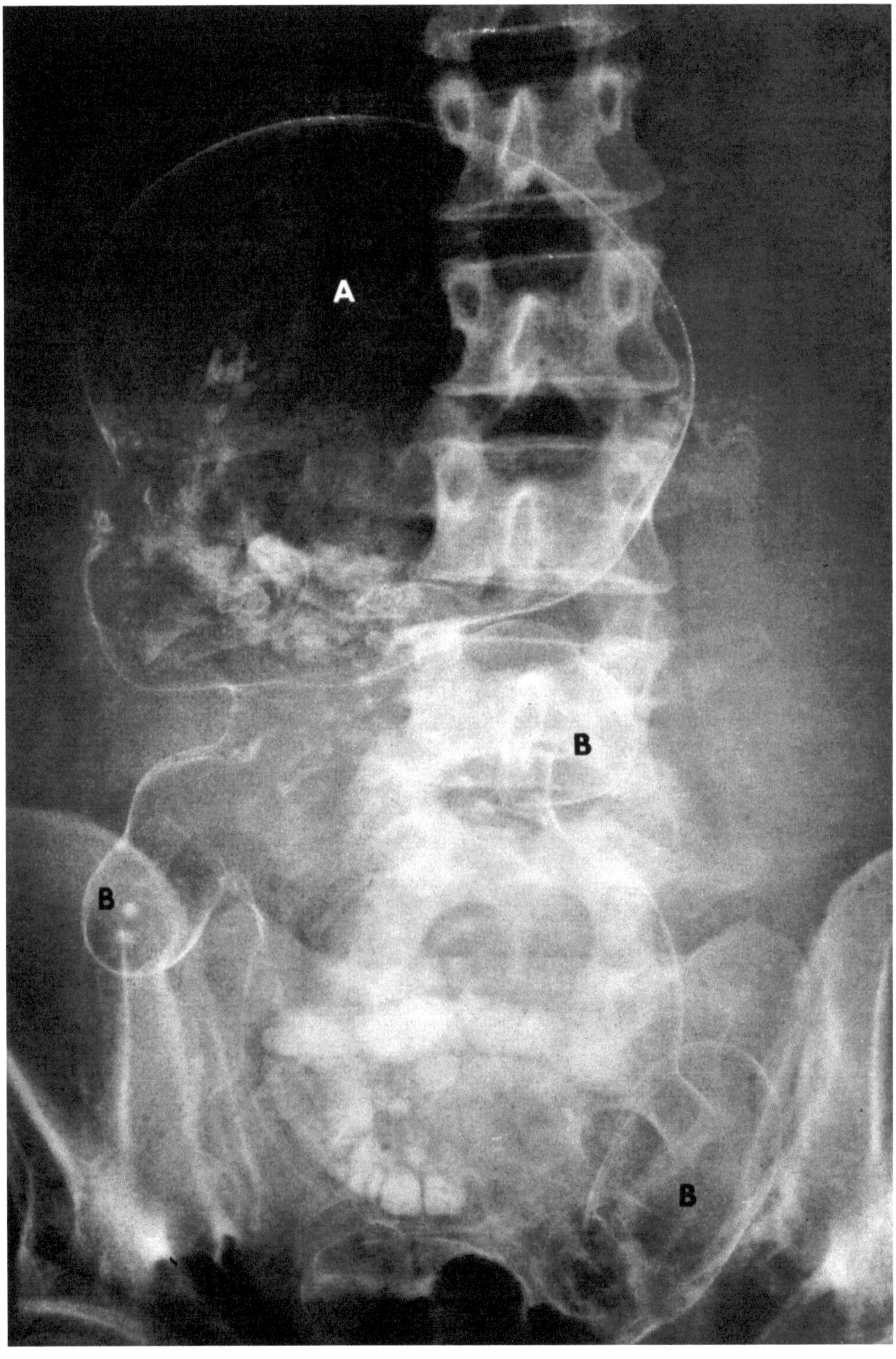

Patient H.C./83, 25 years, second gravidity, one parturition.
**Record:** One clinically intact child.
**Clinical findings:** 36th week of pregnancy; polyhydramnion.
**Ultrasonic findings:** Polyhydramnion; hydrops fetus universalis; internal hydrocephalus.
**Indication for AFG:** Polyhydramnion; search for malformations.
**AFG findings** (Fig. 12: foetogram 24 hours from injection): Female foetus; breech presentation; polyhydramnion; hydrops fetus universalis; shortened and ungainly extremities (B); no ribs detectable; no gastro-intestinal passage of contrast medium detectable; clearly visible protrusion of

**Case 8**

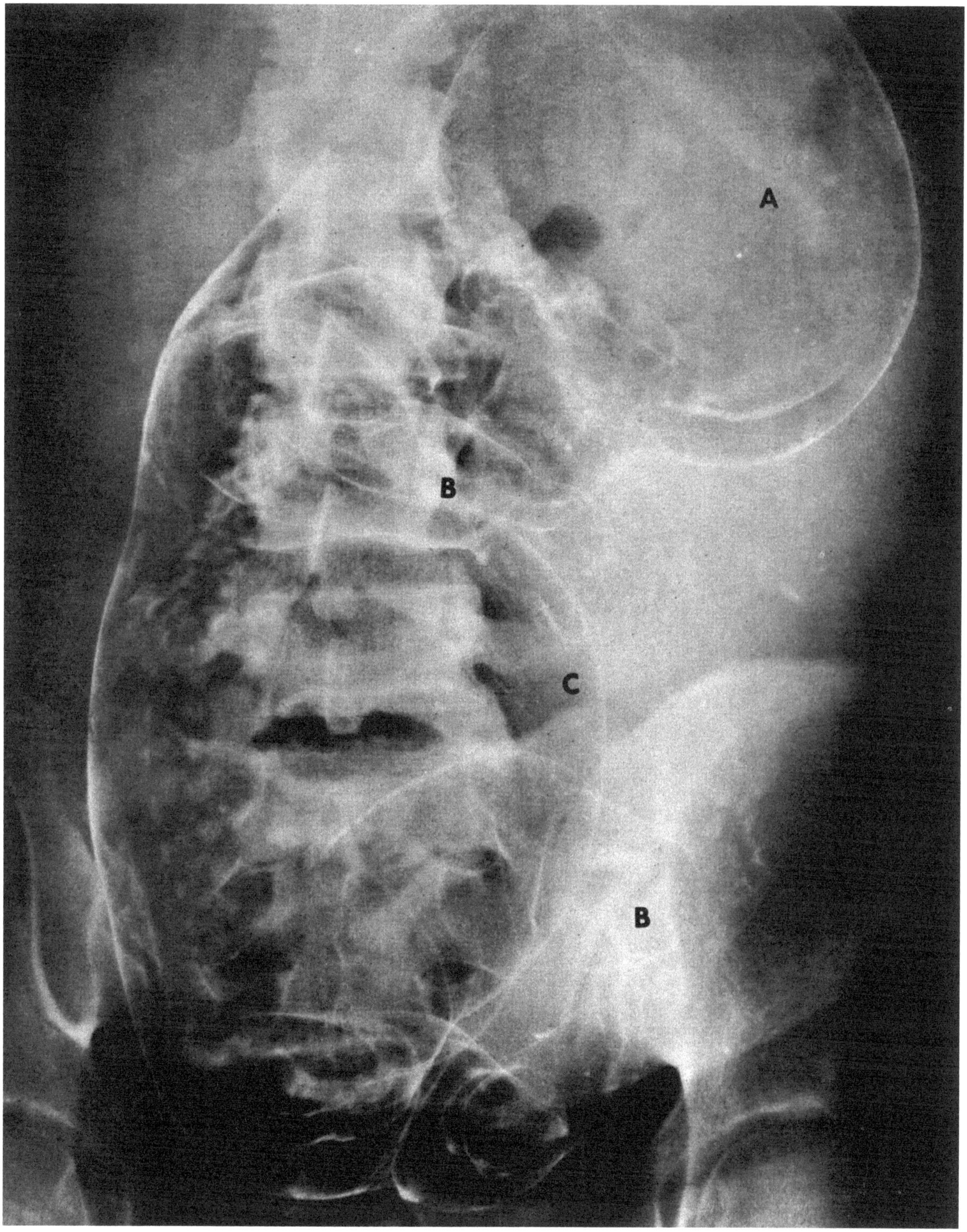


Fig. 12

Case 8 abdominal region ascits (C); incomplete calcification of skull cap reflecting internal hydrocephalus (A).
**Prenatal summary diagnosis:** Hydrops fetus universalis; internal hydrocephalus; skeletal dysplasia.
**Clinical course:** Termination of pregnancy in 36th week; 3,360 g, 50 cm.

**Radiogram** (Fig. 13) and **post-mortem findings:** Short-rib polydactyly syndrome (Saldino-Noonan); internal hydrocephalus; univentricular heart; aortic hypoplasia and aortic valve hypoplasia; four accessory (supernumerary) spleens; mesenterium ileocolicum commune; hydrops fetus universalis (230 ml ascites). ◁

Fig. 13

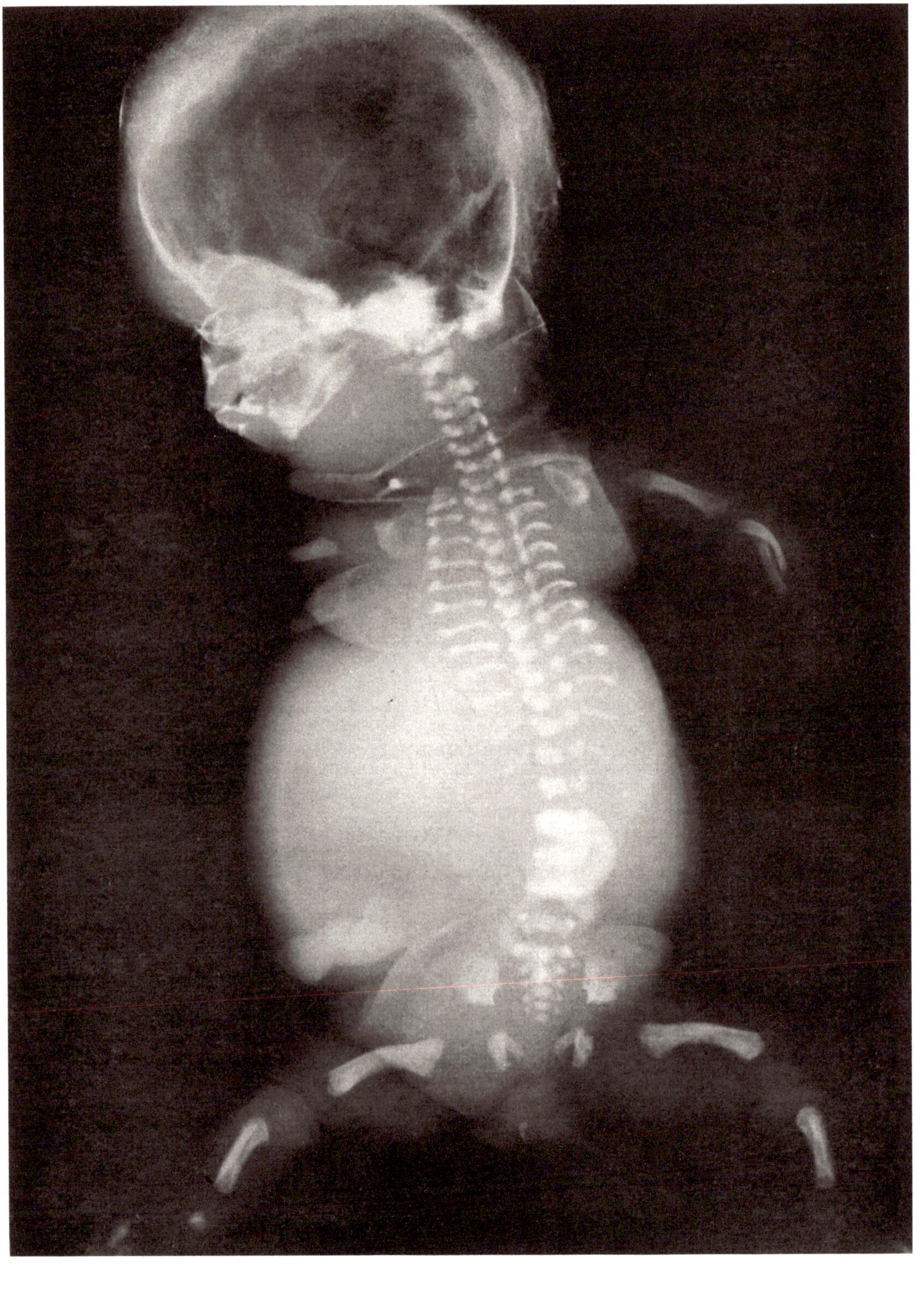

**Patient B.M./82,** 27 years, second gravidity, first parturition.
**Record:** One microcephalic child, postpartum death.
**Clinical findings:** 38th week of pregnancy; no contributory findings.
**Ultrasonic findings:** No prenatal ultrasonic diagnosis.

**Indication for AFG:** Infavourable record.
**AFG findings** (Fig. 14a: foetogram 24 hours from injection; Fig. 14b: 48 hours from injection): Male foetus; cephalic presentation; enlarged head (A); time-adequate gastro-



Fig. 14a

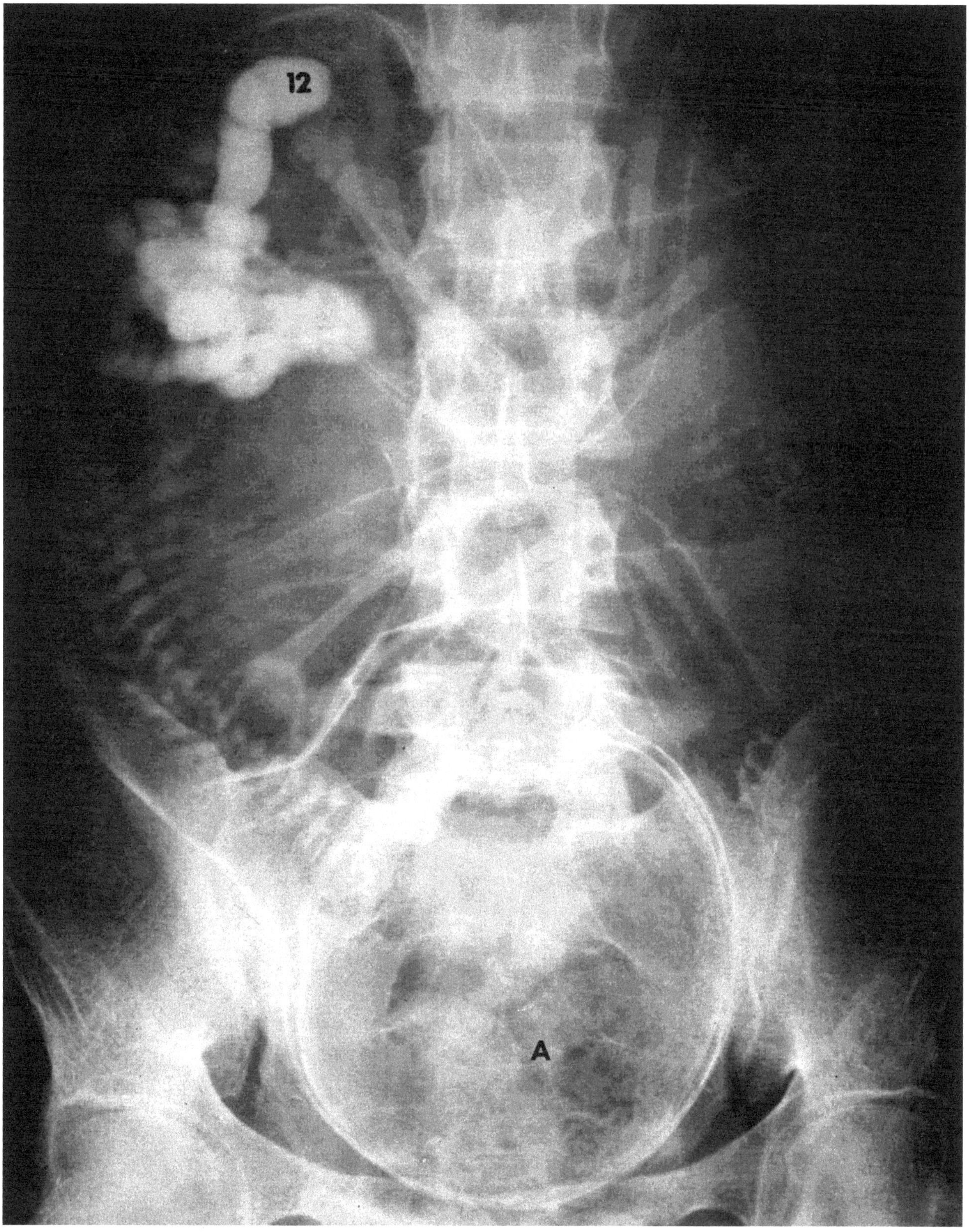

Case 9 intestinal passage of contrast medium up to rectal ampulla; pressure effect on sigma from ventral due to filled urinary bladder in second scan (Fig. 14b).

**Prenatal summary diagnosis:** Suspicion of hydrocephalus.

**Clinical course:** Spontaneous labour after induction in 38th week of pregnancy; newborn, 3,250 g, 54 cm, died at birth.

**Post-mortem diagnosis:** Internal hydrocephalus; cleft lip face palate. ◁

Fig. 14b

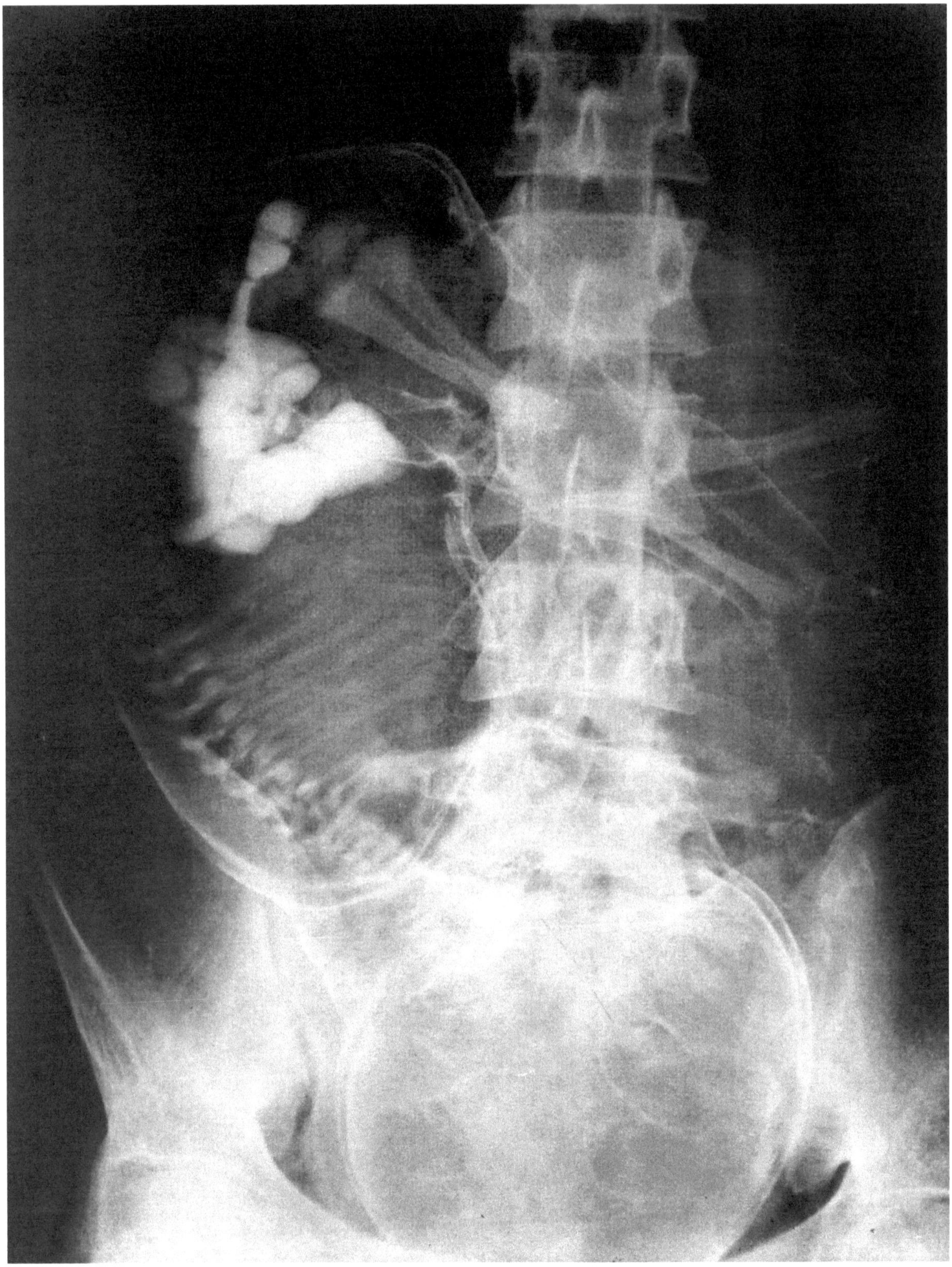

**Patient H.B./85,** 21 years, first gravidity.
**Clinical findings:** 24th week of pregnancy; oligohydramnion.
**Ultrasonic findings:** Oligohydramnion; detection of incompletely developed skull cap, with primordium restricted to occipital arc, so that brain reaches into amniotic cavity like tumour and is in direct contact with amniotic fluid; suspicion of dorsal amniotic cord; no additional malformations detectable.

**Case 10**

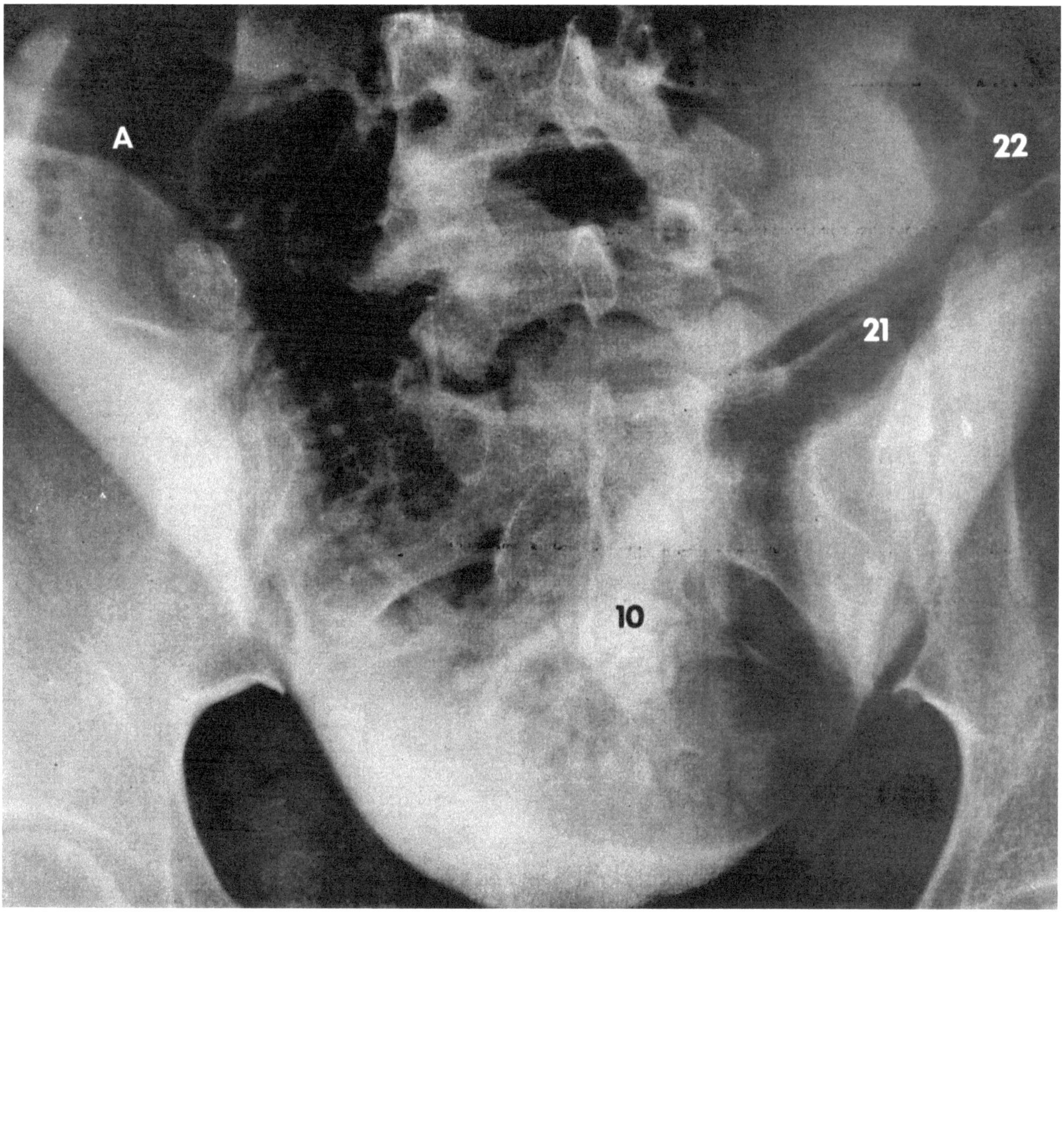


Fig. 15

Case 10 **Indication for AFG:** Oligohydramnion; confirmation of ultrasonic findings; signs indicative of additional malformations.

**AFG findings** (Fig. 15: amniogram 30 minutes from injection): Probable sex is female; breech presentation; oligohydramnion; calcification of skull cap limited to occipital bone; detection of exencephalia stretching ventrally beyond orbit and visceral cranium (A); contrast medium in stomach

Fig. 16a

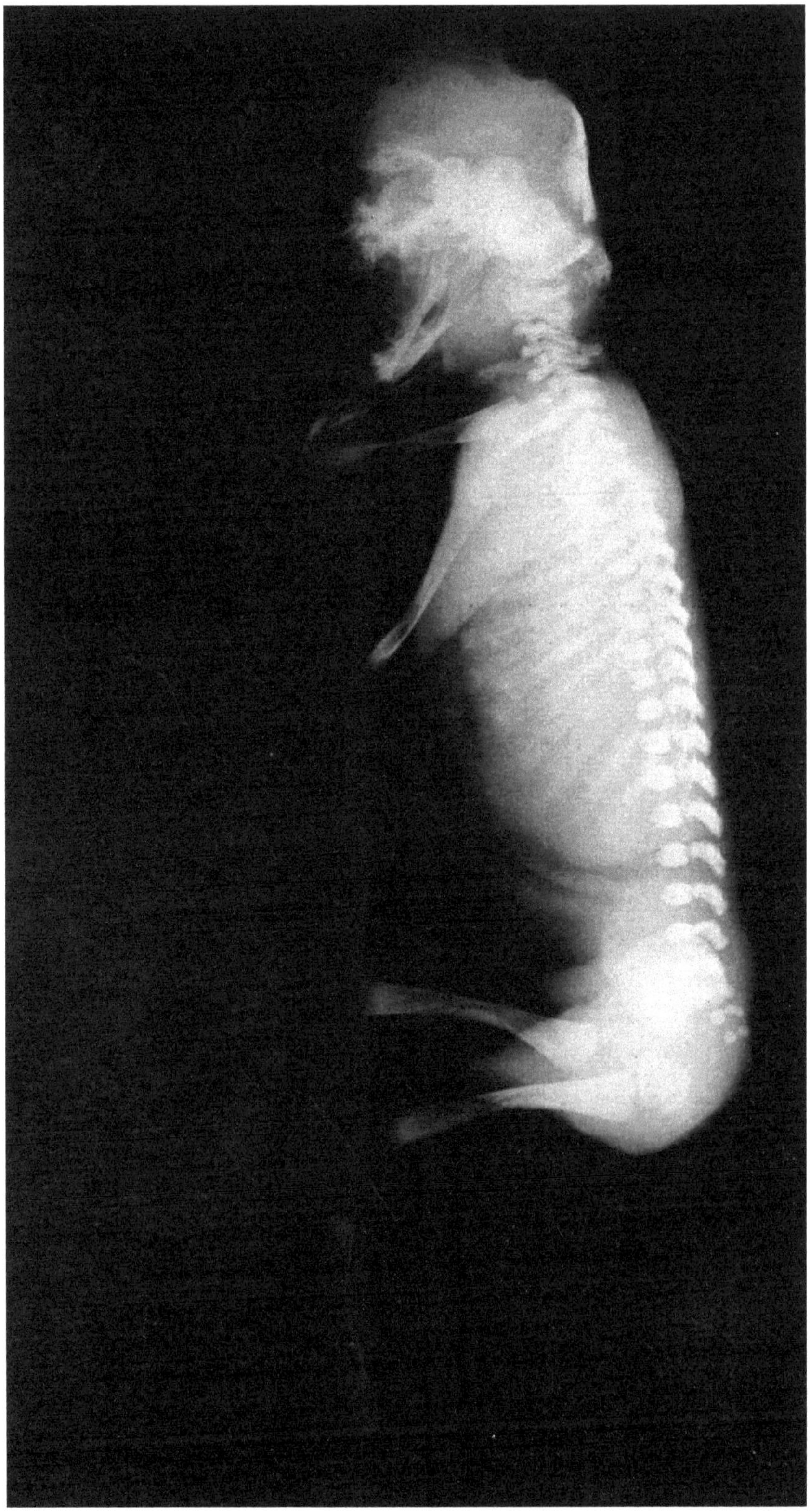

and small intestine; no additional malformations.
**Prenatal summary diagnosis:** Acranius with exencephalia.
**Clinical course:** Termination of gravidity at end of 24th week; female; 480 g, 27 cm.

**Radiogram** (mammography technique; Fig. 16a) and **post-mortem findings:** Confirmation of prenatal diagnosis; clinical aspect shows Figure 16b. ◁

Case 10

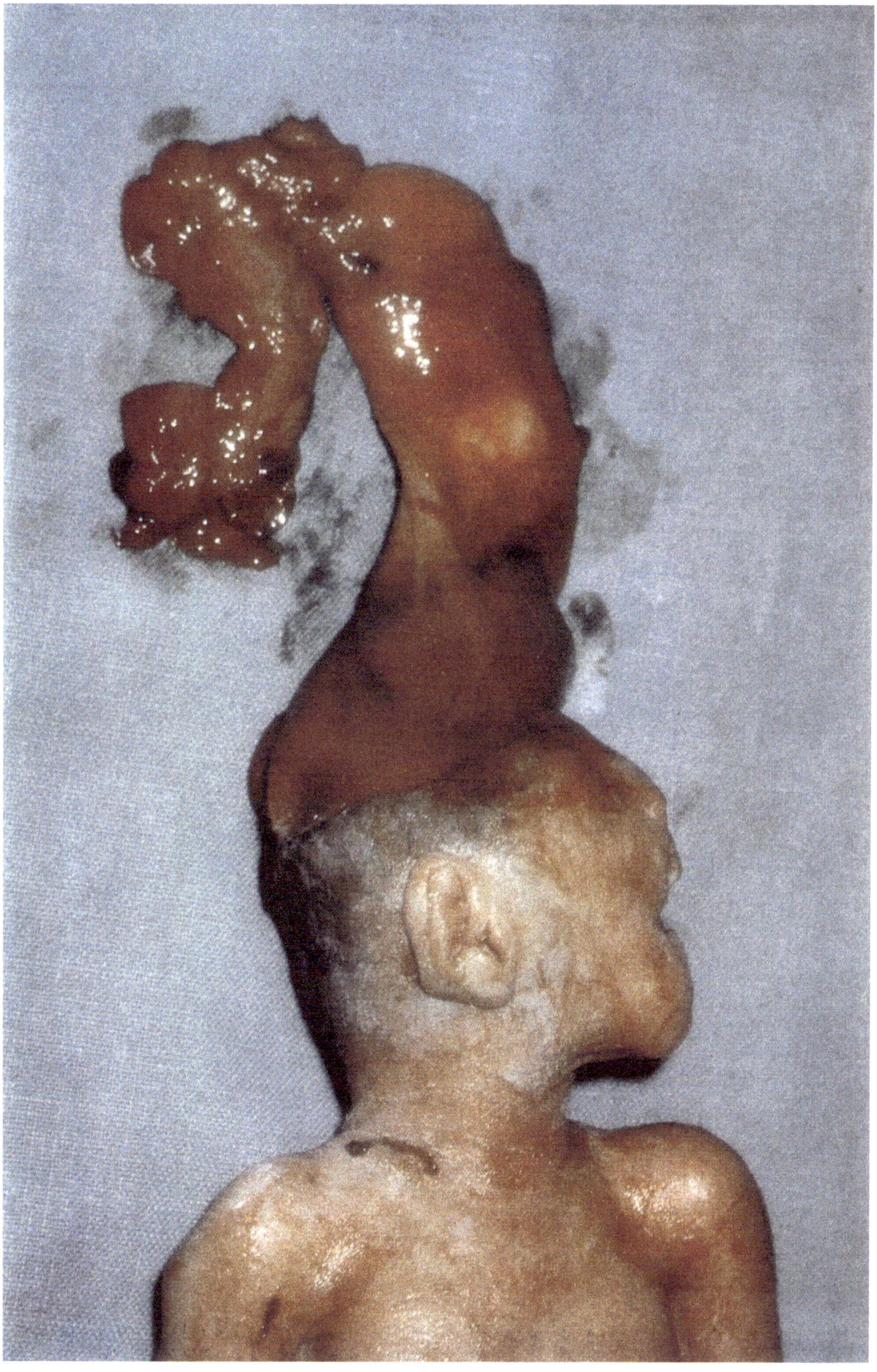

Fig. 16b

**Case 11** **Patient J.G./76,** 26 years, third gravidity, one parturition.
**Record:** One clinically intact child; one interruption.
**Clinical findings:** 36th week of pregnancy; no contributory findings.
**Ultrasonic findings:** Echoless tumour, ca. 8 cm in size, in occipital region; suspicion of meningo-encephalocele; bi-parietal head diameter 8.2 cm; no additional malformations detectable.
**Indication for AFG:** Verification of ultrasonic findings; signs indicative of additional malformations.
**AFG findings** (Fig. 17: amniogram 30 minutes from injection): Sex of foetus not determinable; cephalic presentation;

Fig. 17

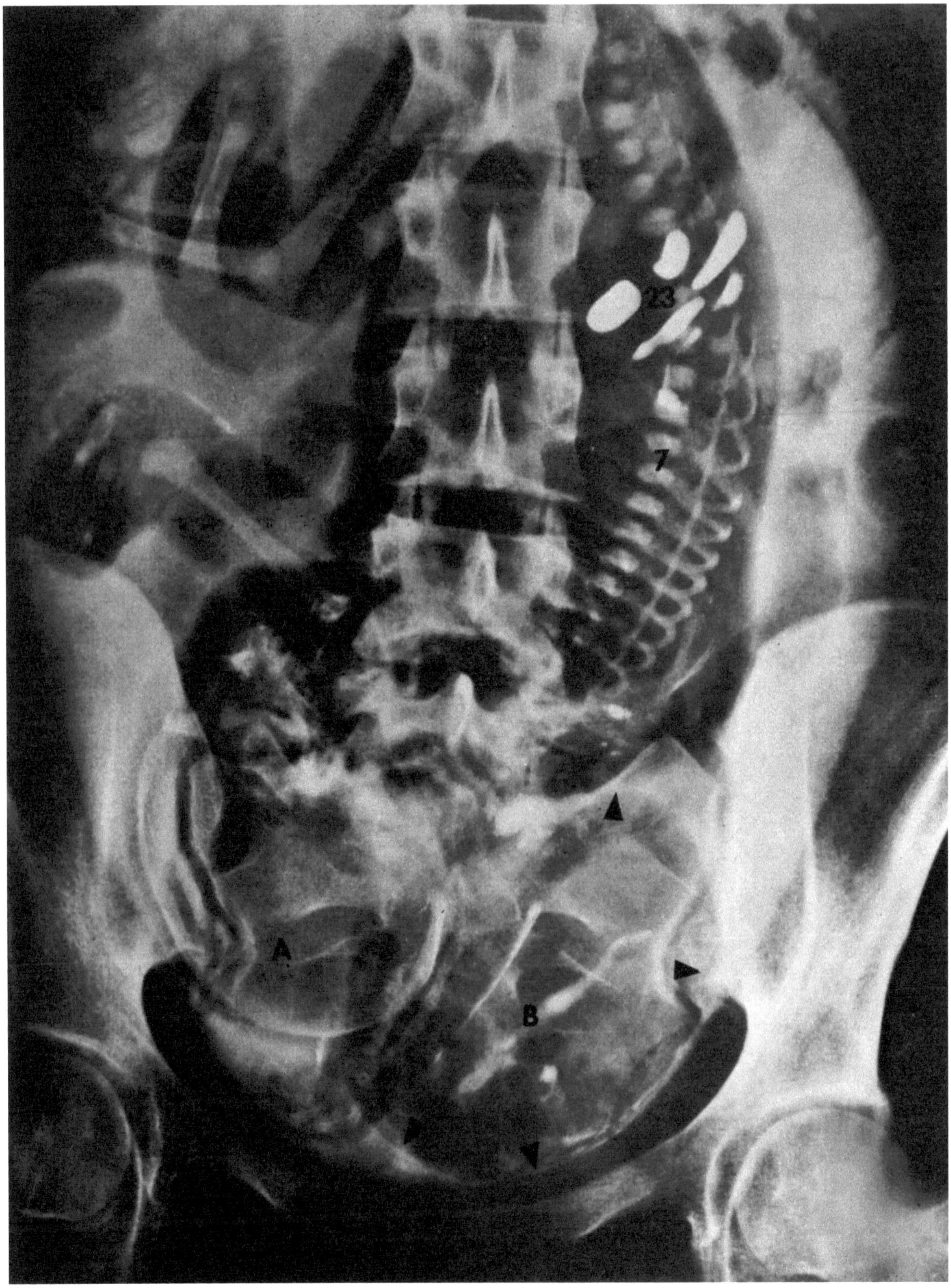

microcephalus (A); oval recess in contrast medium, 12 cm, in nuchal region (B; arrows); no additional malformations detectable.
**Prenatal summary diagnosis:** Large meningo-encephalocele; microcephalia.

Case 11

**Clinical course:** Spontaneous labour in 37th week; delivery of boy, 3,290 g, 50 cm; death of child after birth.
**Radiogram** (Fig. 18): Occipital soft-tissue tumour, 12 cm; extensive osseous occipital defect.
**Post-mortem findings:** Confirmation of prenatal diagnosis. ◁

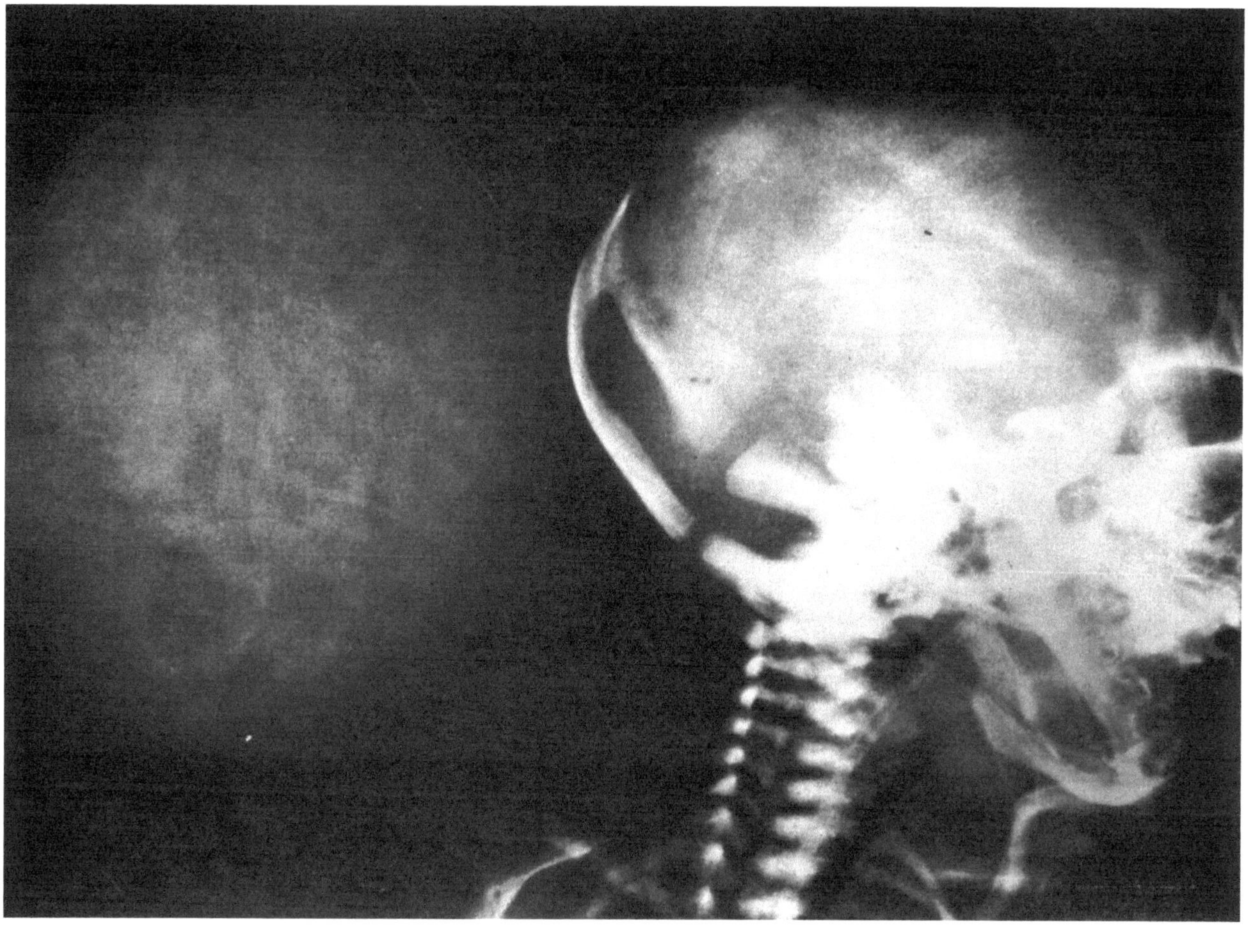

Fig. 18

**Case 12** **Patient S.P./84,** 32 years, third gravidity, one parturition.
**Record:** One abortion; one stillbirth (unknown cause); diabetes mellitus on insulin medication.
**Clinical findings:** 35th week of pregnancy; no contributory findings.
**Ultrasonic findings** (Fig. 19): Both lateral ventricles slightly enlarged since 27th week of pregnancy; no occipital meningocele in earlier tests, but 7-cm meningocele (diameter) in 35th week of pregnancy; no solid structures in cele (×); arachnoid floating in synchronicity with pulsation was the only finding recordable from osseous defect of occipital

Fig. 19

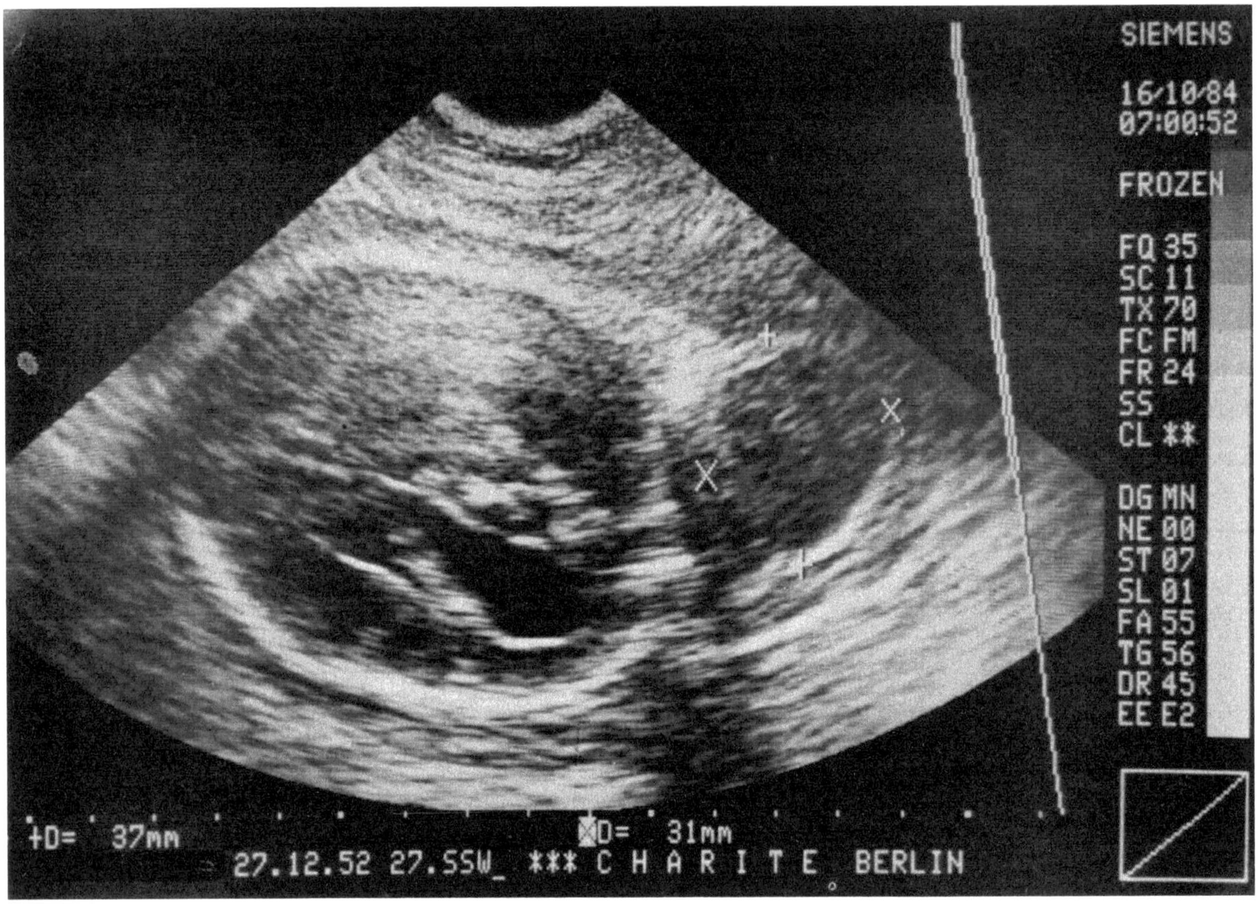

bone; no additional malformations; inconspicuous movement of extremities.
**Indication for AFG:** Search for additional malformations.
**AFG findings** (Fig. 20a: amniogram 120 minutes from injection; Fig. 20b: foetogram 24 hours from injection):

Female foetus; cephalic presentation; amniogram shows occipital cele as recess in contrast-imaged amniotic fluid with Lipiodol marking (A); contrast of stomach and small intestine; foetogram shows occipital cele, 6 cm in size; complete gastro-intestinal passage of contrast medium up



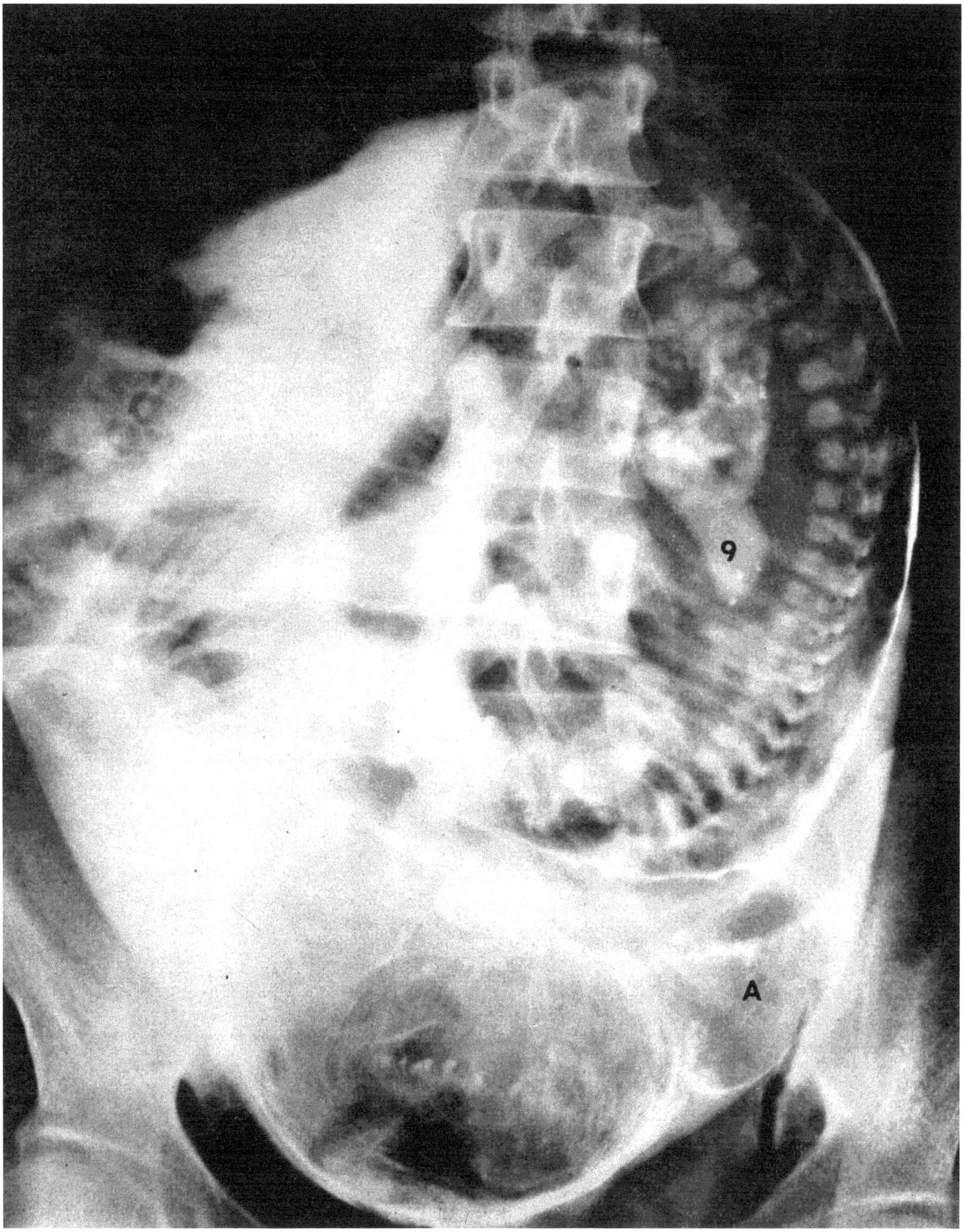


Fig. 20a

Case 12 to rectal ampulla; inconspicuous skeletal configuration; no additional malformations.

**Computed tomography:** No additional findings were obtained from computed tomography of foetal cranium conducted in parallel with AFG.

**Prenatal summary diagnosis:** Slight internal hydrocephalus; genuine occipital meningocele.

**Clinical course:** Delivery by caesarean section in 36th week of pregnancy; 2,890 g, 50 cm; operation on meningocele on second day of age; no intraoperative complications. ◁

Fig. 20b

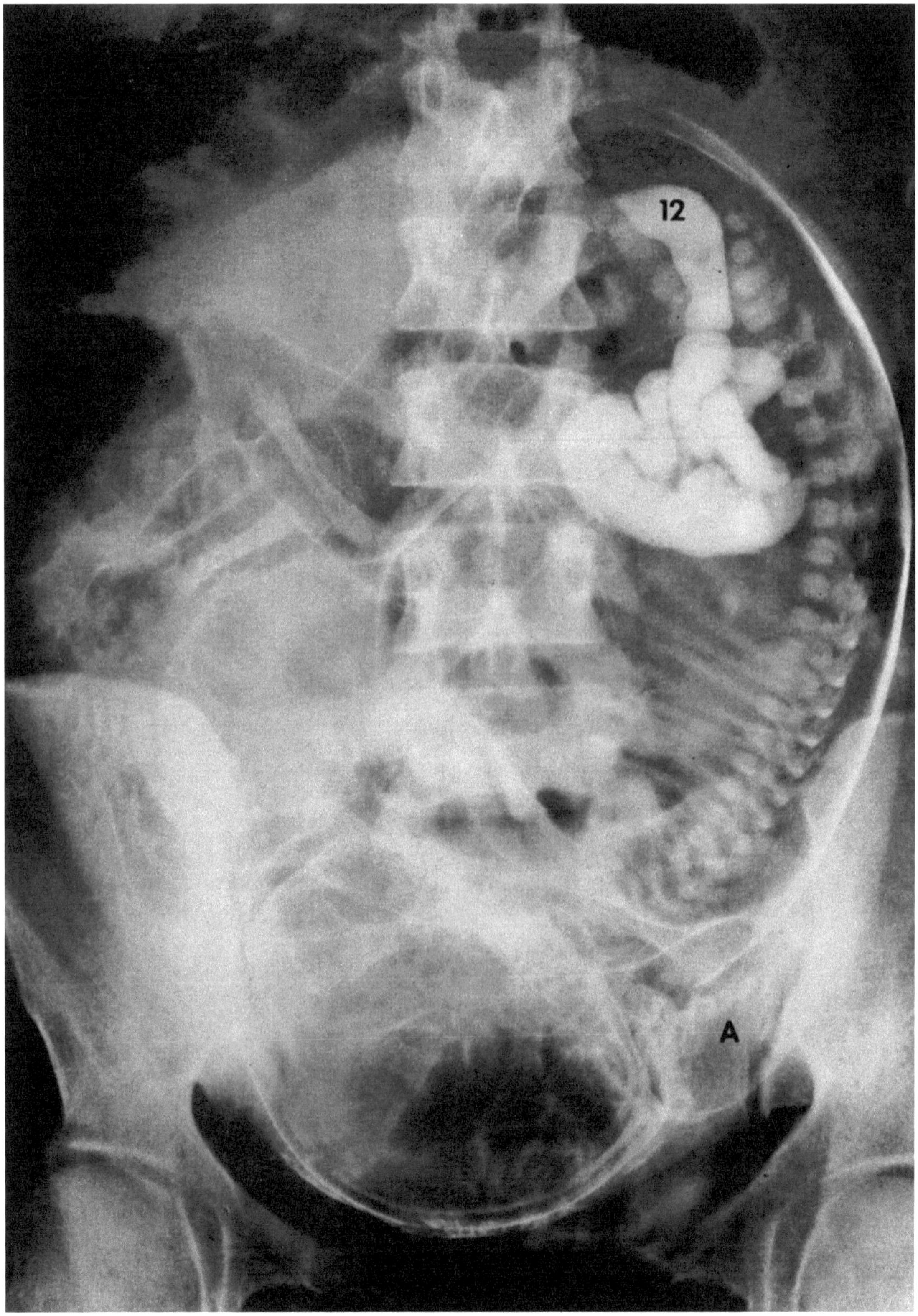

**Patient S.A./85,** 28 years, second gravidity, one parturition.
**Record:** One anencephalic child.
**Clinical findings:** 32nd week of pregnancy; no contributory findings.
**Ultrasonic findings:** Internal hydrocephalus, 15 mm in maximum pallium thickness; gibbus at levels of cervical and thoracic spine; neural tube defect with 7-cm cele containing cystic and solid components; normal motility of all extremities; normophagia.

**Case 13**

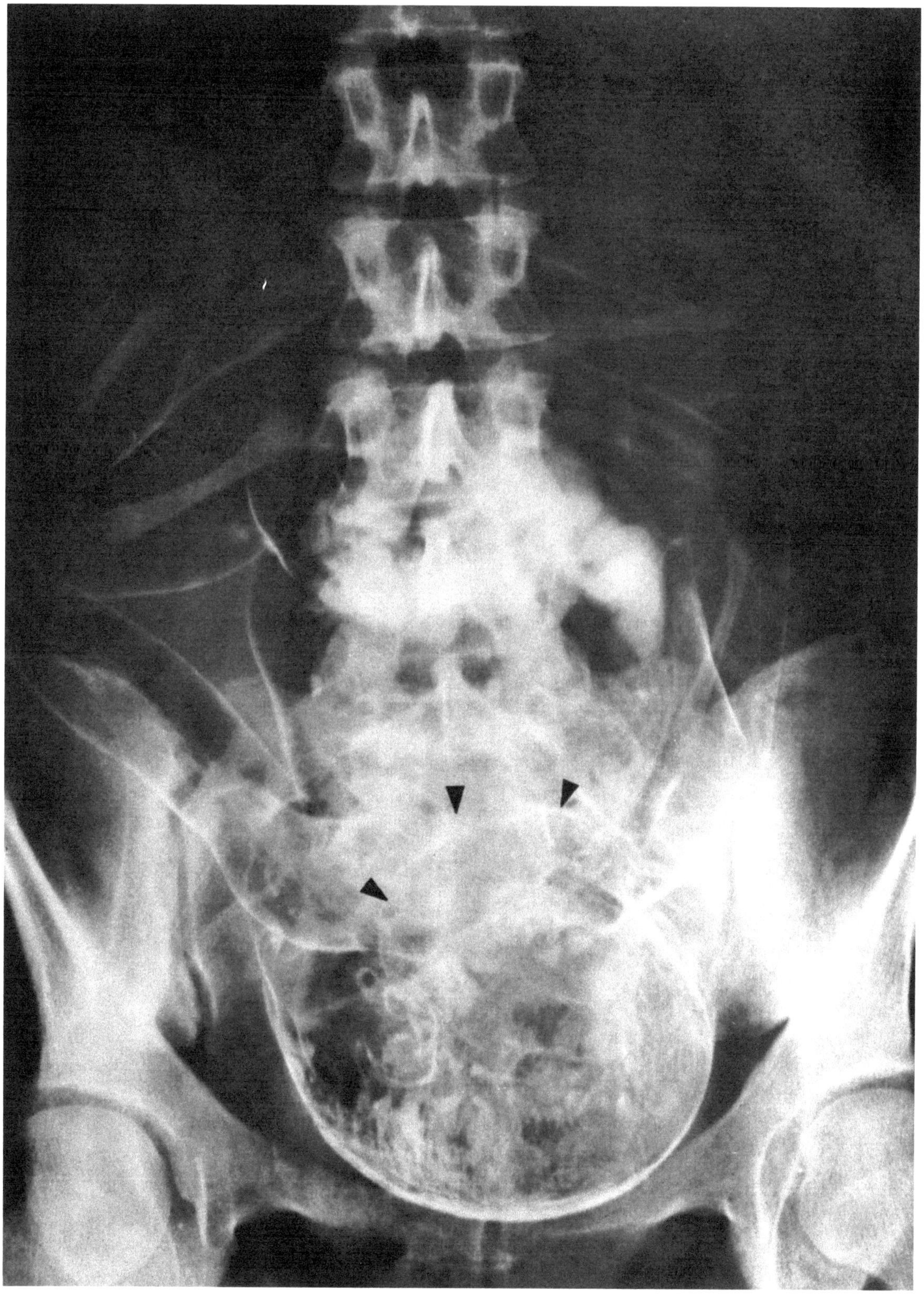

Fig. 21

Case 13 **Indication for AFG:** Confirmation of ultrasonic findings; search for additional malformations.
**AFG findings** (Fig. 21: foetogram 24 hours from injection): Sex of foetus not determinable; cephalic presentation; arcuate contour in cervical region (arrows); vertebral column cannot be assessed for superimposition by maternal skeleton; vague calcification of skull cap; regular gastro-intestinal passage of contrast medium; no clue to club-feet.

Fig. 22a

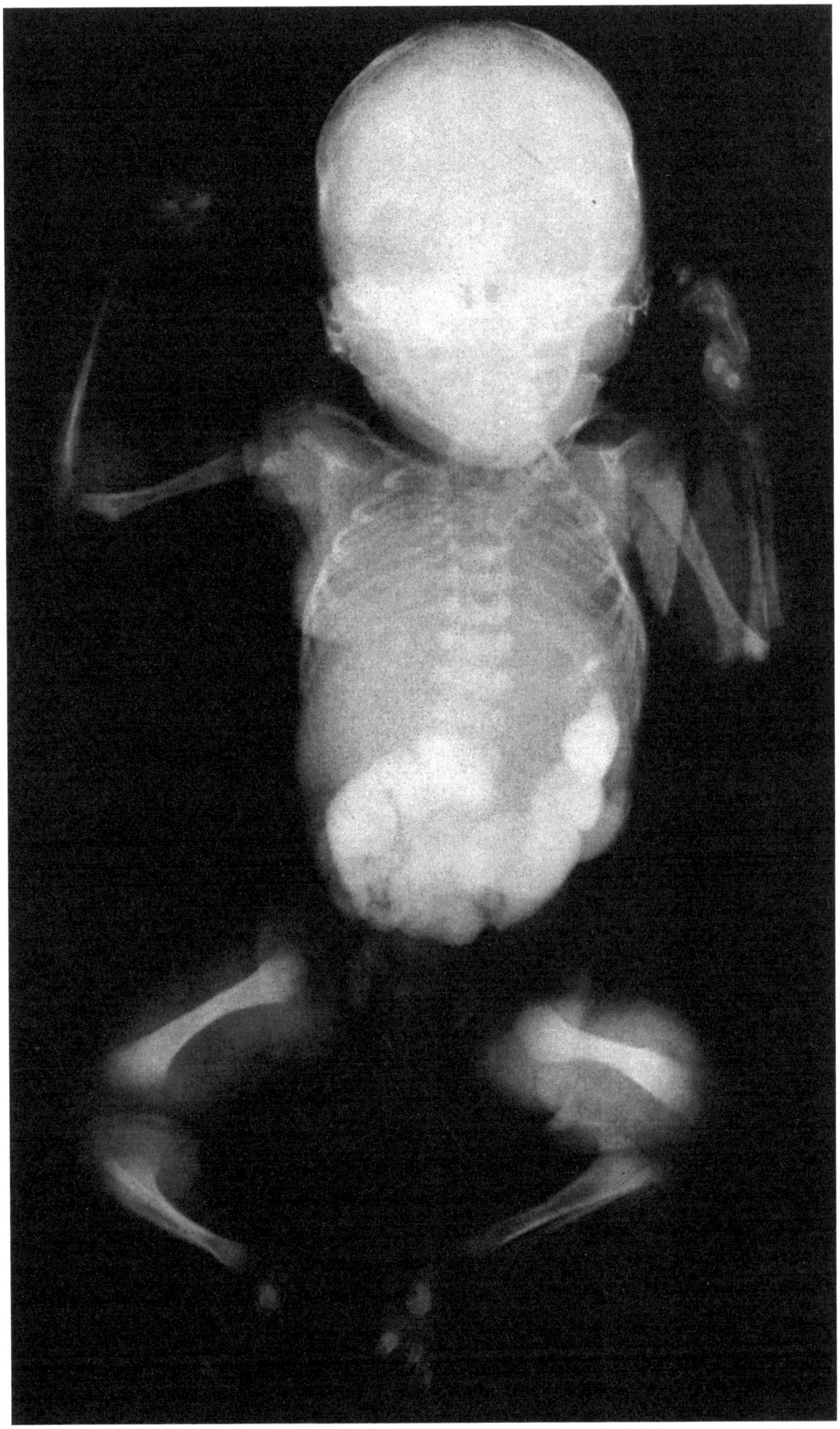

**Prenatal summary diagnosis:** Internal hydrocephalus; thoracic myelomeningocele; no paraplegic symptoms.
**Clinical course:** Termination of pregnancy in 32nd week; female foetus, 2,400 g, 44 cm; intrapartum death.

**Radiogram** (Fig. 22a, b) and **post-mortem findings:** Internal hydrocephalus; myelomeningocele of thoracic spine (arrows); multiple malformations of vertebral bodies of thoracic spine; transposition of large vessels. ◁

Case 13

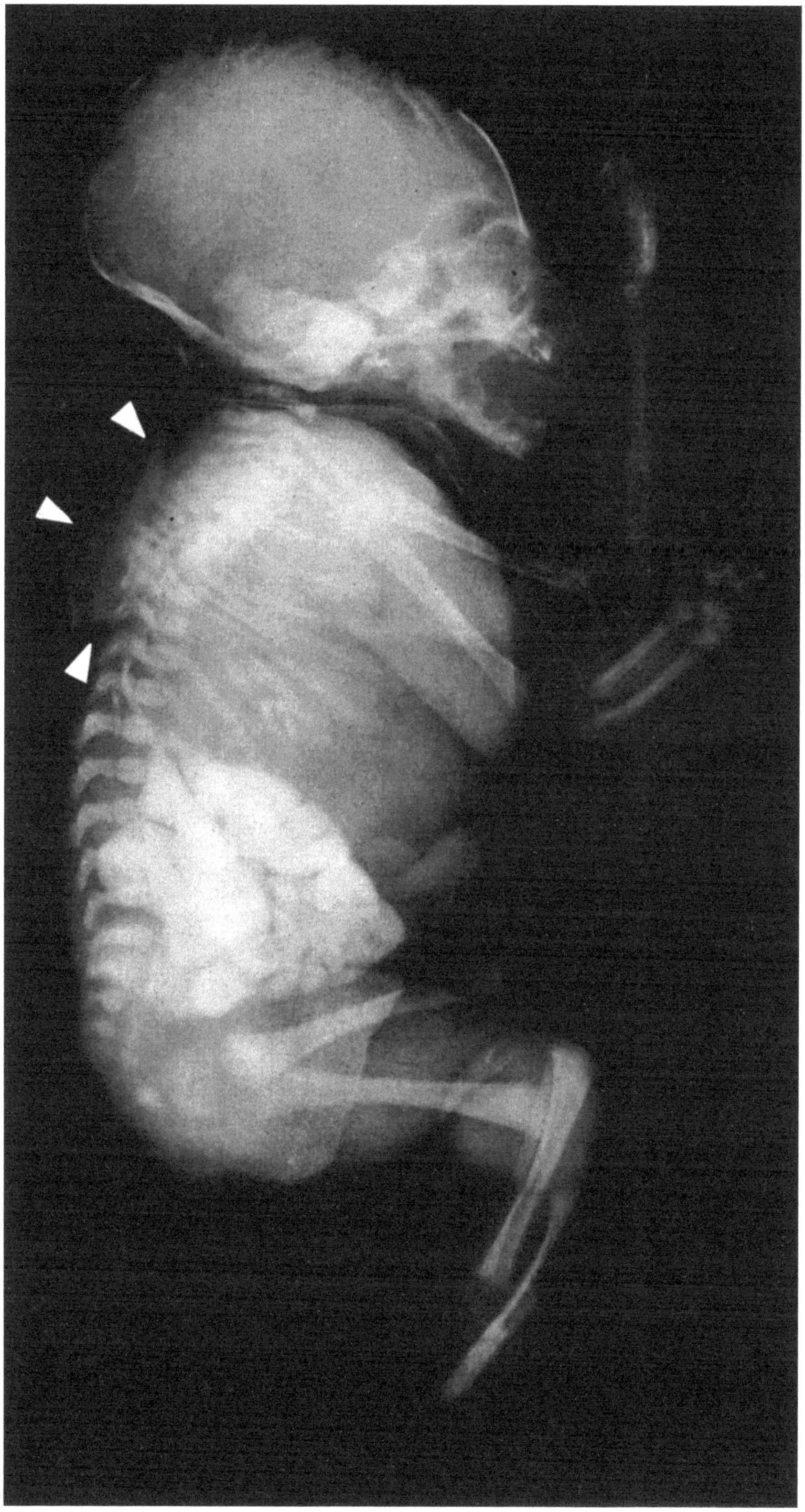

Fig. 22 b

**Case 14** **Patient M.C./84,** 20 years, first gravidity.
**Clinical findings:** 37th week of pregnancy; no contributory findings.

**Ultrasonic findings:** Biparietal head diameter 10.7 cm; ventricular diameter 7.6 cm; suspicion of lumbar neural tube defect with celes; assessment impaired by oligohydramnion.

Fig. 23a

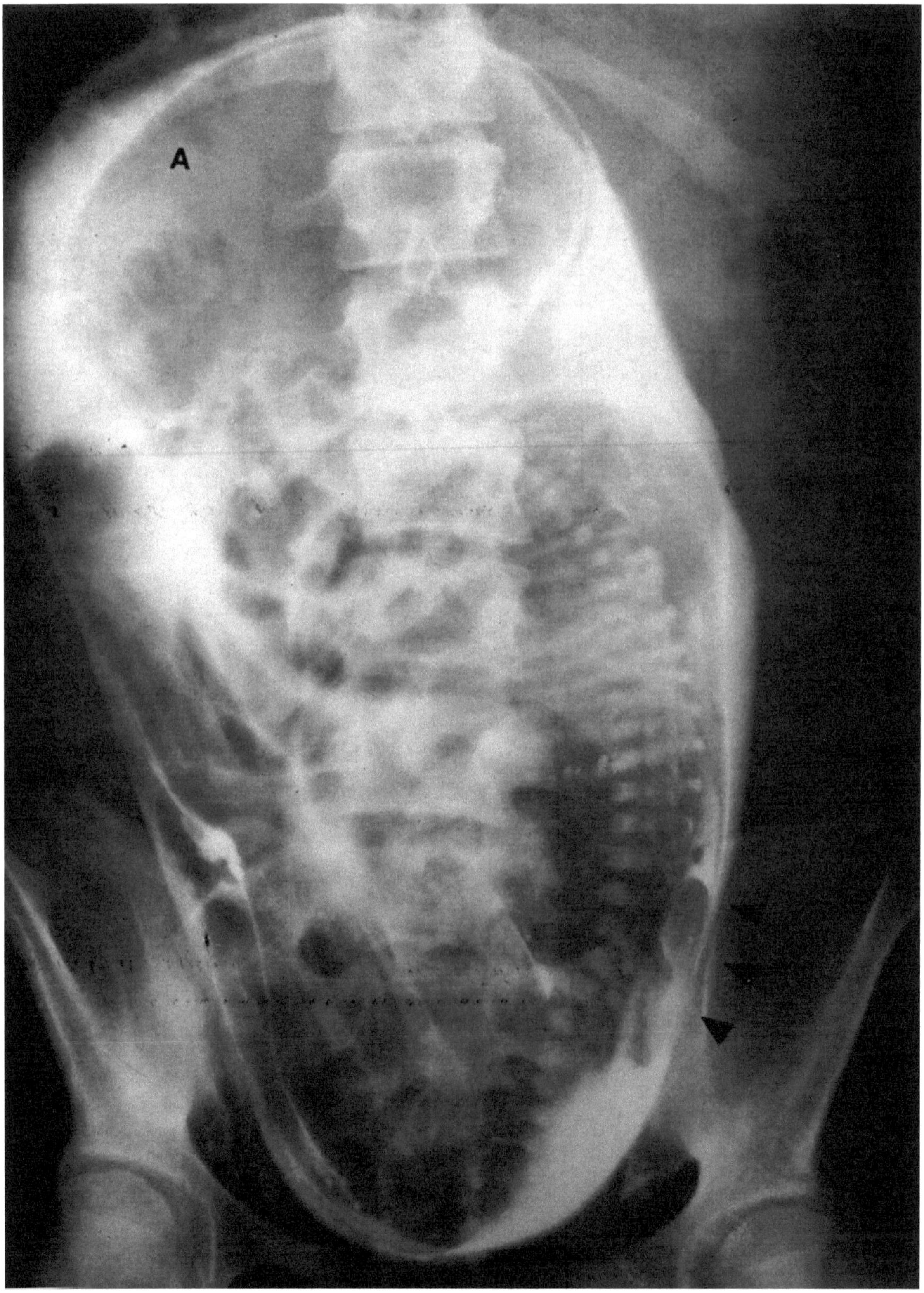

**Indication for AFG:** Verification of ultrasonic findings; oligohydramnion; search for additional malformations.
**AFG findings** (Fig. 23a: amniogram 30 minutes from injection; Fig. 23b: foetogram 24 hours from injection): Sex of foetus not safely determinable; breech presentation; oligohydramnion; no change in foetal position after 24 hours;

Case 14

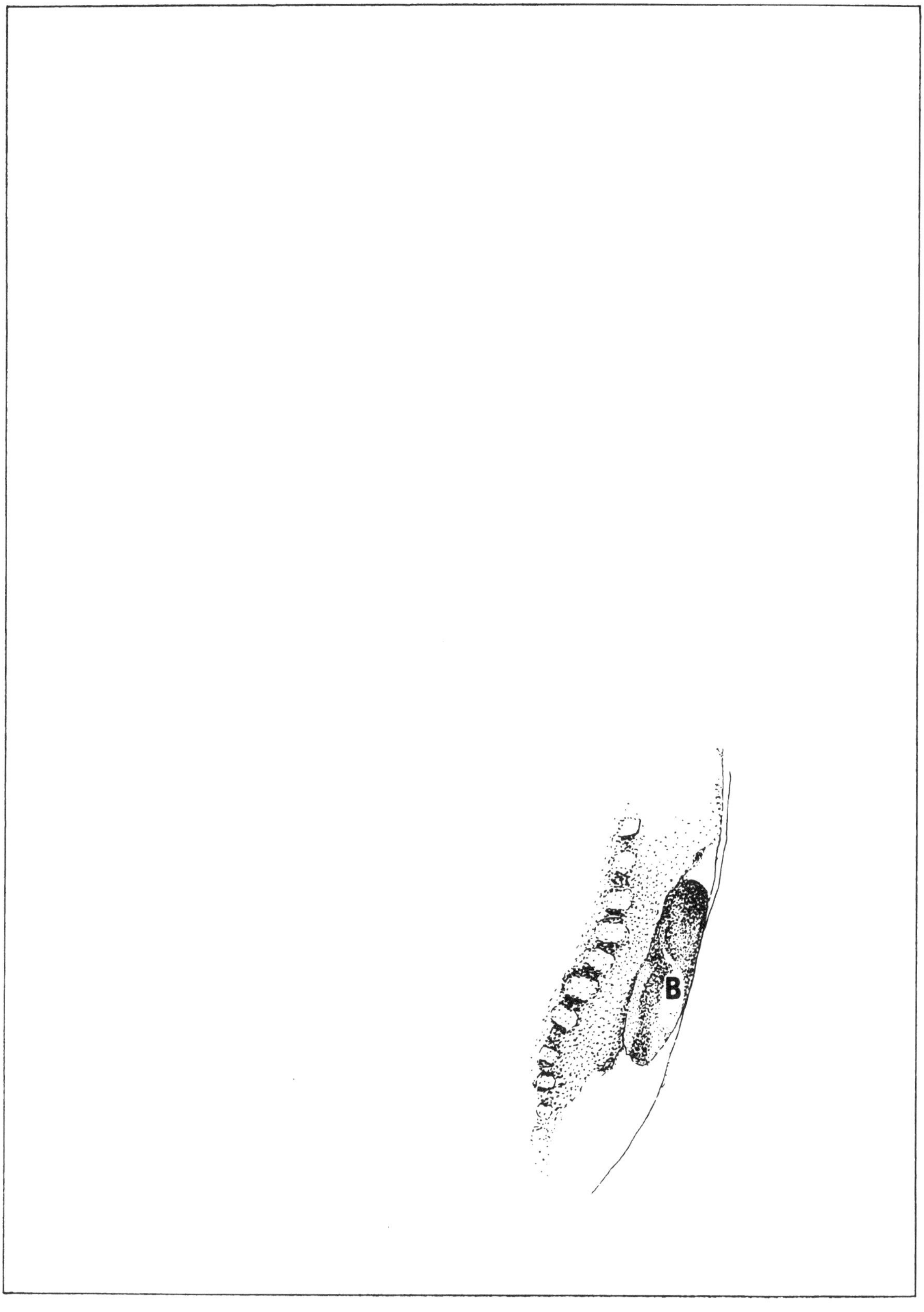


Fig. 23a

**Case 14** **macrocephalus** with incomplete calcification of skull cap (A); **recess of contrast medium** in amniotic fluid, 5.5 cm in length, **at lumbar level** shown in amniogram (Fig. 23a); same cele less clearly visible in foetogram (Fig. 23b; B; arrows); no additional malformation.

**Prenatal summary diagnosis:** Internal hydrocephalus; lumbar

Fig. 23b

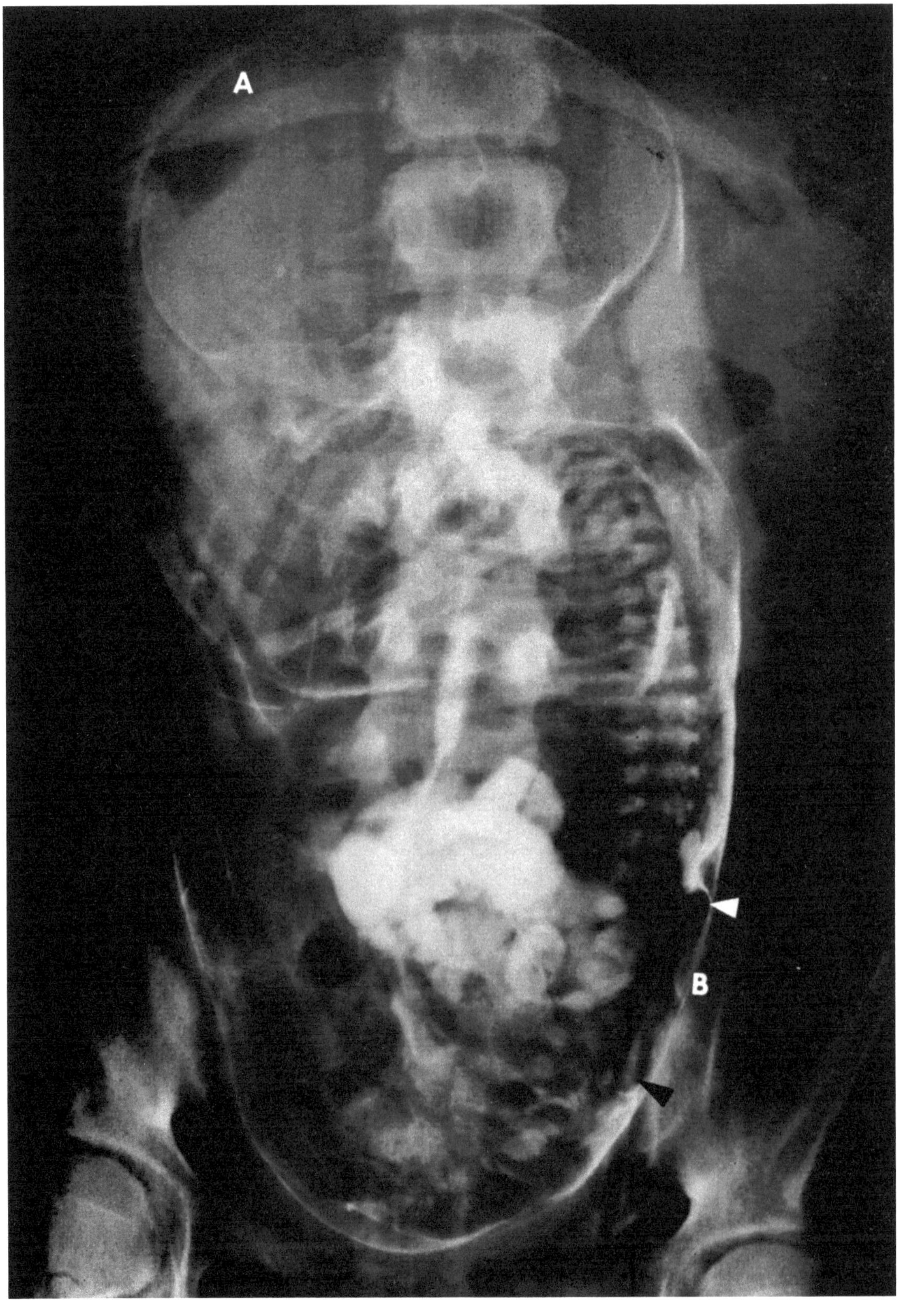

neural tube defect with cele.
**Clinical course:** Termination of pregnancy in 37th week; male, 3,000 g, 53 cm; intrapartum death (craniotomy).

**Radiogram** (Fig. 24) and **post-mortem findings:** Confirmation of prenatal diagnosis. ◁

**Case 14**

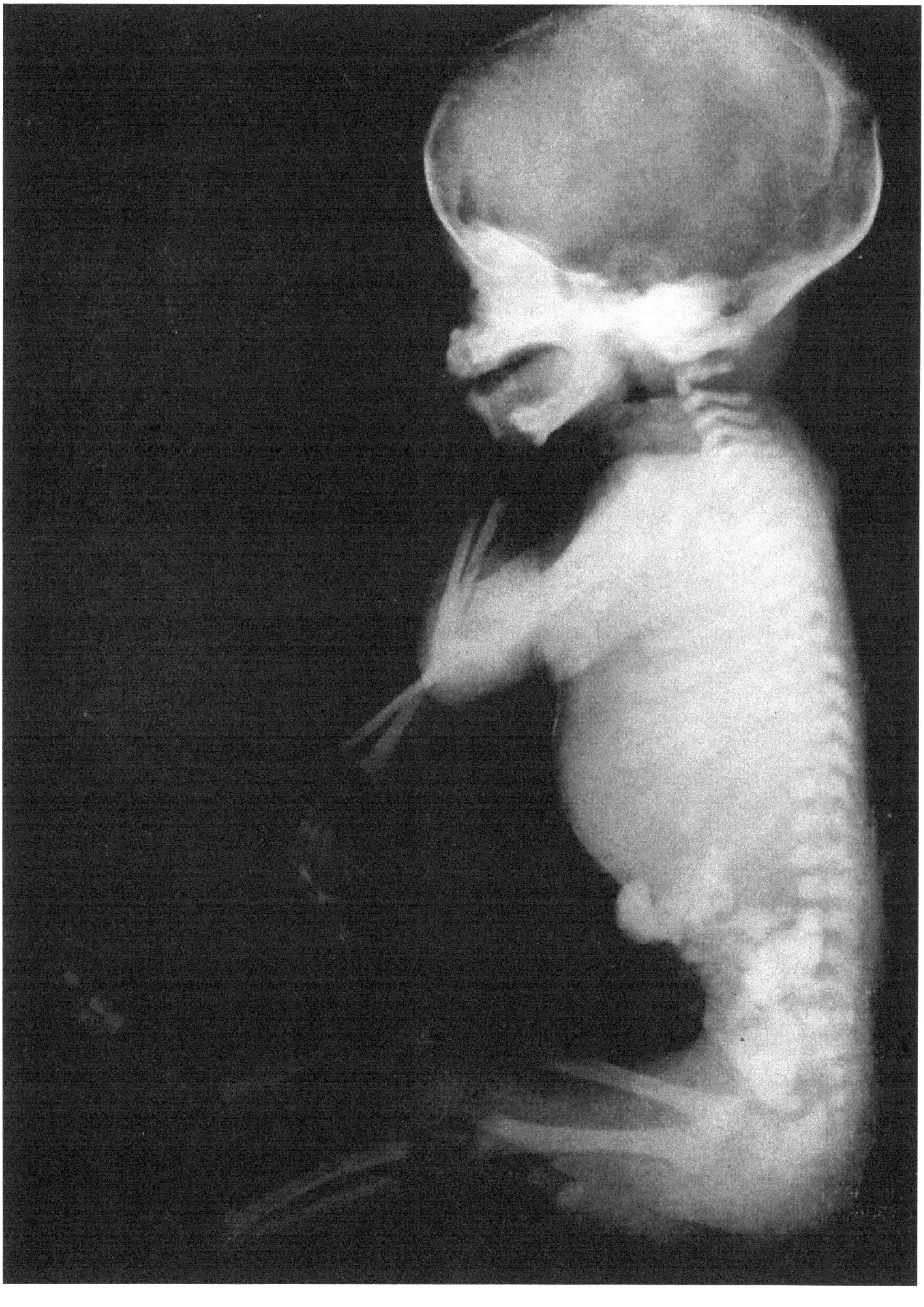

Fig. 24

**Case 15** **Patient D.M./85**, 23 years, second gravidity, one parturition.
**Record:** One clinically intact child.
**Clinical findings:** 36th week of pregnancy; no contributory findings.

**Ultrasonic findings:** Asymmetrical enlargement up to 25 mm of first and second cerebral ventricles; pallium of 12 mm in thickness; thoracolumbar open neural tube defect without cele, 6.5 cm in length, 3 cm in width (Fig. 25a, b; arrows);

Fig. 25a

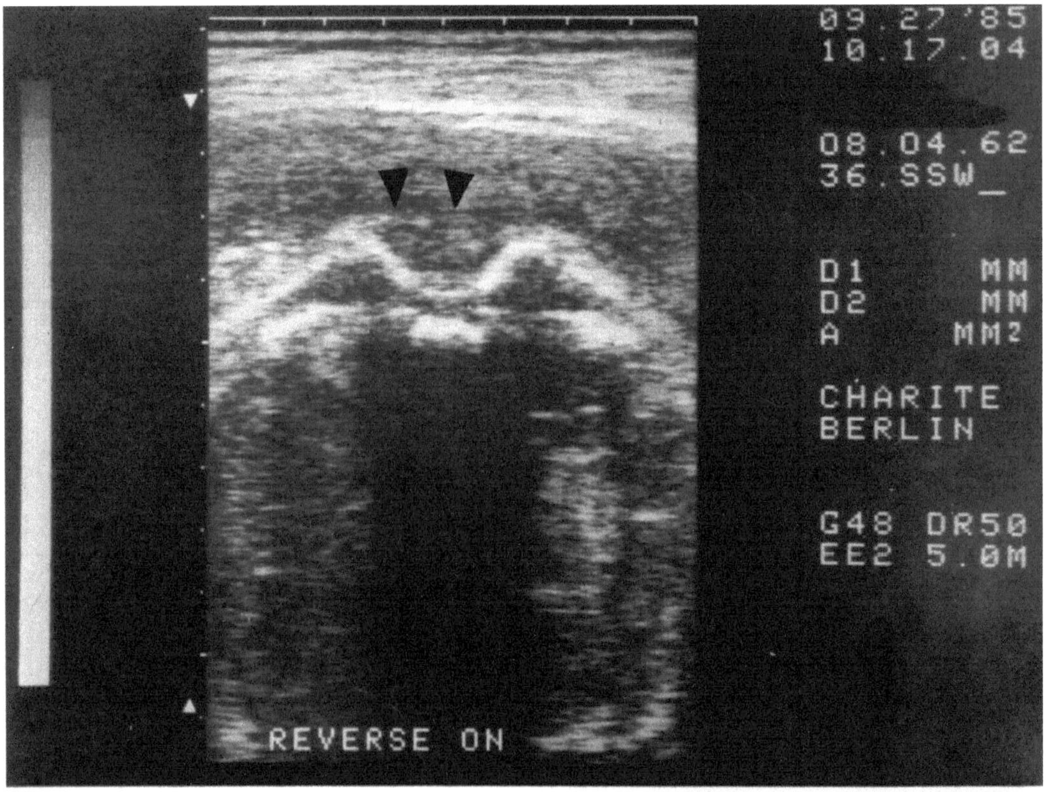


Fig. 25b

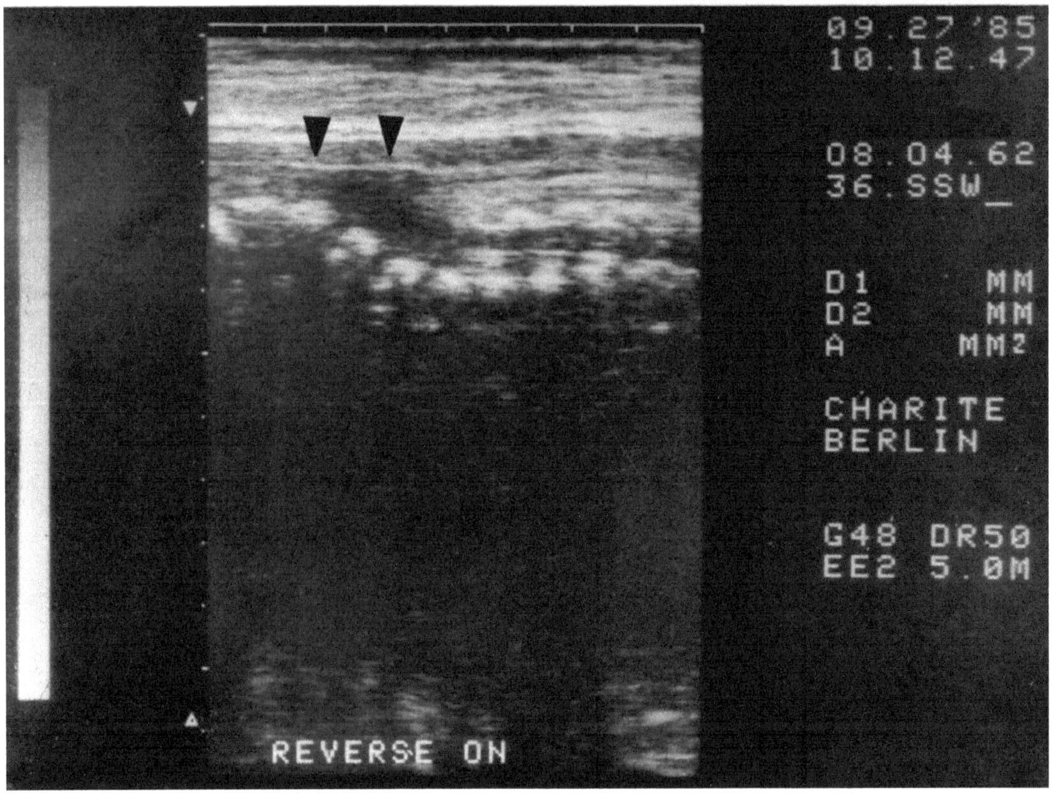

gibbus caudal from defect; no spontaneous or provokable mobility of lower extremities; malformations of thoracic vertebral bodies.

**Indications for AFG:** Verification of ultrasonic findings; signs indicative of additional malformations.

**AFG findings** (Fig. 26 a: amniogram 30 minutes from injection; Fig. 26 b: foetogram 24 hours from injection): Female foetus; cephalic presentation; amniogram shows

Case 15

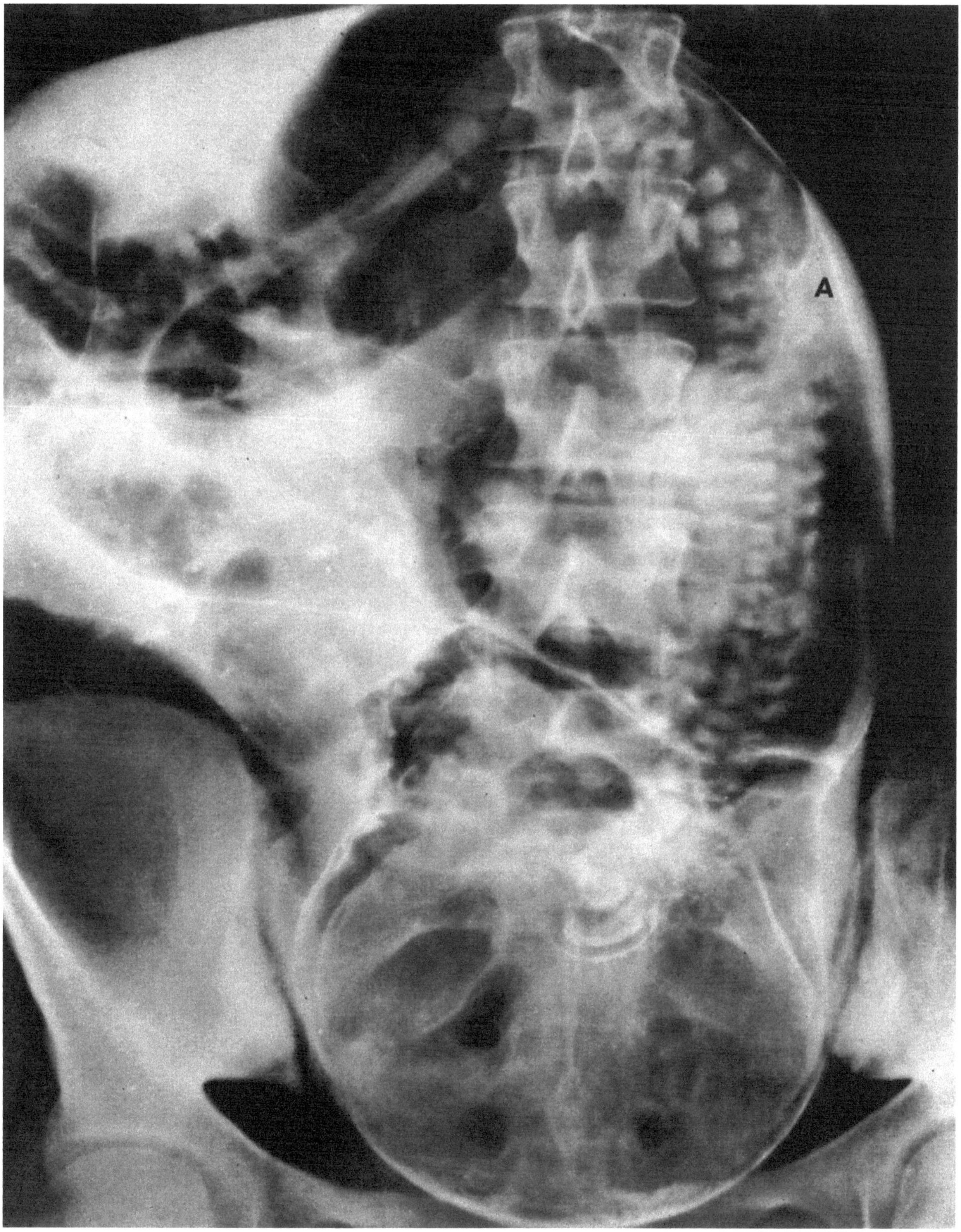


Fig. 26a

**Case 15** disruption of dorsal skin contour in thoracolumbar region, with defect filled up with amniotic fluid containing contrast medium (A); malformation of at least two vertebral bodies in upper section of thoracic spine (B; arrow); gibbus beneath schisis; foetogram shows almost identical position of foetus, reflecting impaired vitality; contour defect close to schisis

Fig. 26b

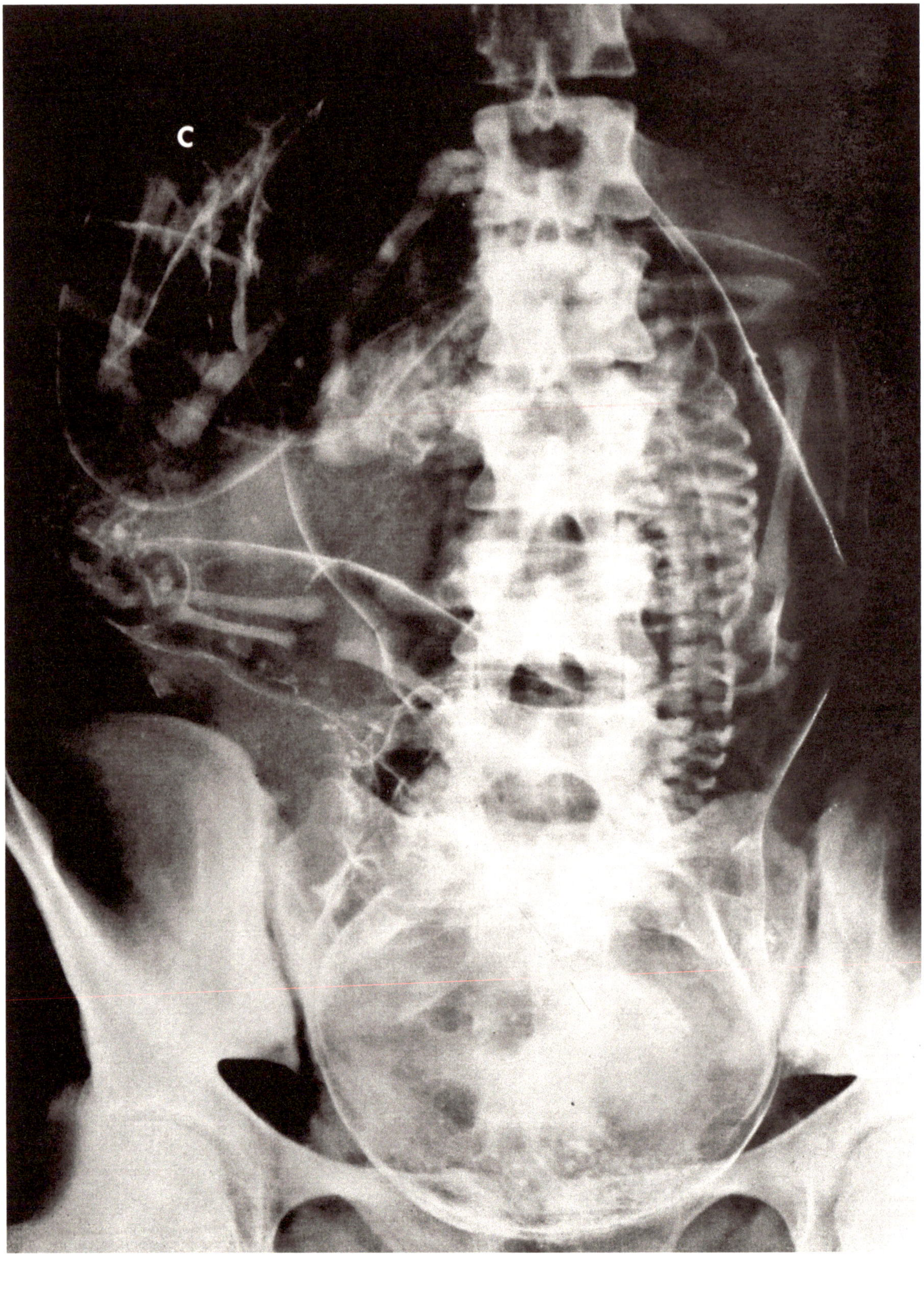

hard to detect for dorsal position not being in strictly tangential focus; club-foot posture (C); inadequate calcification of parietal skull cap indicative of hydrocephalus.

**Prenatal summary diagnosis:** Hydrocephalus; neural tube defect without cele; paraplegic symptoms.

**Clinical course:** Spontaneous labour after induction in 36th

Case 15

Fig. 27a

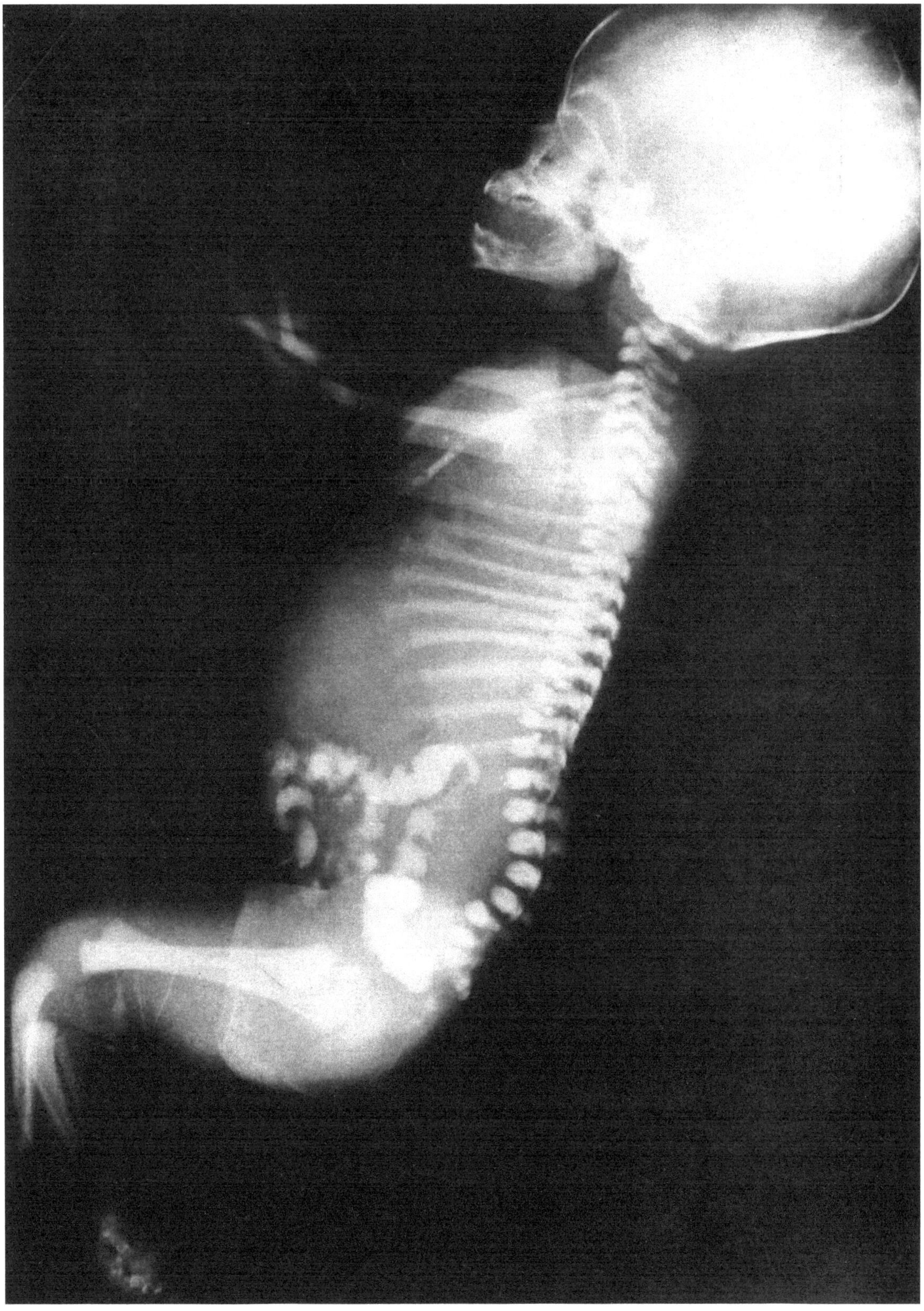

Case 15 week of pregnancy; death of newborn at birth; 2,950 g, 46 cm.

**Radiogram** (Fig. 27 a): Confirmation of prenatal findings; conspicuous spasm of colon in contrast image; clinical aspect shows Figure 27 b.

**Post-mortem findings:** Arnold-Chiari syndrome with caudal displacement of cerebellar tissue, in addition to above findings. ◁

Fig. 27 b

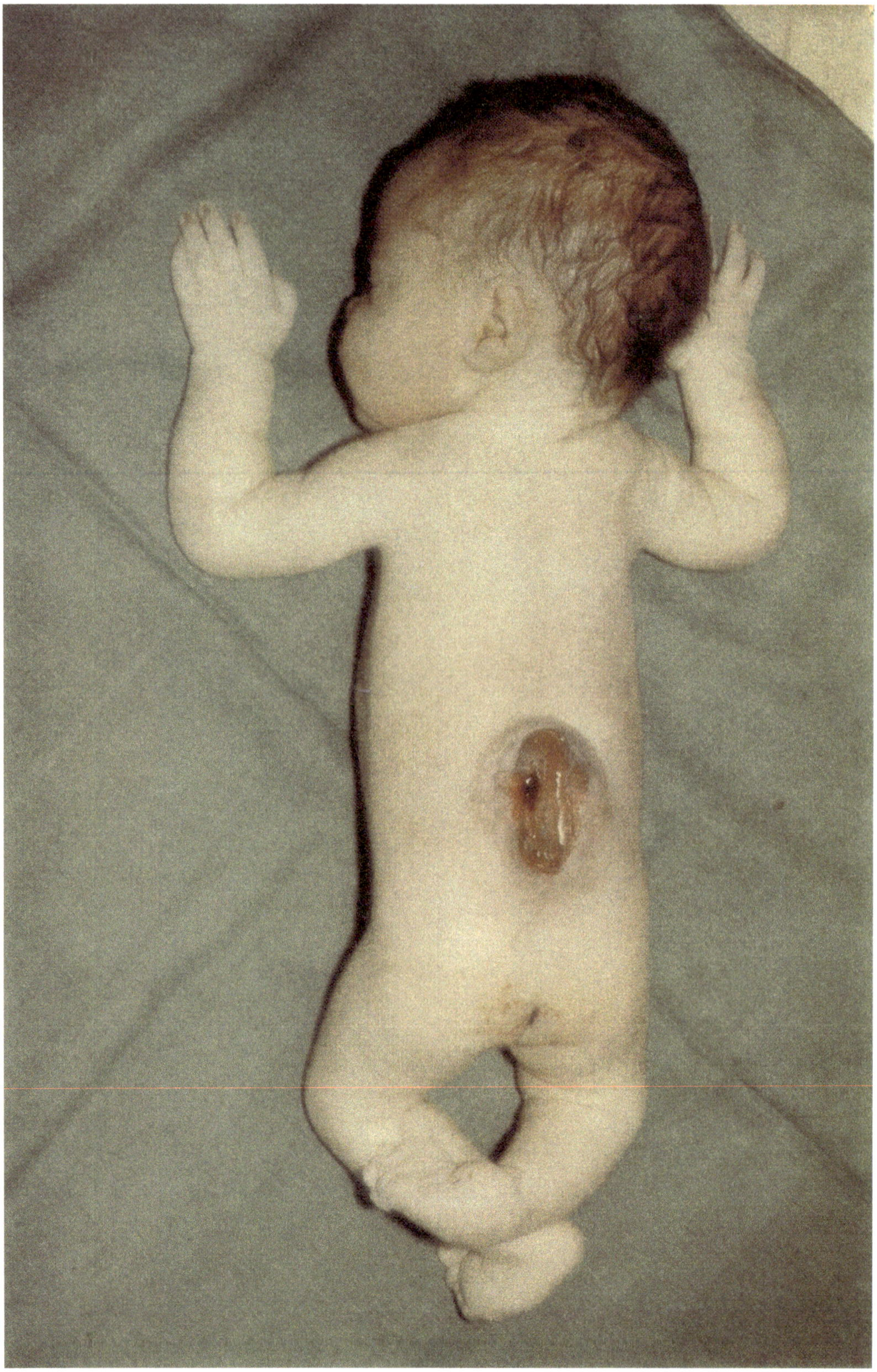

**Patient L.M./78,** 22 years, first gravidity.
**Clinical findings:** 34th week of pregnancy; no contributory findings.
**Ultrasonic findings:** Internal hydrocephalus; no additional foetal malformation detectable.
**Indication for AFG:** Verification of ultrasonic findings; search for additional malformations.
**AFG findings** (Fig. 28a: amniogram 30 minutes from injection; Fig. 28b: foetogram 24 hours from injection): Female foetus; breech presentation; clearly visible enlargement of head and protrusion of forehead; no calcification of skull cap (A); foetogram shows gibbus in lower section of

**Case 16**

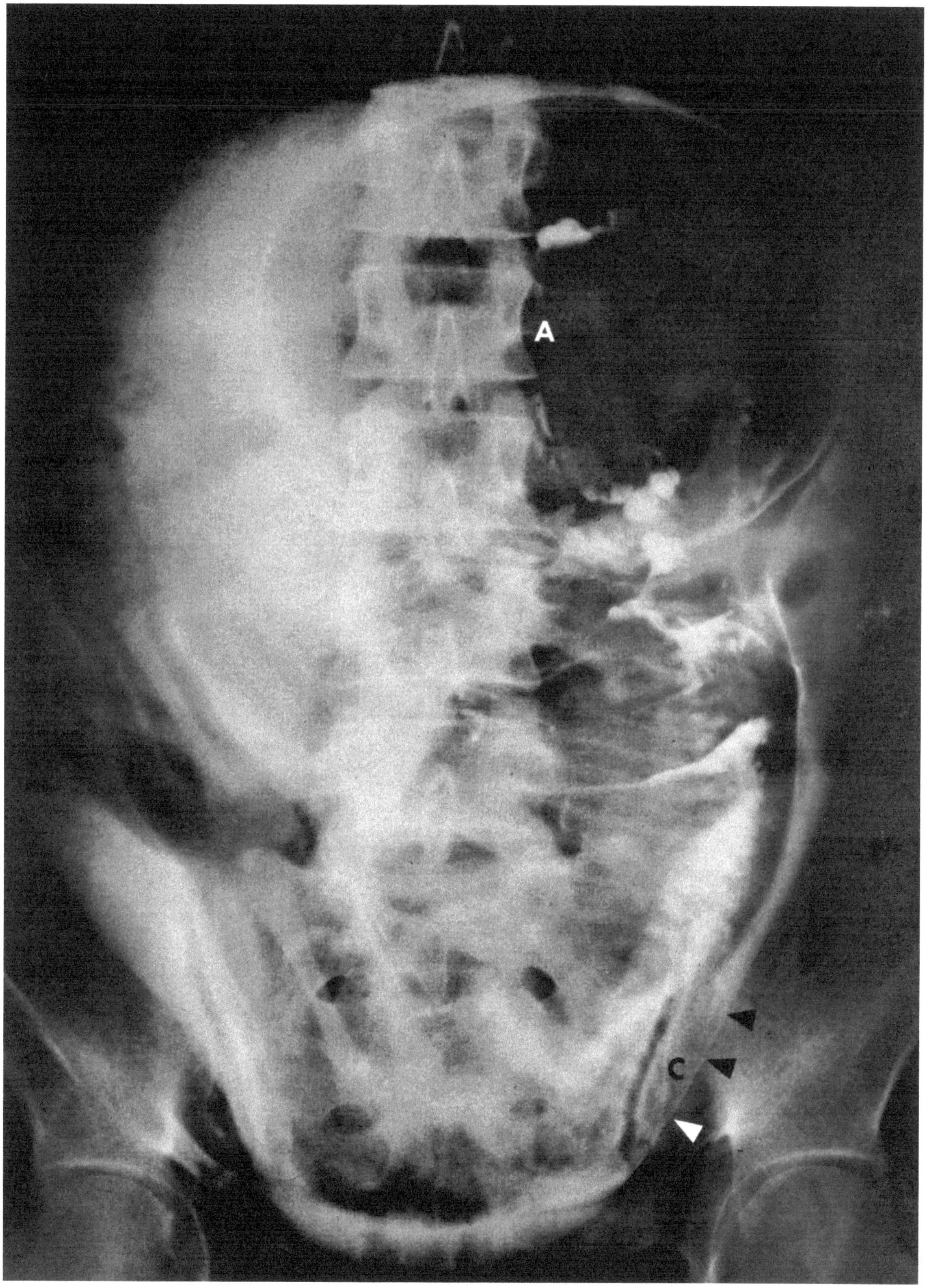


Fig. 28a

Case 16 lumbar spine (B; arrows); amniogram and foetogram show flat lumbosacral cele, ca. 6 cm in length (C; arrows); clearly visible deceleration of gastro-intestinal passage of contrast medium; convolution of small intestine not detectable until 24 hours from injection.

**Prenatal summary diagnosis:** Hydrocephalus; lumbosacral neural tube defect; impaired intestinal motility.
**Clinical course:** Premature termination of pregnancy in 35th week of pregnancy; craniotomy; 2,600 g, 51 cm.
**Post-mortem diagnosis:** Hydrocephalus; myelomeningocele. ◁

Fig. 28b

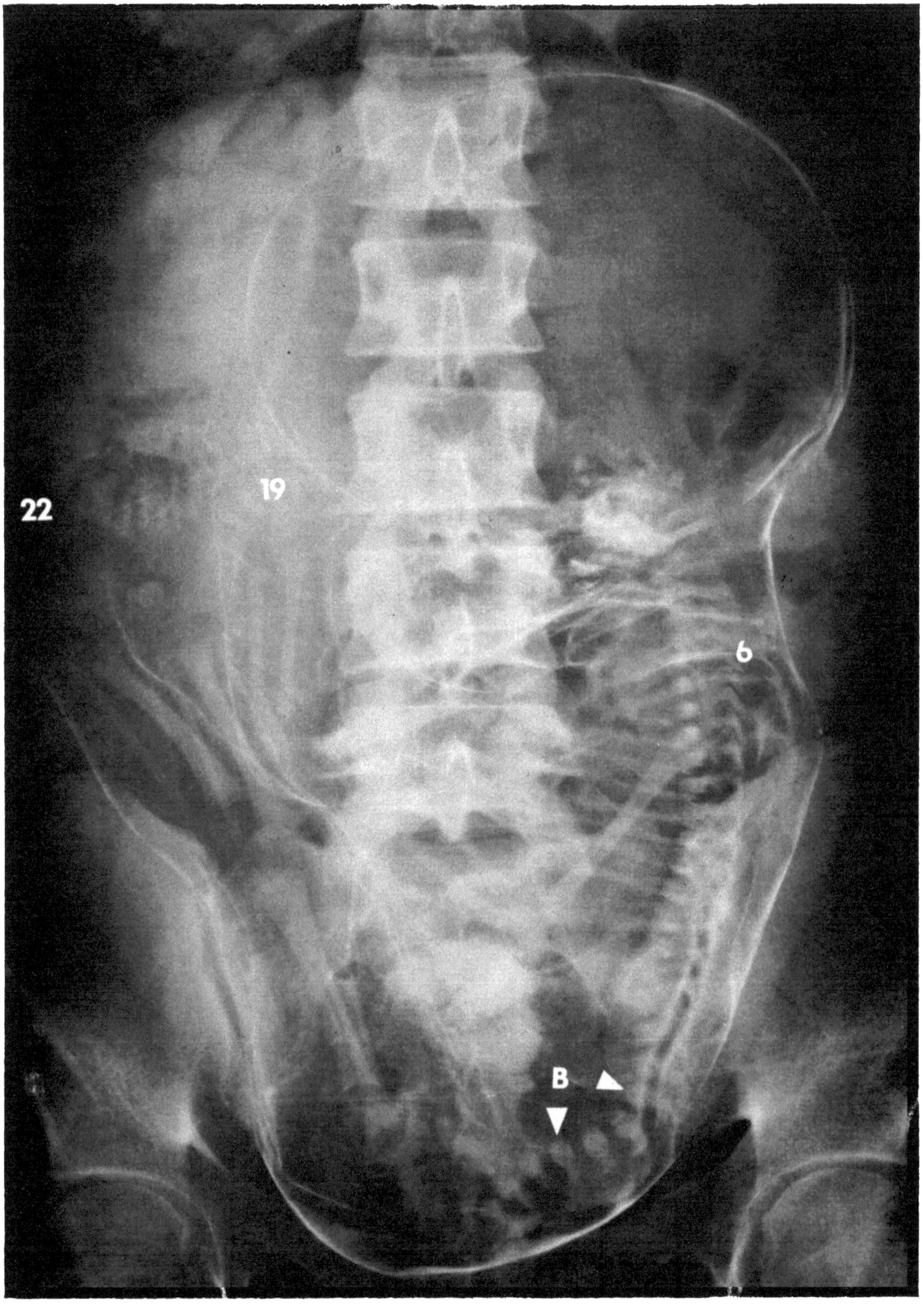

**Case 17**

**Patient D.C./85,** 29 years, fourth gravidity, second parturition.
**Record:** One clinically intact child; one child with anencephalus; one abortion.
**Clinical findings:** 28th week of pregnancy; no contributory findings.
**Ultrasonic findings** (Fig. 29a, b): Bifid spine with lumbosacral cele of 25 mm in diameter (arrows); spontaneous movement of lower extremities following provocation; no hydrocephalus; no additional malformations.
**Indication for AFG:** Confirmation of ultrasonic findings; infavourable record; signs indicative of additional malformations.
**AFG findings** (Fig. 30: foetogram 24 hours from injection): Sex of foetus not safely determinable; cephalic presentation; spinal contour disrupted by celes (A, arrows); time-adequate

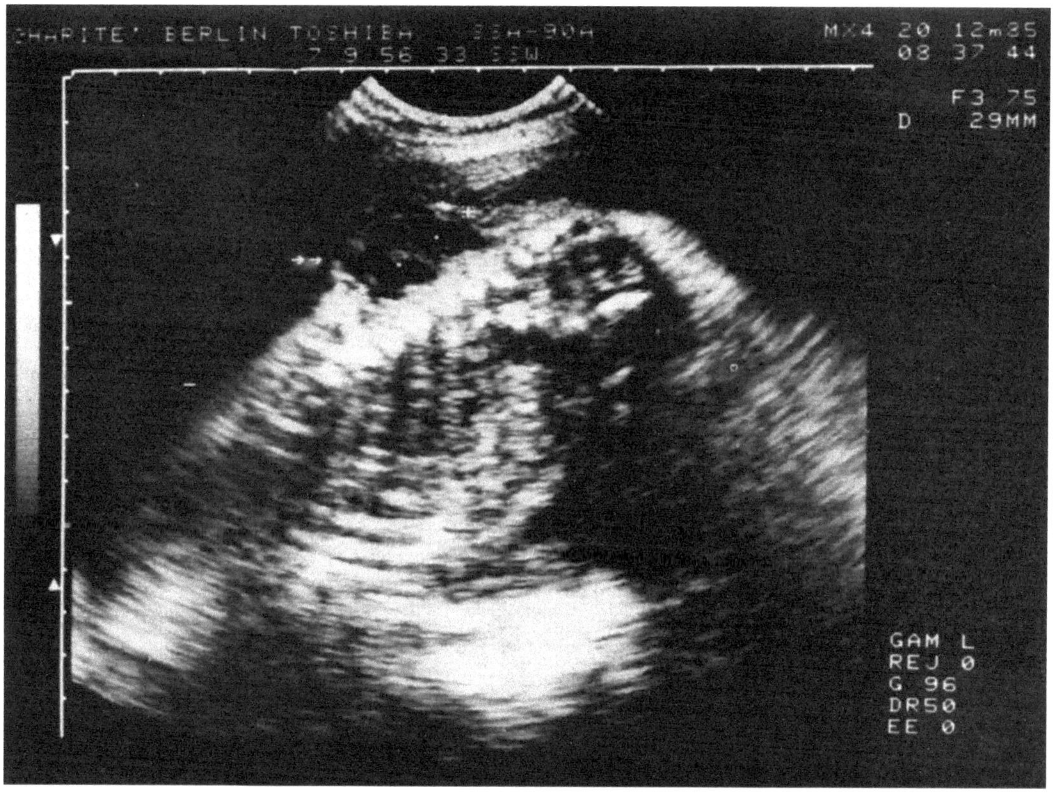


Fig. 29a

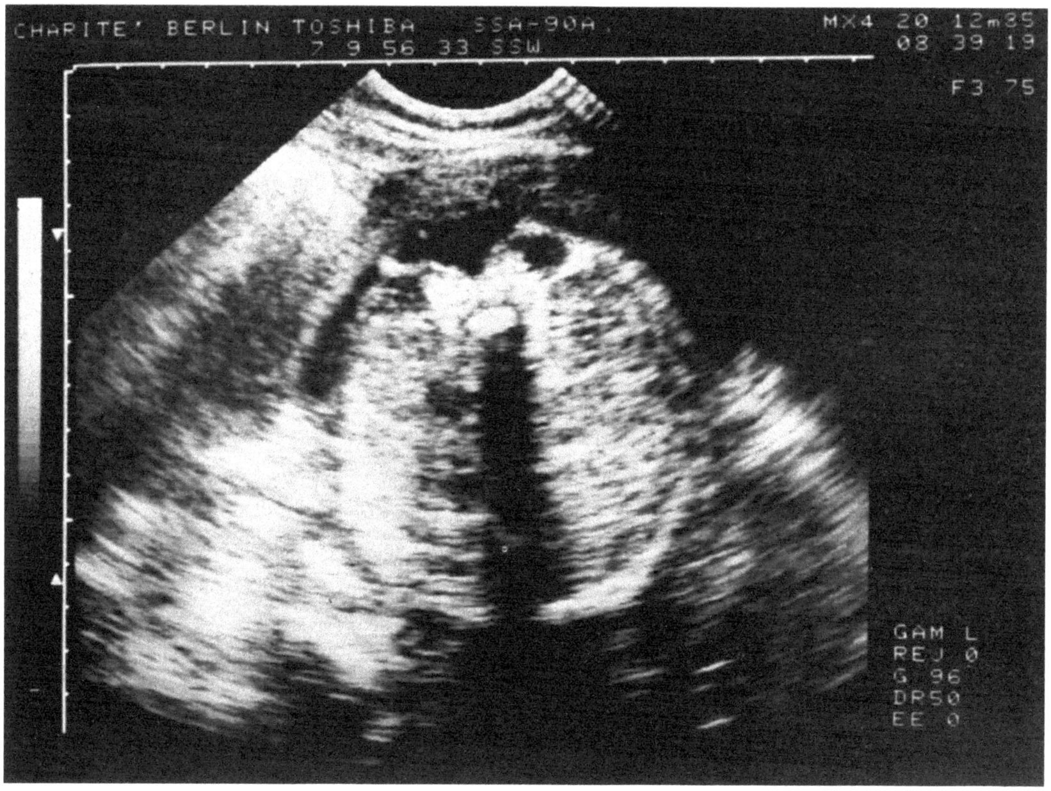


Fig. 29b

Case 17 complete gastrointestinal passage of contrast medium; thoracic spine not assessable; no signs indicative of club-feet; no signs of hydrocephalus nor other malformations.

**Prenatal summary diagnosis:** Neural tube defect with celes in sacral region; no paraplegic symptoms.

**Clinical course:** Spontaneous labour in 36th week of pregnancy; male, 2,970 g, 45 cm; neurosurgery for myelomeningocele immediately after birth; subsequent development of internal hydrocephalus; valve implantation; detection by micturition cysto-urethrography of bilateral fifth-degree vesico-ureteral reflux; neurogenic bladder voiding disorder; partial temporary anal sphincteric paralysis; prenatally undetected malformation of three vertebral bodies in upper part of thoracic spine. ◁

Fig. 30

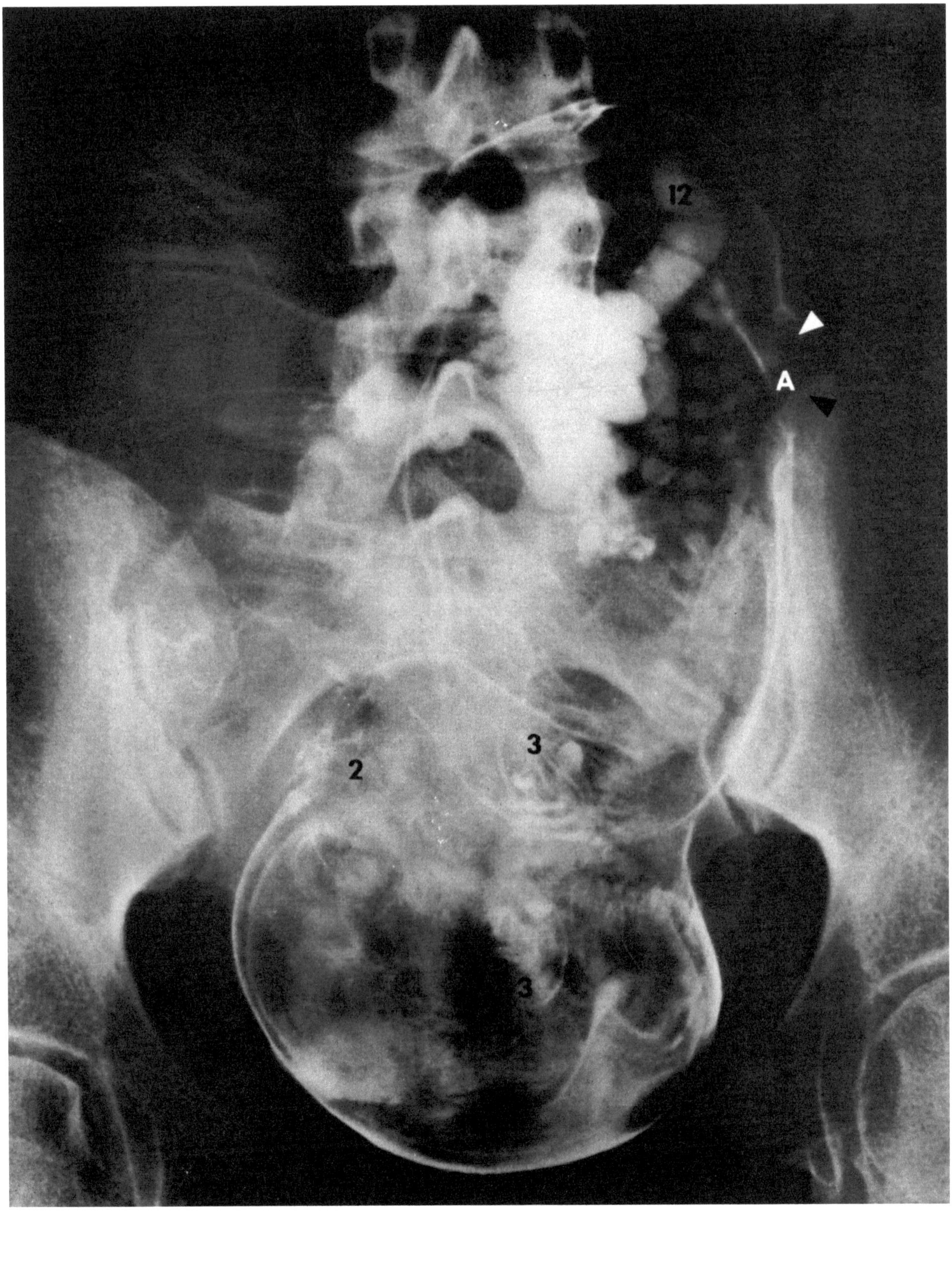

**Patient A.B./84,** 38 years, fourth gravidity, first parturition.
**Record:** One clinically intact child; two abortions.
**Clinical findings:** 36th week of pregnancy; no contributory findings.
**Ultrasonic findings:** Suspicion of bifid spine with cele in sacral region; no spontaneous or provocable movement of lower extremities. Fig. 31 a: Club-foot; 31 b: Cele (arrows).
**Indication for AFG:** Confirmation of ultrasonic findings; signs indicative of additional malformations.
**AFG findings** (Fig. 31 c: foetogram 24 hours from injection): Male foetus; breech presentation; club-feet both sides (B); time-adequate gastro-intestinal passage of contrast medium

**Case 18**

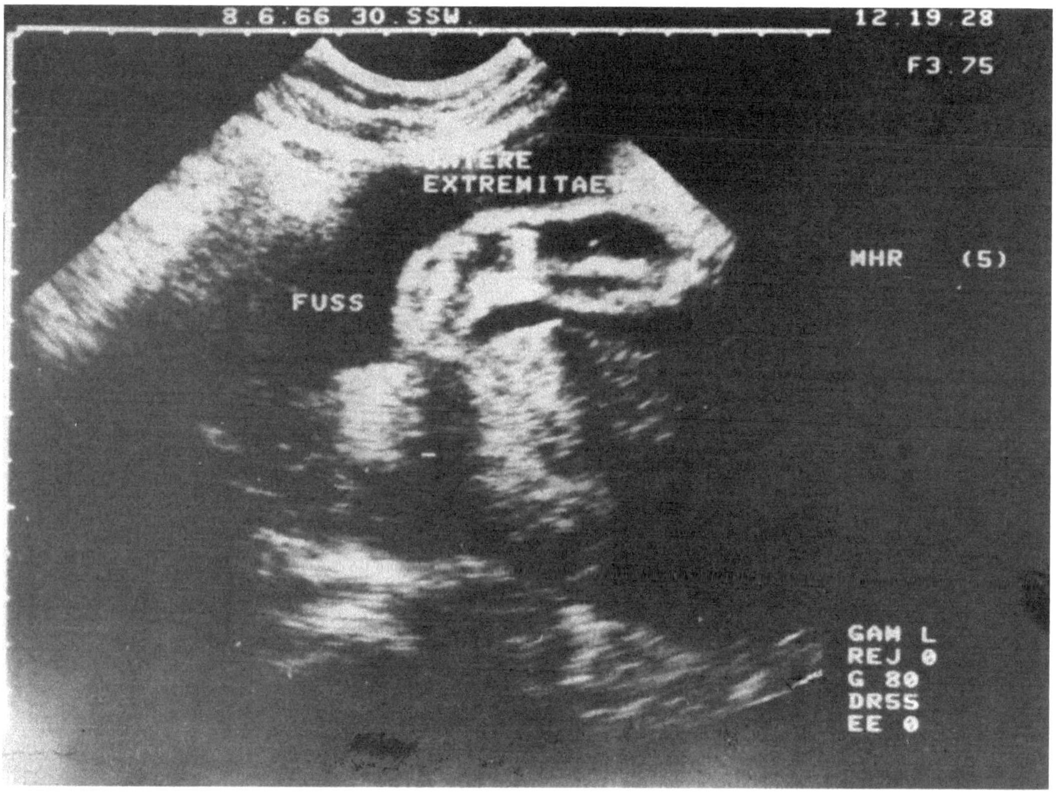


Fig. 31 a

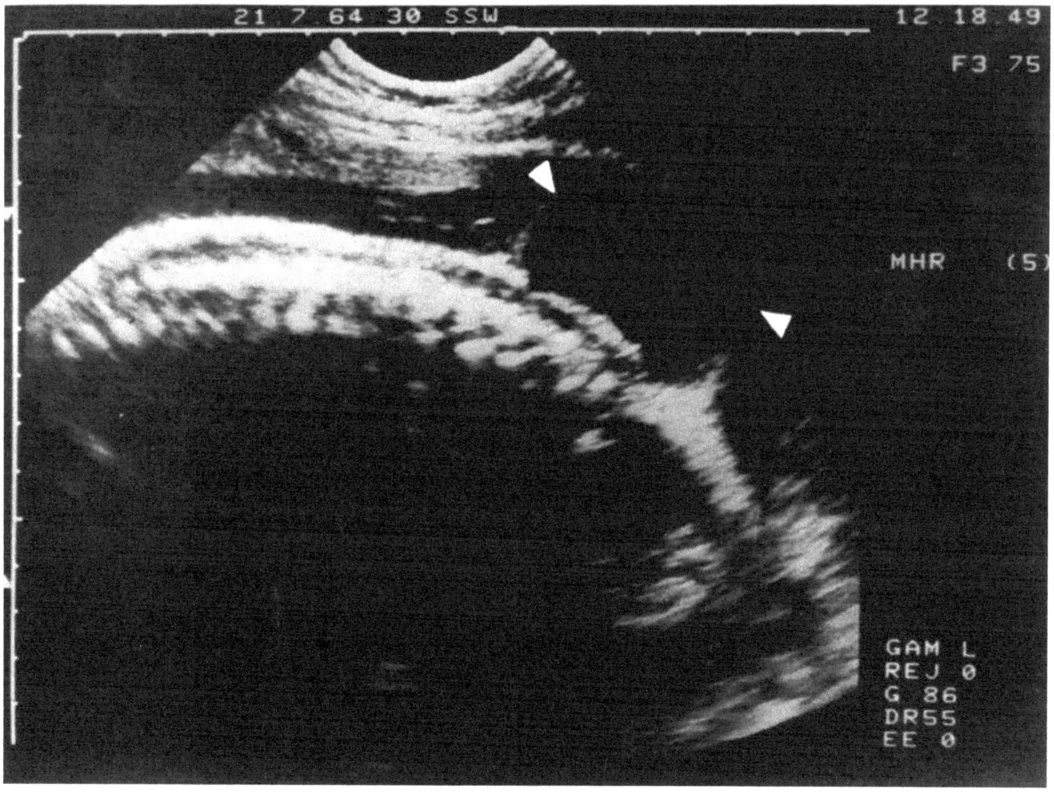


Fig. 31 b

Case 18 without visualisation of rectal ampulla; round contrast medium pattern, 42 mm in diameter, below intestinal convolution at sacral level (A; arrows); lower part of vertebral column not assessed for superimposition of maternal skeleton; no signs of hydrocephalus or additional malformations.

**Prenatal summary diagnosis:** Neural tube defect with cele in sacral region, with signs indicative of paraplegic symptoms.
**Clinical course:** Spontaneous labour in 37th week of pregnancy; 48 cm, 2,630 g; meningocele in sacral region; clubfeet with spastic paralysis of legs. ◁

Fig. 31 c

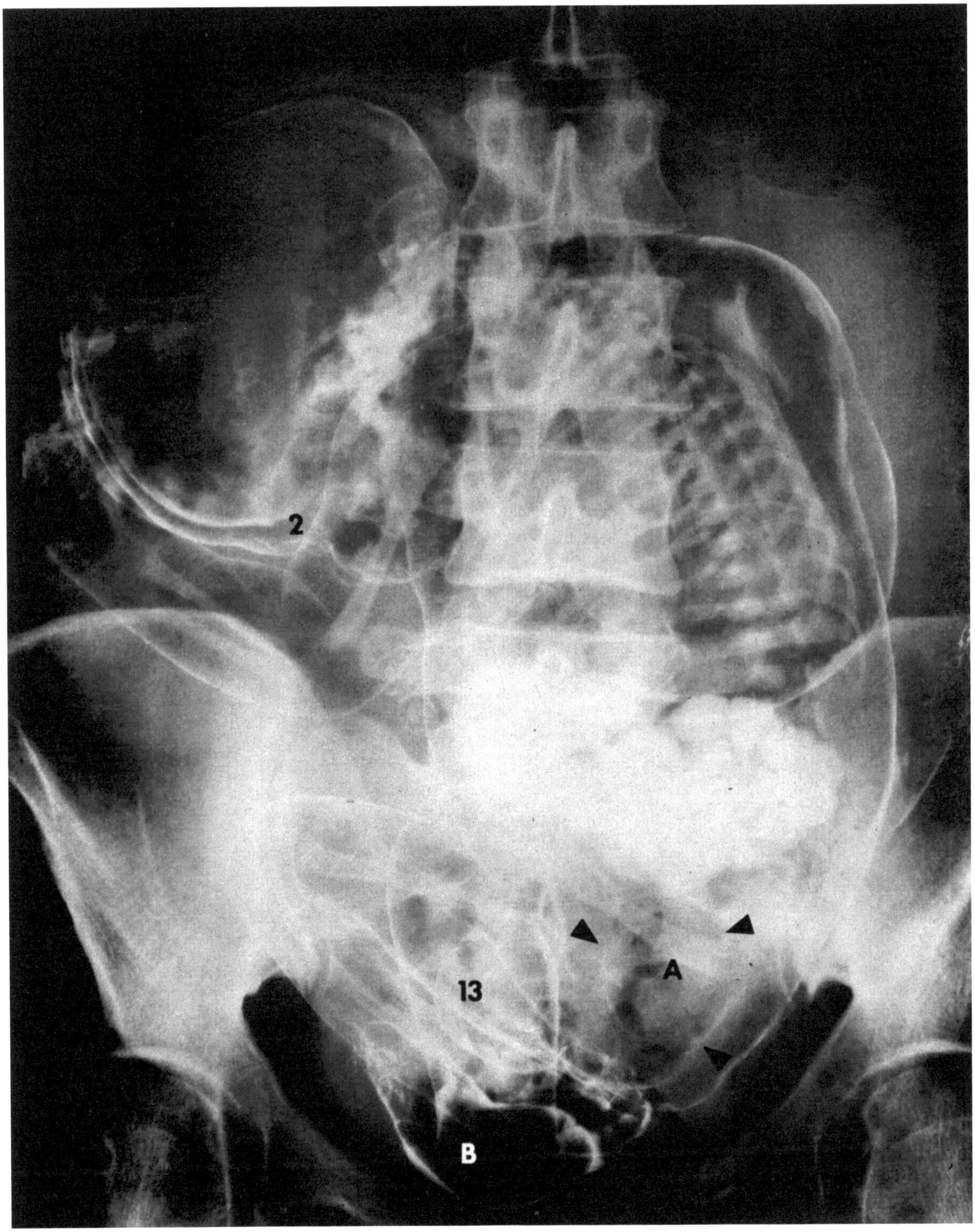

**Patient M.S./85,** 20 years, first gravidity.
**Clinical findings:** 33rd week of pregnancy; no contributory findings.
**Ultrasonic findings:** Clearly detectable hydrocephalus internus, 10 mm maximum in pallium thickness; no detectable neural tube defect; no sign indicative of additional malformations.
Pallium thickness reduced to 7 mm after seven days; therefore, puncture of cerebral ventricle; clearly pathological value recorded by brain pressure measurement; sampling



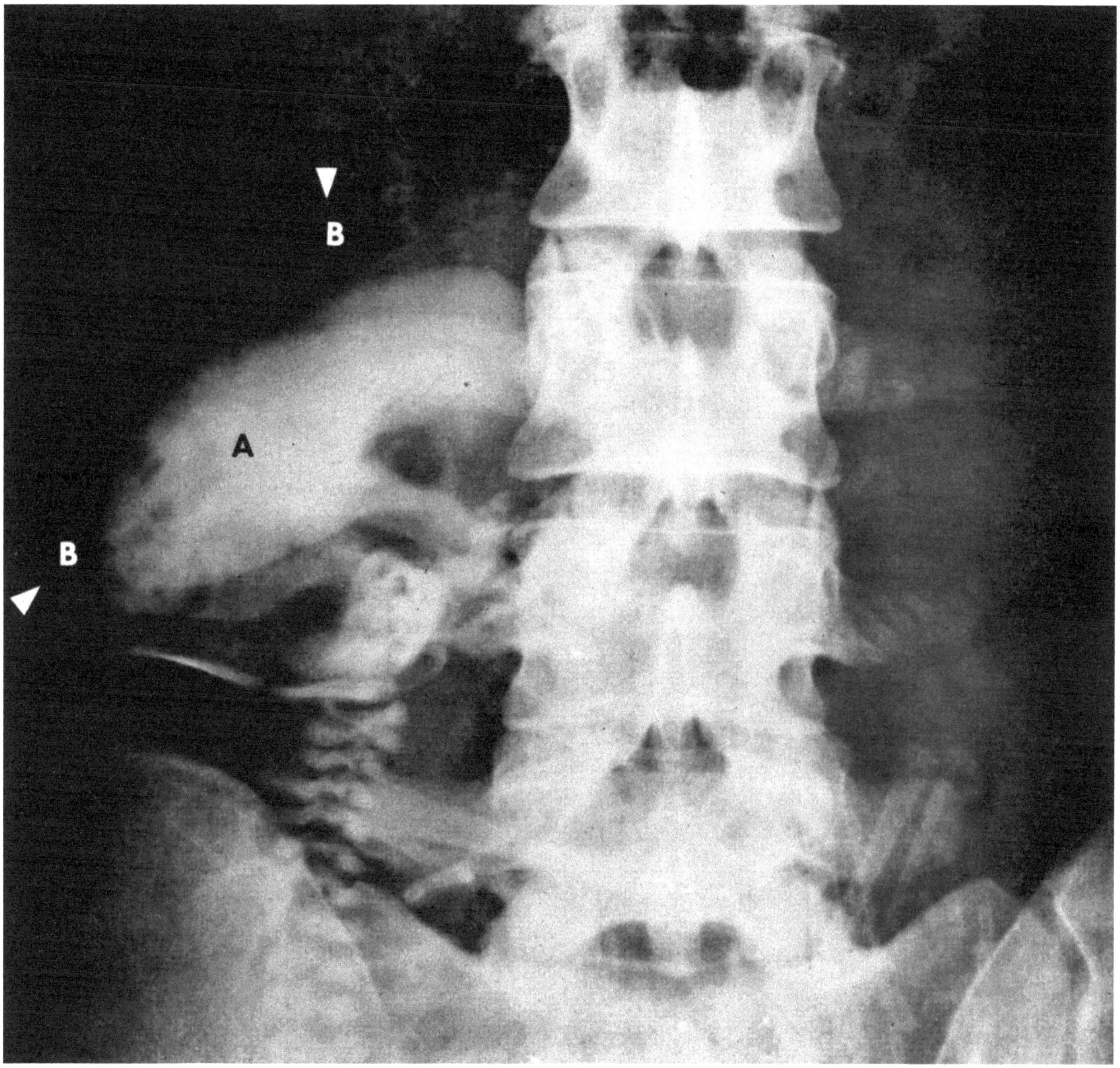


Fig. 32

Case 19 of 35 ml of cerebrospinal liquor and instillation of 5 ml contrast medium (Amipaque); no parallel AFG.

**Radiological findings** (Fig. 32: scan 15 minutes after injection): Fluoroscopic examination of cranium shows massive broadening of both lateral ventricles (A); no imaging of third and fourth ventricles; incomplete calcification of skull cap (B; arrow).

**Prenatal summary diagnosis:** Occlusive hydrocephalus; no additional malformations.

**Clinical course:** Spontaneous labour in 34th week of pregnancy, after induction, for immediate postnatal attention to

Fig. 33a

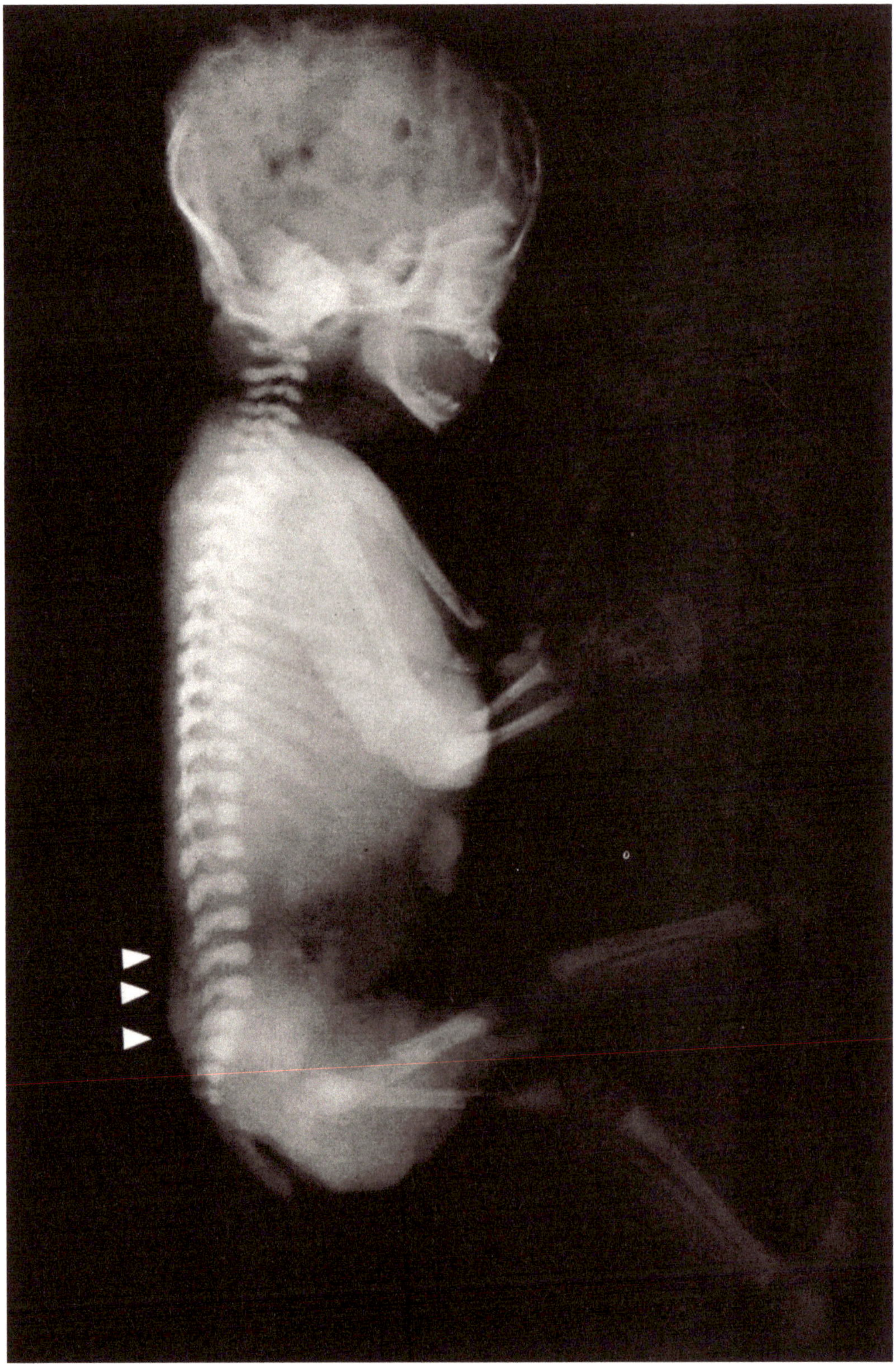

rapidly progressing hydrocephalus; female foetus, 1,950 g, 43 cm; death of newborn on second day of age of severe immaturity of lung; flat lumbosacral neural tube defect (Fig. 33a: **radiogram**) which had been prenatally undetected. **Post-mortem findings:** Internal hydrocephalus; lumbosacral myelomeningocele; clinical aspect shows Figure 33b. Above lumbosacral neural tube defect for irregularity of skin surface would have been detected with high probability by AFG and would have prompted repetitive target-oriented prenatal ultrasonic check-up. ◁

Case 19

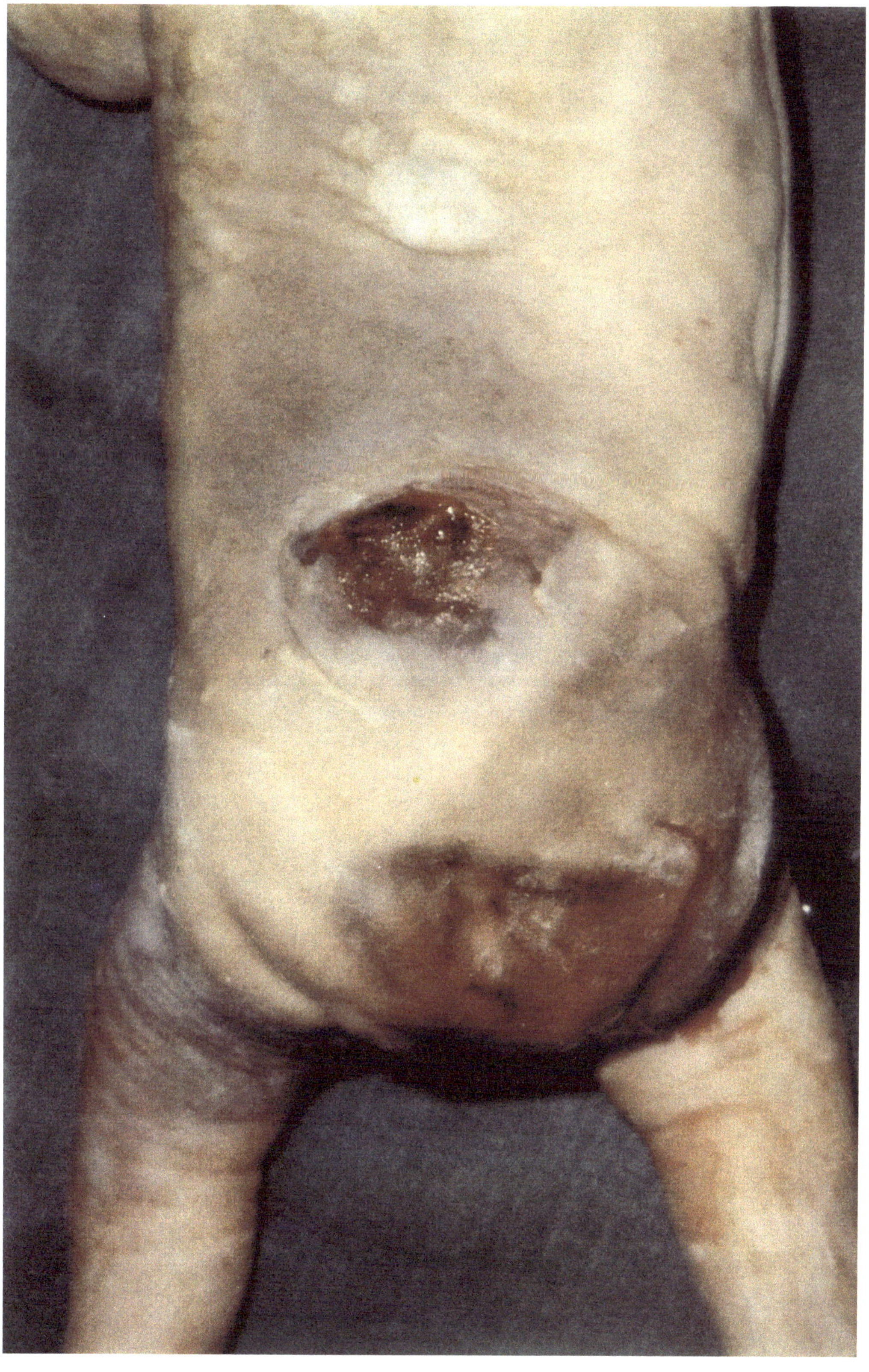

Fig. 33b

**Case 20** **Patient C.T./85,** 20 years, first gravidity.
**Clinical findings:** 27th week of pregnancy; no contributory findings.
**Ultrasonic findings** (Fig. 34a, b): Ultrasonic screening revealed presence of multiple cystic growths in thorax (CY); suspicion of diaphragmatic defect with herniation of intrathoracic intestinal sections; differential diagnosis revealed cystic pulmonary malformation.

Fig. 34a

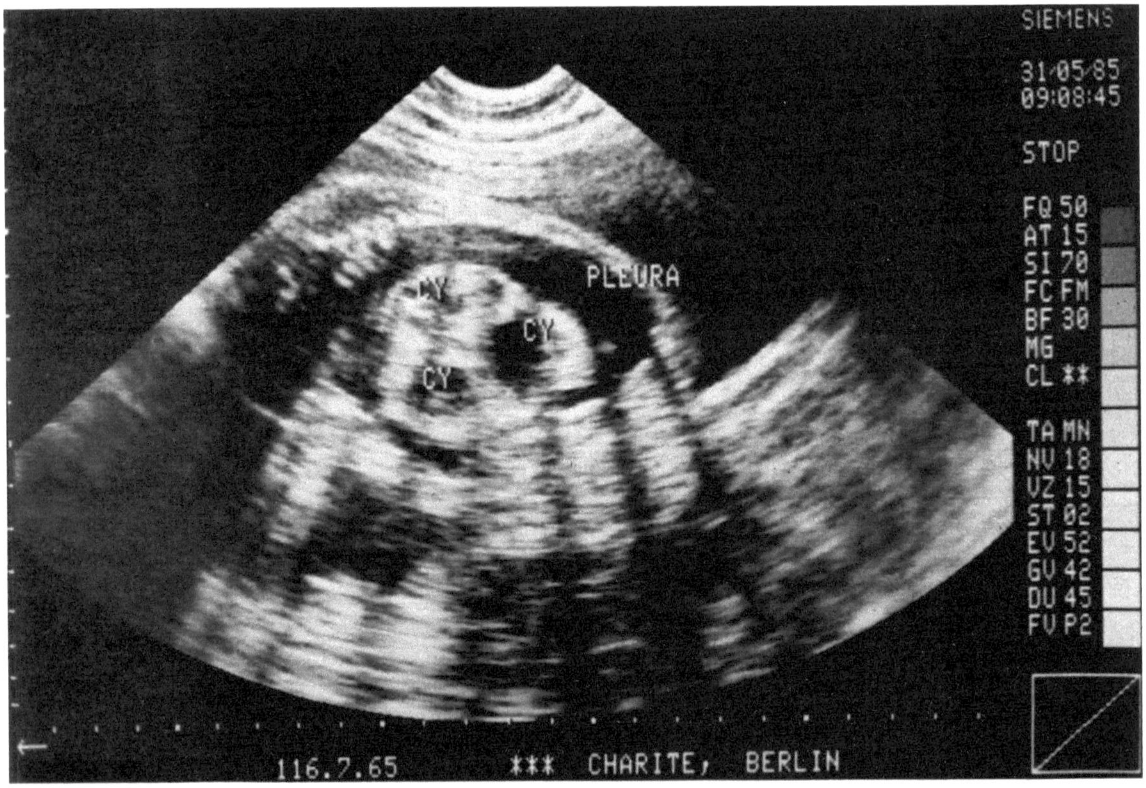


Fig. 34b

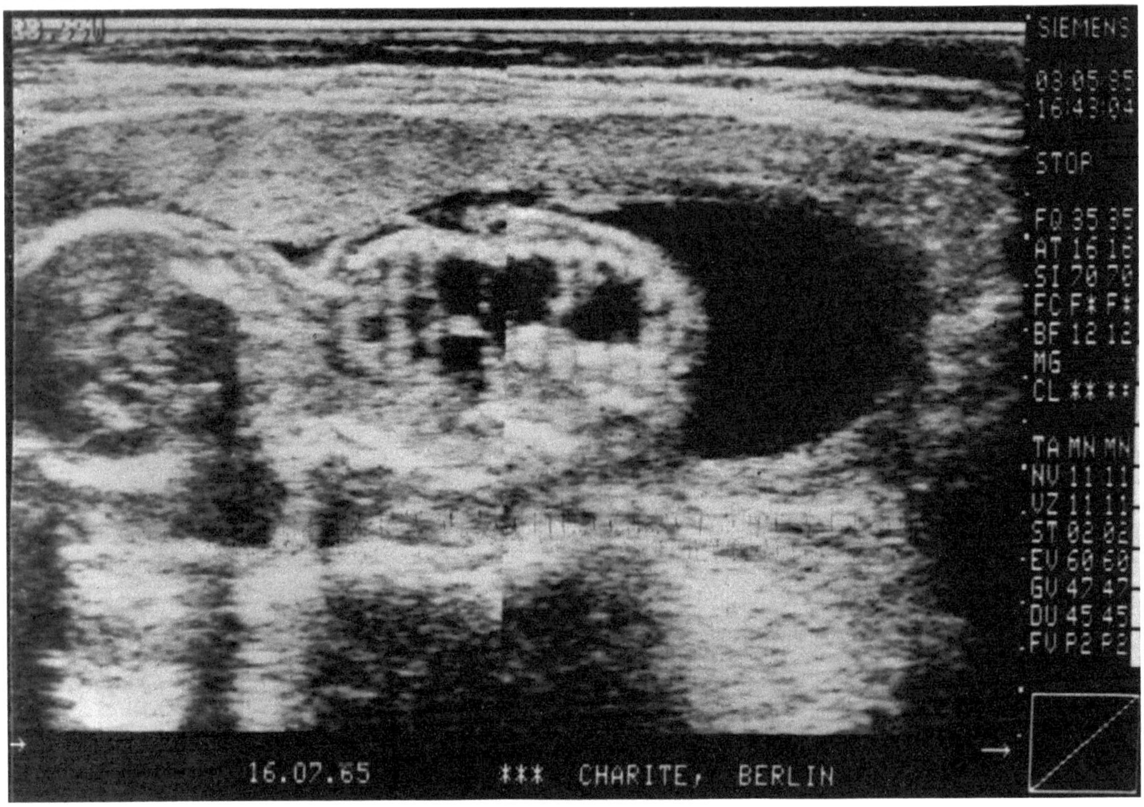

**Indication for AFG:** Elucidation of sonographic suspicious diagnosis; verification of malformations.
**AFG findings** (Fig. 35: foetogram 24 hours from injection): Female foetus; cephalic presentation; time-adequate gastro-intestinal passage of contrast medium up to rectal amuplla; orthotopic position of intestinal loops; no detectable malformation.
Repetitive targeted sonographic check-up to clear up intra-

Case 20

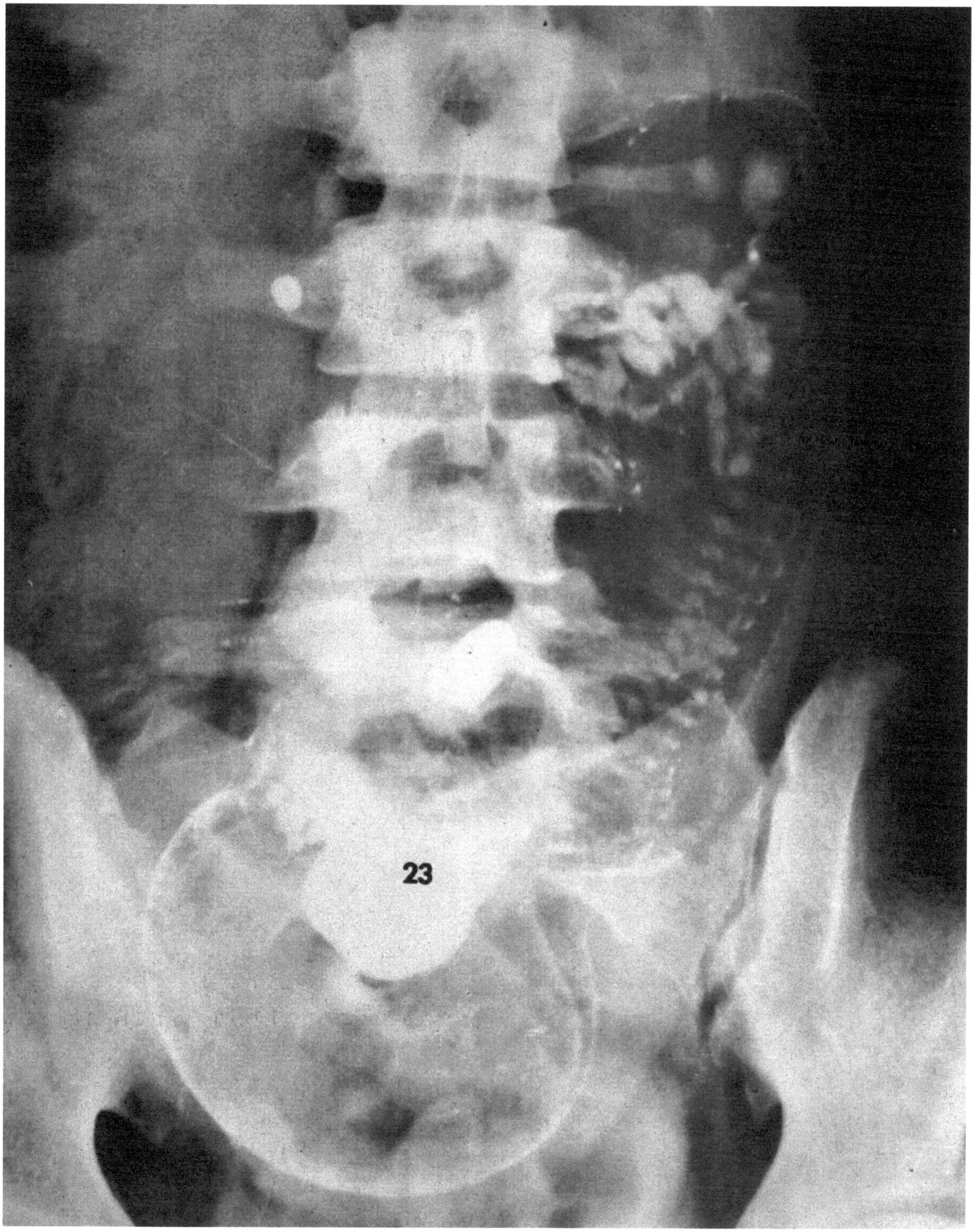


Fig. 35

Case 20 thoracic AFG findings; peristaltic movements of intrathroracic cystic growths were not even observed after intravenous application to the mother of 0.02 g of Cerucal* (metoclopramide hydrochloride).

**Prenatal summary diagnosis:** Cystic pulmonary malformation. Cystic area was punctured and water-soluble contrast

Fig. 36

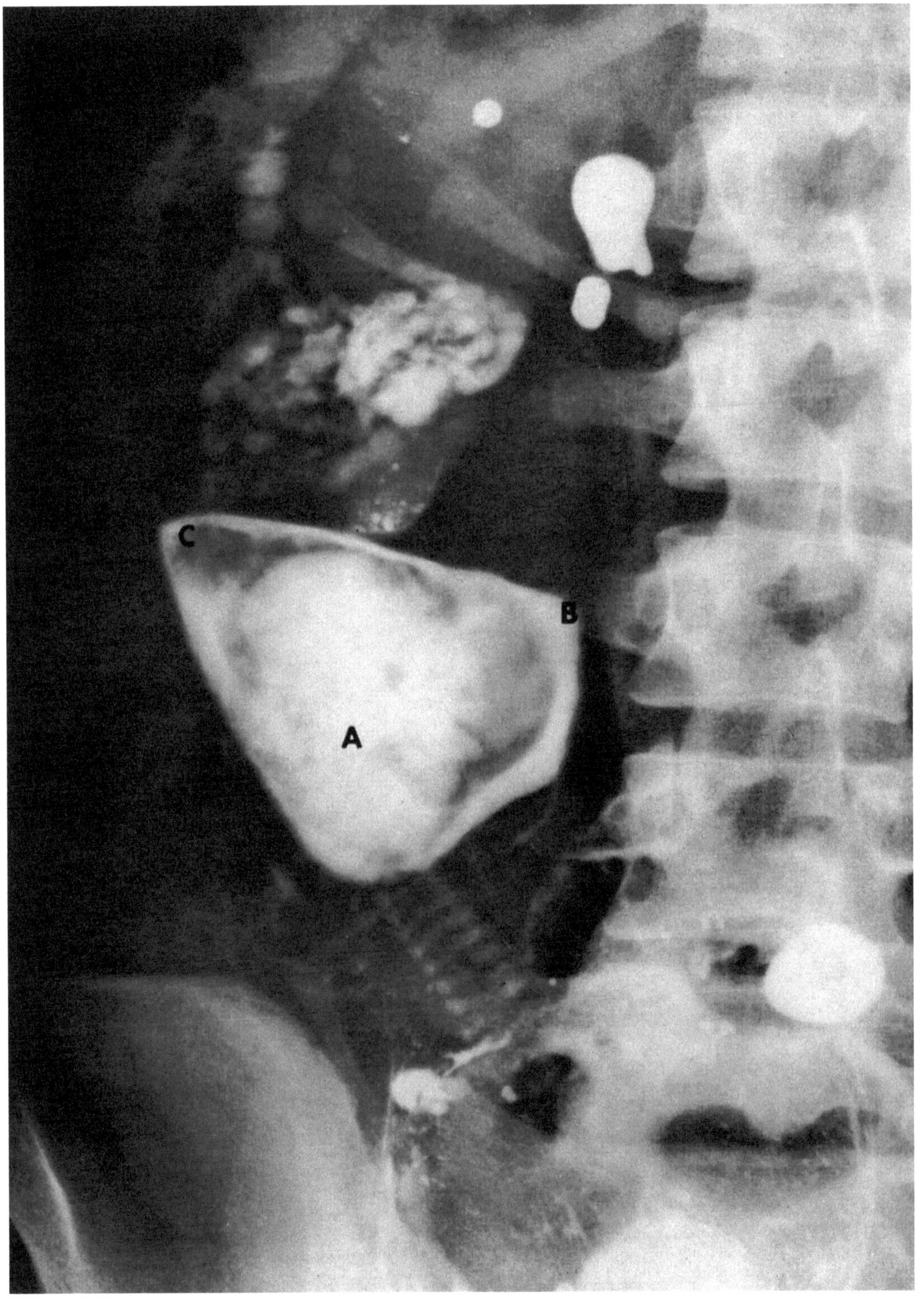

medium instilled under sonographic control for complementary quantitative assessment of cystic pulmonary malformation; large communicative cysts were fluoroscopically (Fig. 36) detected to cover the greater part of the thoracic cavity (A); contrast medium in pleural cavity (B); residual lung (C) in caudal direction (Fig. 36b).

Case 20

Fig. 36

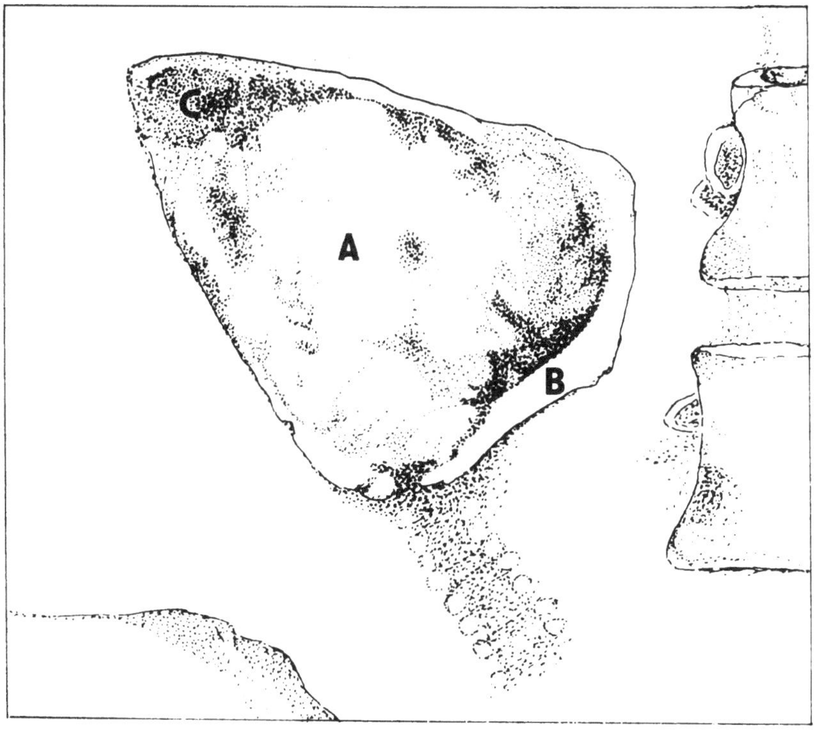

Case 20 **Clinical course:** Spontaneous labour in 31st week of pregnancy; 1,750 g, 43 cm; not resuscitable after brief period of spontaneous breathing.
**Radiogram** (Fig. 37): Bilateral pneumothorax; pulmonary dysplasia with large cysts; residual lung in caudal direction; retrieval of contrast medium in intestine by AFG four weeks before.
**Post-mortem findings:** Confirmation of prenatal diagnosis. ◁

Fig. 37

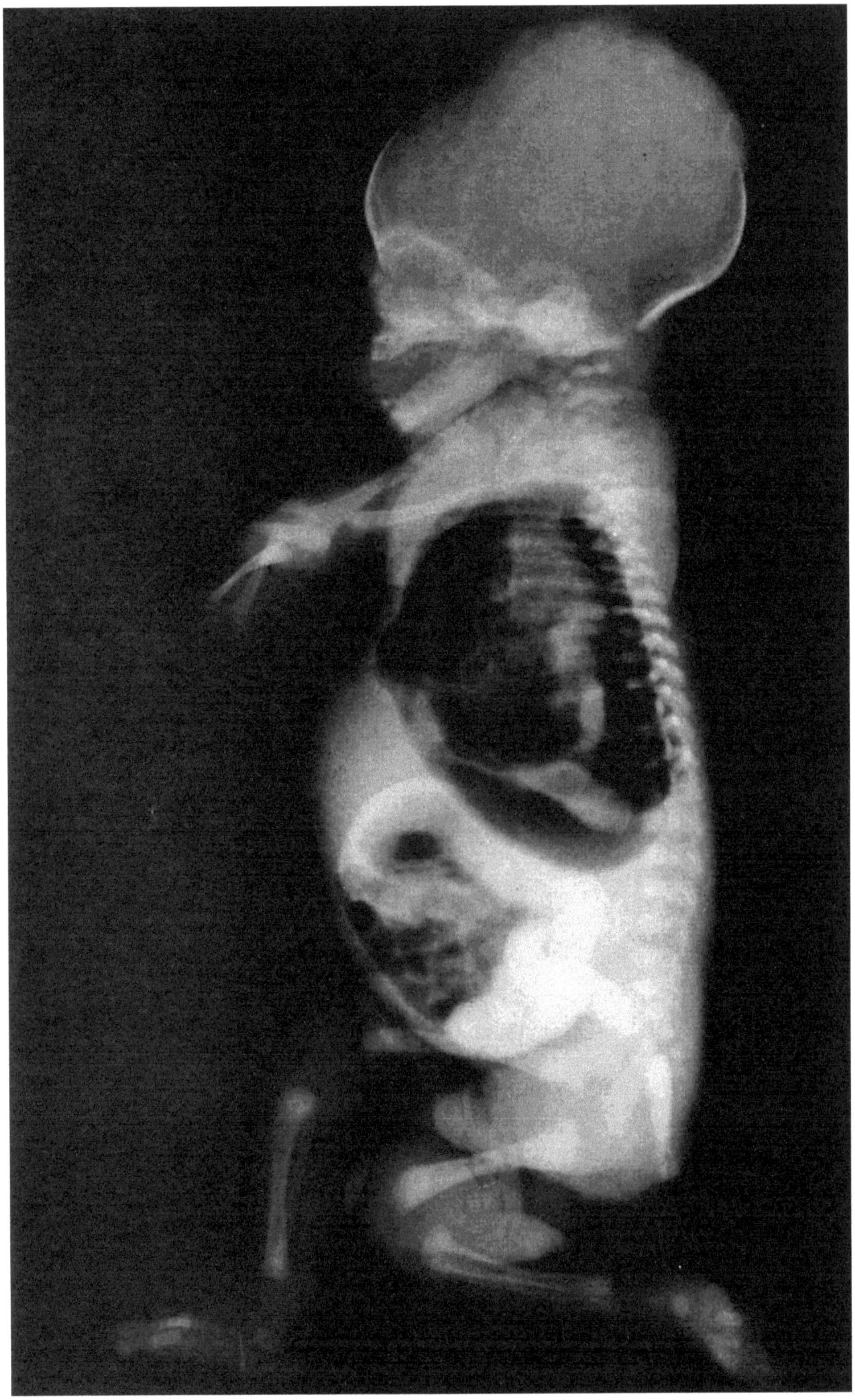

Patient K.R./85, 30 years, fourth gravidity, one parturition.
**Record:** One clinically intact child; two abortions in third and fourth months.
**Clinical findings:** 34th week of pregnancy; polyhydramnion.
**Ultrasonic findings:** Polyhydramnion; struma colli of the foetus; no signs indicative of malformations.

**Indication for AFG:** Polyhydramnion; search for malformations.
**AFG findings** (Fig. 38a: amniogram 30 minutes from injection; Fig. 38b: foetogram 24 hours from injection): Sex of foetus not safely determinable; breech presentation; polyhydramnion (A); slightly retarded gastro-intestinal passage

**Case 21**

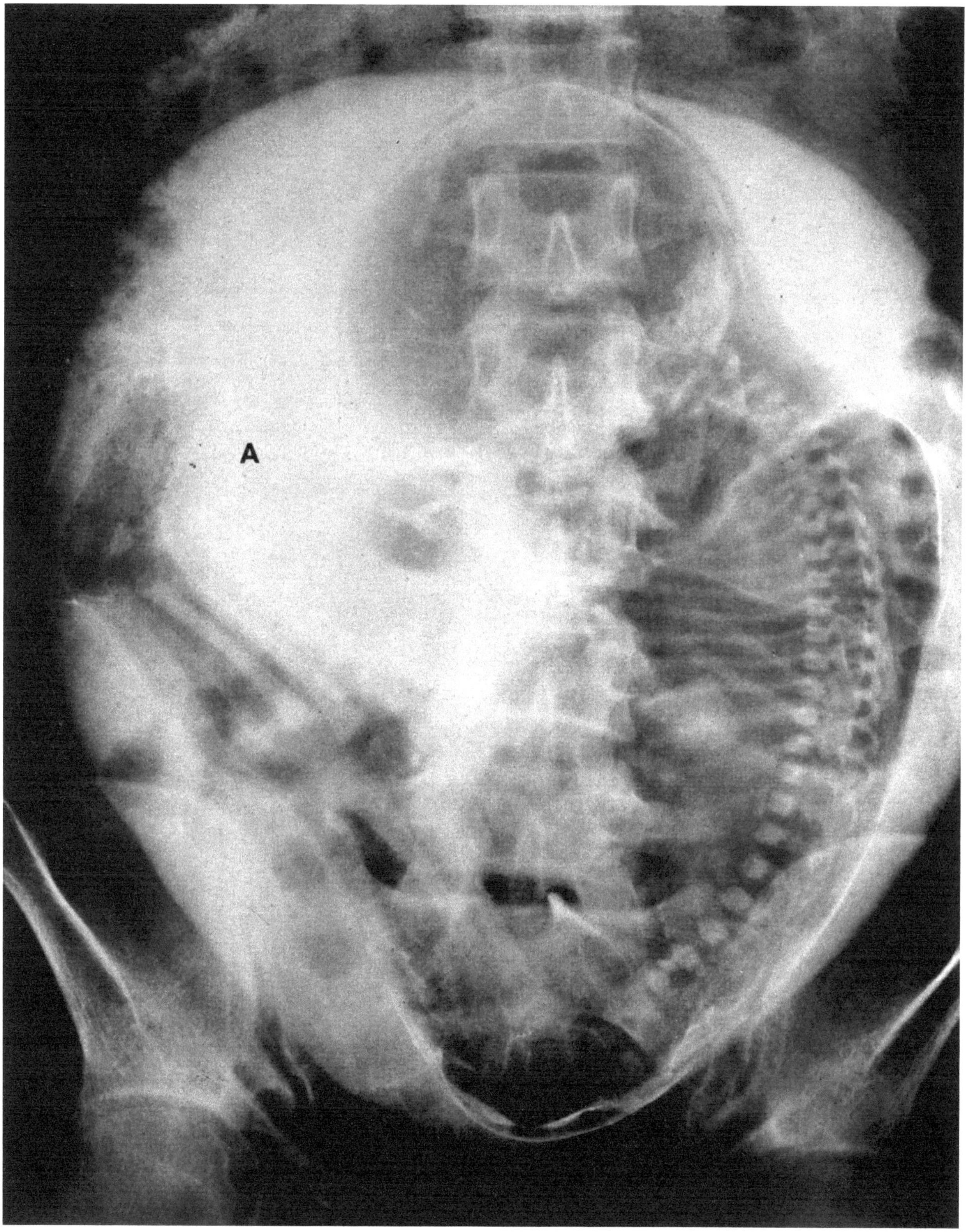


Fig. 38a

Case 21 of contrast medium; almost unchanged position of foetus in foetogram; no detectable malformation.

**Prenatal summary diagnosis:** Struma colli congenita; hypokinesia; retarded gastro-intestinal passage; suspicion of hypothyreosis.

**Clinical course:** Spontaneous labour in 36th week of pregnancy; girl, 2,610 g, 50 cm; paediatric hospitalisation on fifth day of age for icterus, hypogastric oedema, muscular hypotension, and inadequate drinking; treatment of hypothyreosis with good success; child in good condition. ◁

Fig. 38b

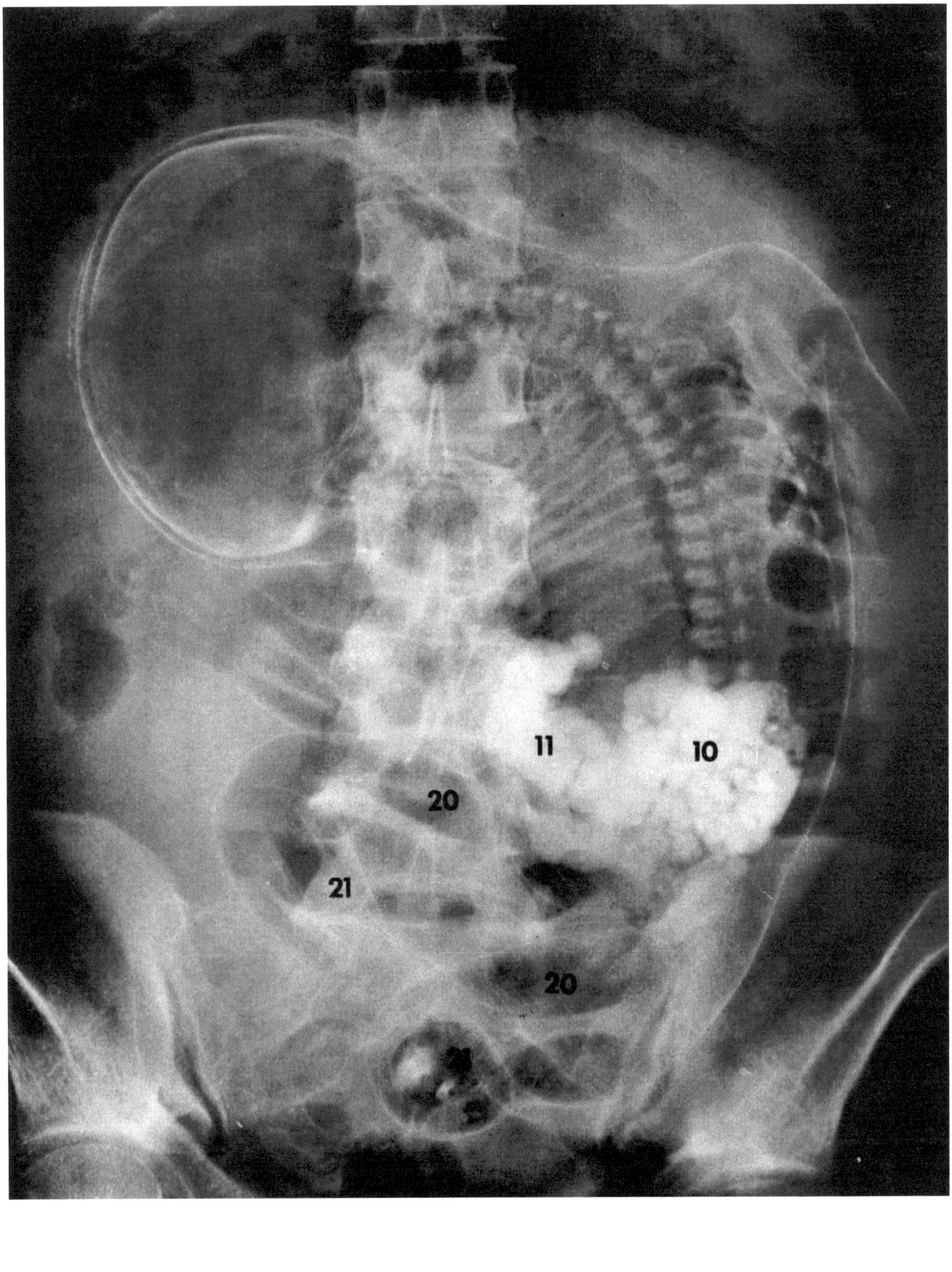

**Patient B.S./85,** 27 years, third gravidity, two parturitions.
**Record:** One stillbirth in 35th week of pregnancy; placental insufficiency; one child clinically intact.
**Clinical findings:** 32nd week of pregnancy; polyhydramnion.
**Ultrasonic findings:** Polyhydramnion since 27th week of pregnancy; no detectable malformations; struma colli of the foetus. Fig. 39a, b: Normal lumen of small intestine (DD) and colon.
**Indication for AFG.** Polyhydramnion, infavourable record.
**AFG findings** (Fig. 39c: foetogram 24 hours from injection): Female foetus; cephalic presentation; large amount of free Lipiodol UF; instillation of 10 ml of Lipiodol UF, in other

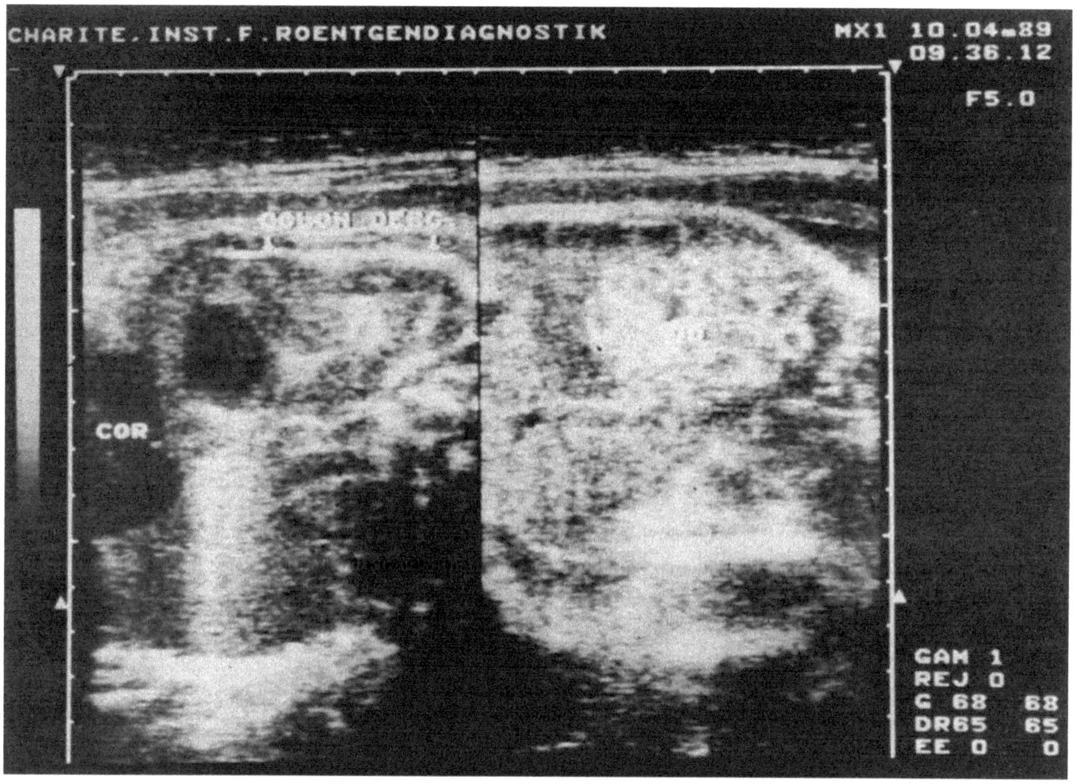


Fig. 39a

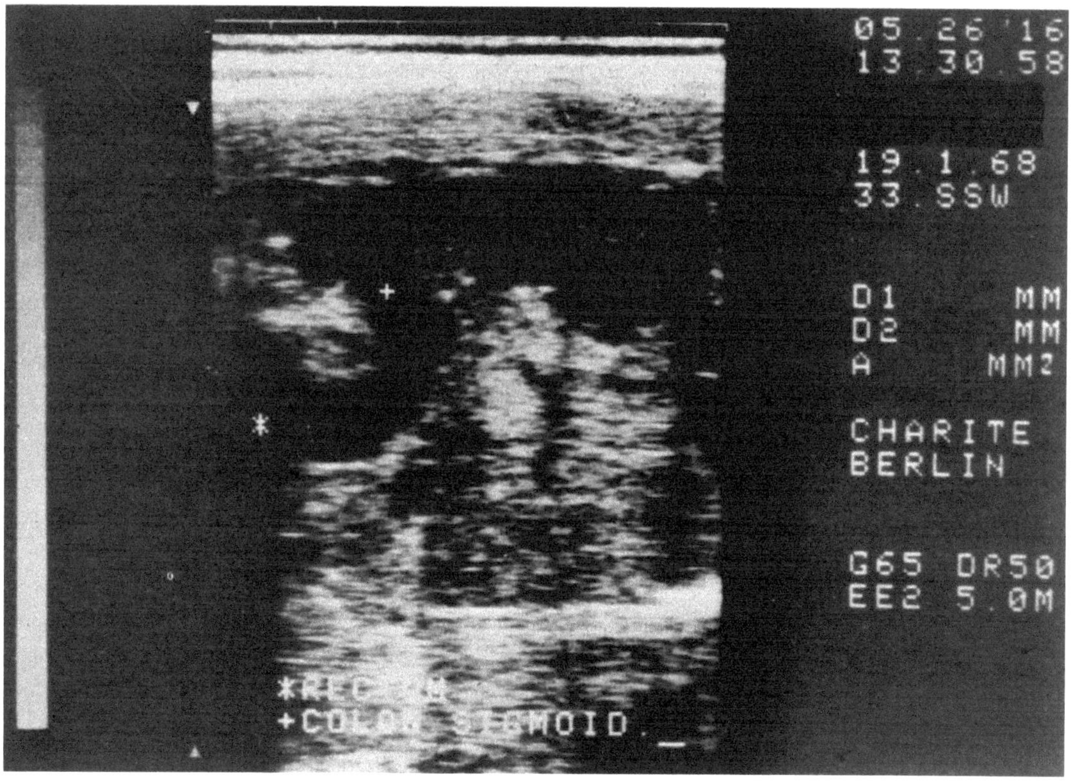


Fig. 39b

Case 22 words, too high quantity for 32nd week of pregnancy; time-adequate gastrointestinal passage of contrast medium up to rectal ampulla; partial contraction of intestinal lumen (A); high-contrast patchy structures in intestinal lumen were Lipiodol flakes.

**Prenatal summary diagnosis:** Spastic colon; no malformation, struma colli congenita.

**Clinical course:** Spontaneous labour in 33rd week of pregnancy; 2,200 g, 45 cm; struma colli congenita which had been detected by prenatal sonography prior to AFG; radiological detection of dolichocolon; first spontaneous defaecation at end of first week of age; gastro-oesophageal reflux. ◁

Fig. 39c

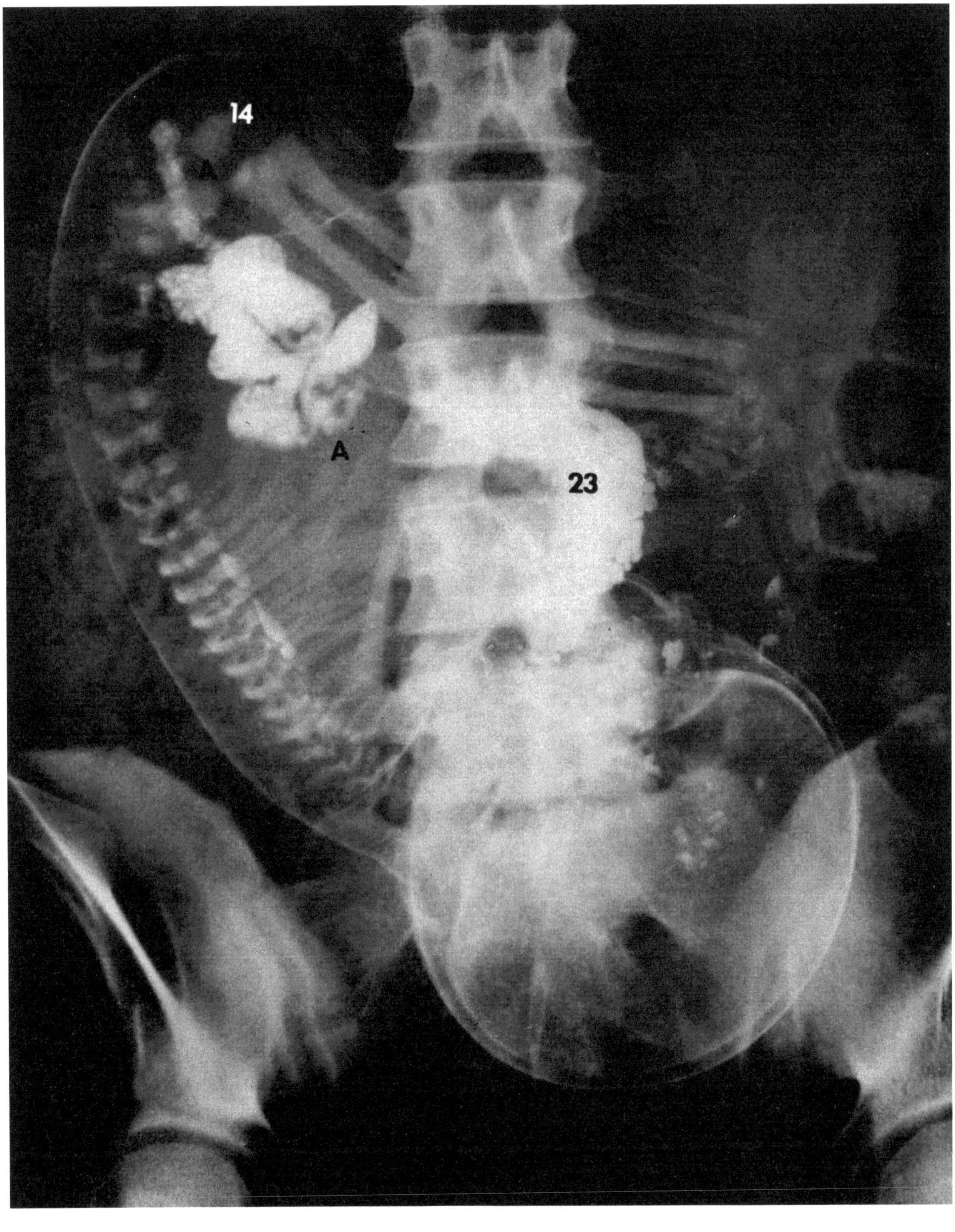

**Patient M.S./75,** 20 years, first gravidity.
**Clinical findings:** 29th week of pregnancy; imminent premature birth for insufficiency of the cervix.
**Ultrasonic findings:** Slight polyhydramnion; conspicuously abnormal thorax with abnormal configuration; intra-uterine tumour not accurately identified.

**Indication for AFG:** To clear up ultrasonic findings; search for malformations.
**AFG findings:** (Fig. 40a: amniogram 30 minutes from injection; Fig. 40b: foetogram 24 hours from injection): Sex of foetus not determinable; cephalic presentation; accumulation of either contrast medium in atypical localisation and

**Case 23**

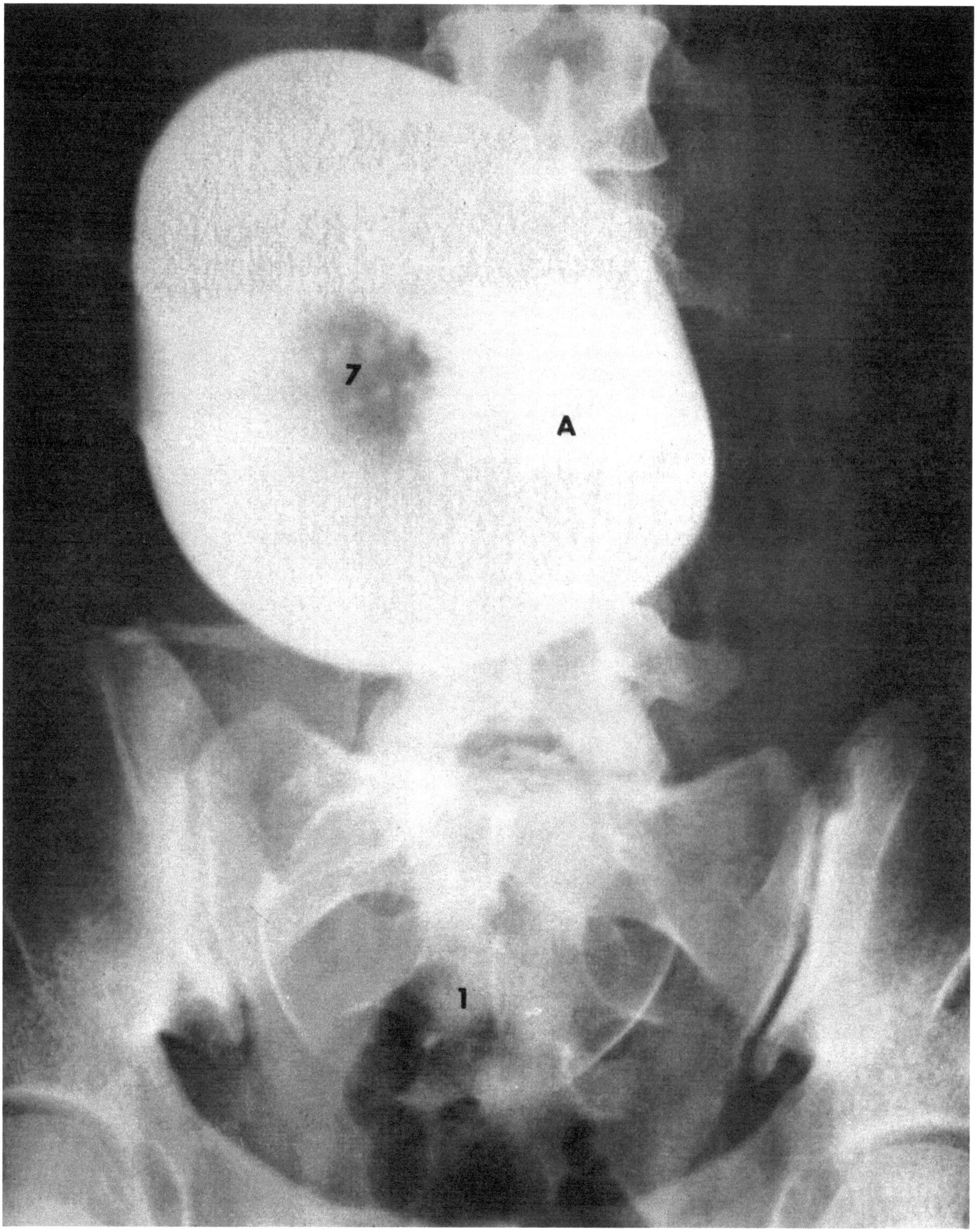


Fig. 40a

Case 23 without amniographic effect (A); foetogram shows conspicuous highcontrast amniotic fluid with foetus imaged in negative contrast; high-contrast umbilical cord (C); hyperlordosis of vertebral column (B; arrows); suspicion of uterus subseptus; fine-drop accumulation of Lipdiodol UF in abdominal wall region (D); maternal excretory urogram.
**Prenatal summary diagnosis:** Hyperlordosis of vertebral column; no unambiguous interpretation of atypical distridistribution of contrast medium.
**Clinical course:** Termination of pregnancy in 3th week;

Fig. 40b

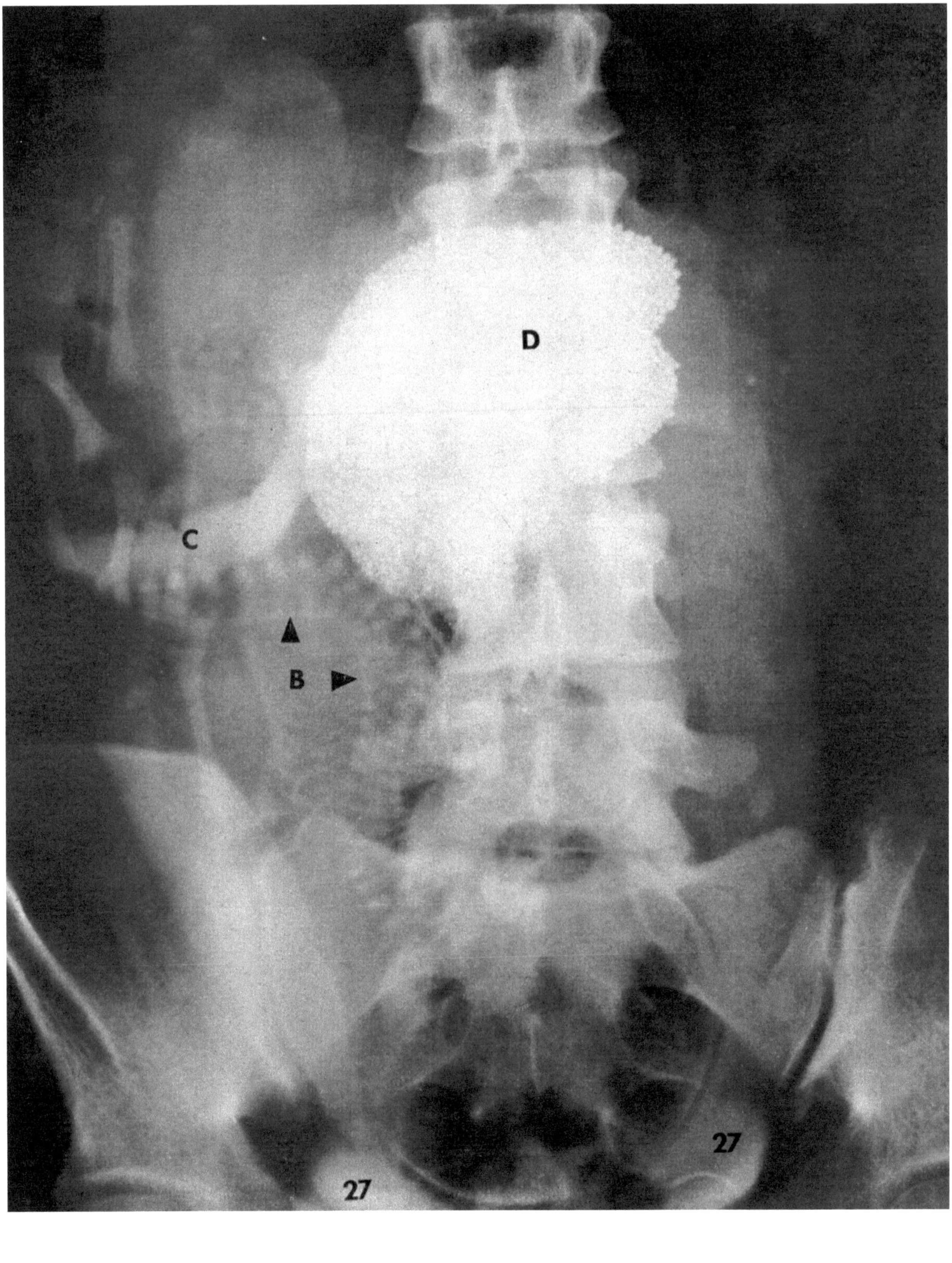

female foetus, 1,000 g, 36 cm; 36 cm; intrapartum death. **Radiogram** (Fig. 41) and **post-mortem findings:** Large omphalocele with destroyed wall; liver, spleen, and large fragments of gastro-intestinal tract in celenic sac; mesenterium ileocolicum commune; dextroposition of stomach; hypoplasia of lungs; 180 torsion of vertebral column with 90 angle; abnormal posture of both feet.
Contrast medium was accidentally instilled into omphalocele, as amniocentesis under permanent sonographic control had not been mandatory at that time (1975). ◁

Case 23

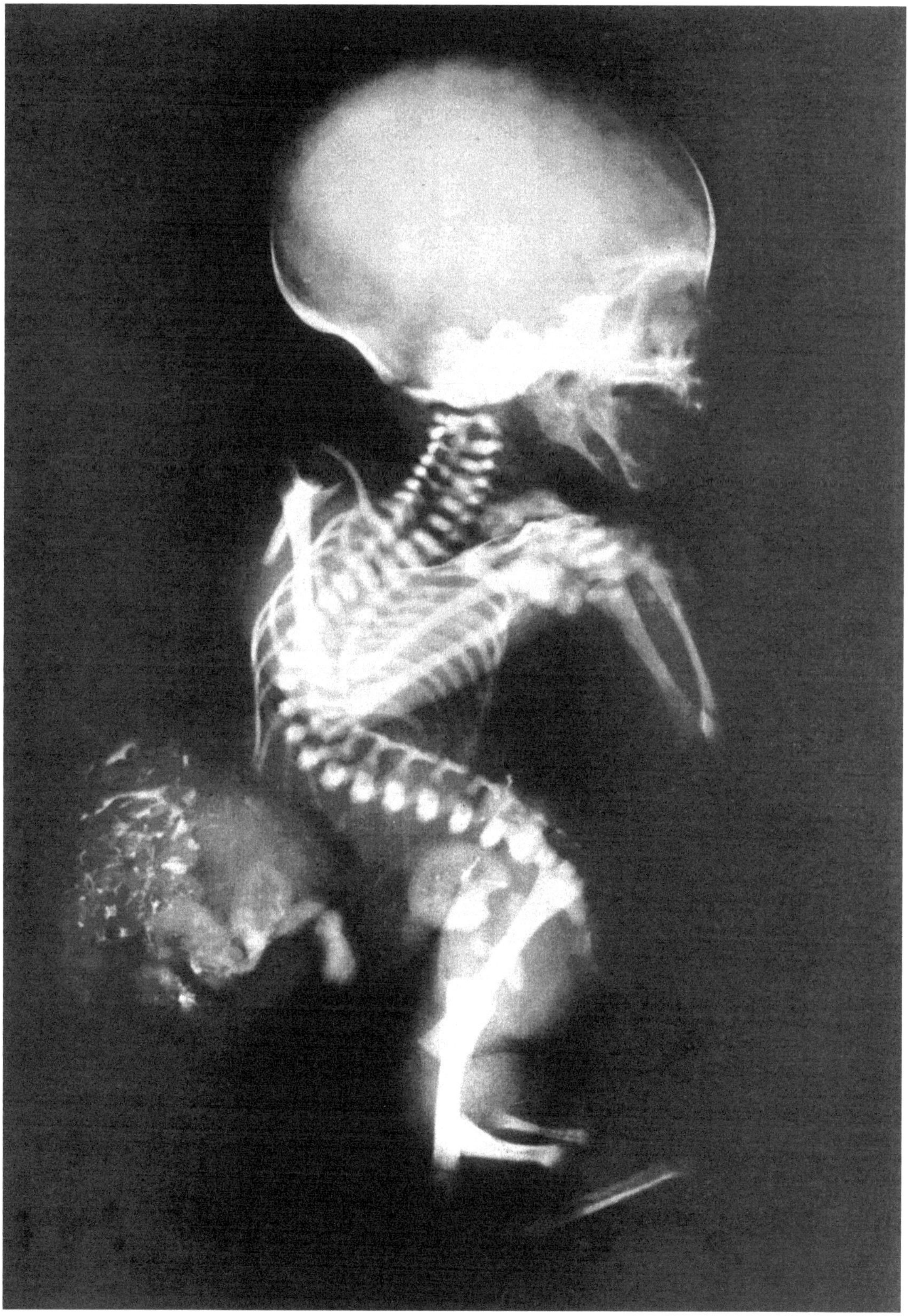

Fig. 41

**Case 24** **Patient S.D./85,** 21 years, first gravidity.
**Clinical findings:** 34th week of pregnancy; polyhydramnion.
**Ultrasonic findings** (Fig. 42a, b): Polyhydramnion; disproportionality between head and thorax; echo structures adjacent to umbilical cord, possibly indicative of omphalocele (arrows).

Fig. 42a

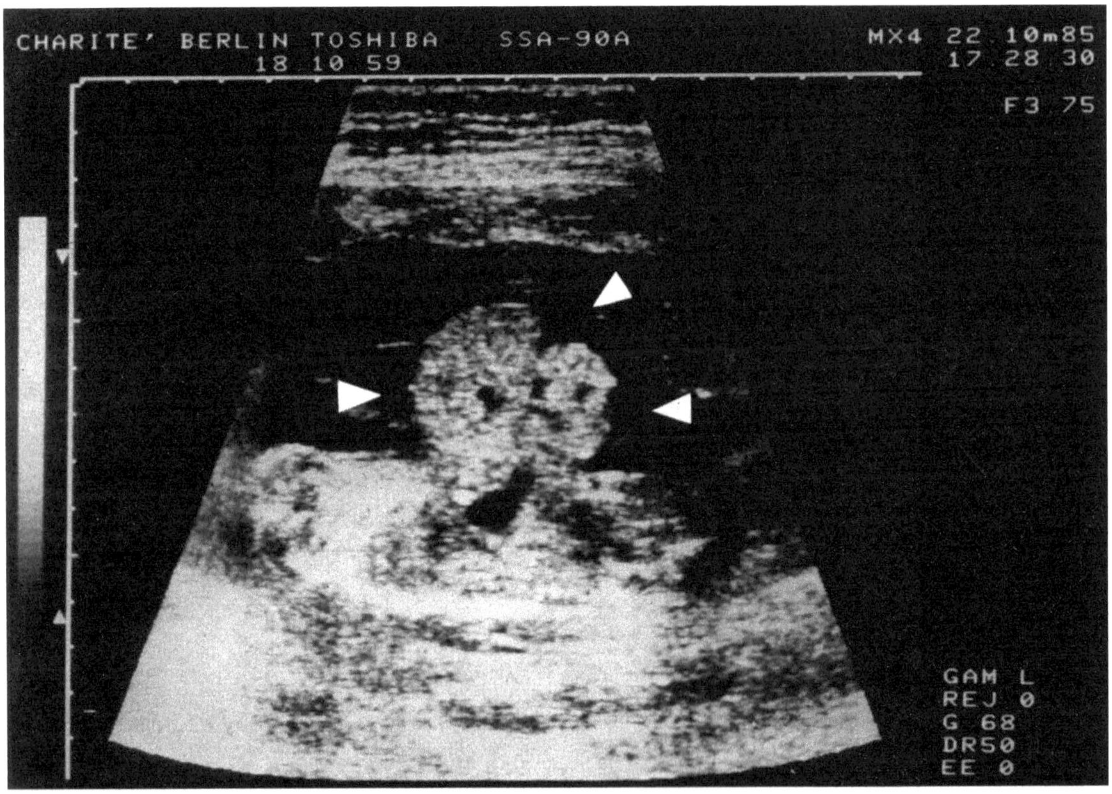


Fig. 42b

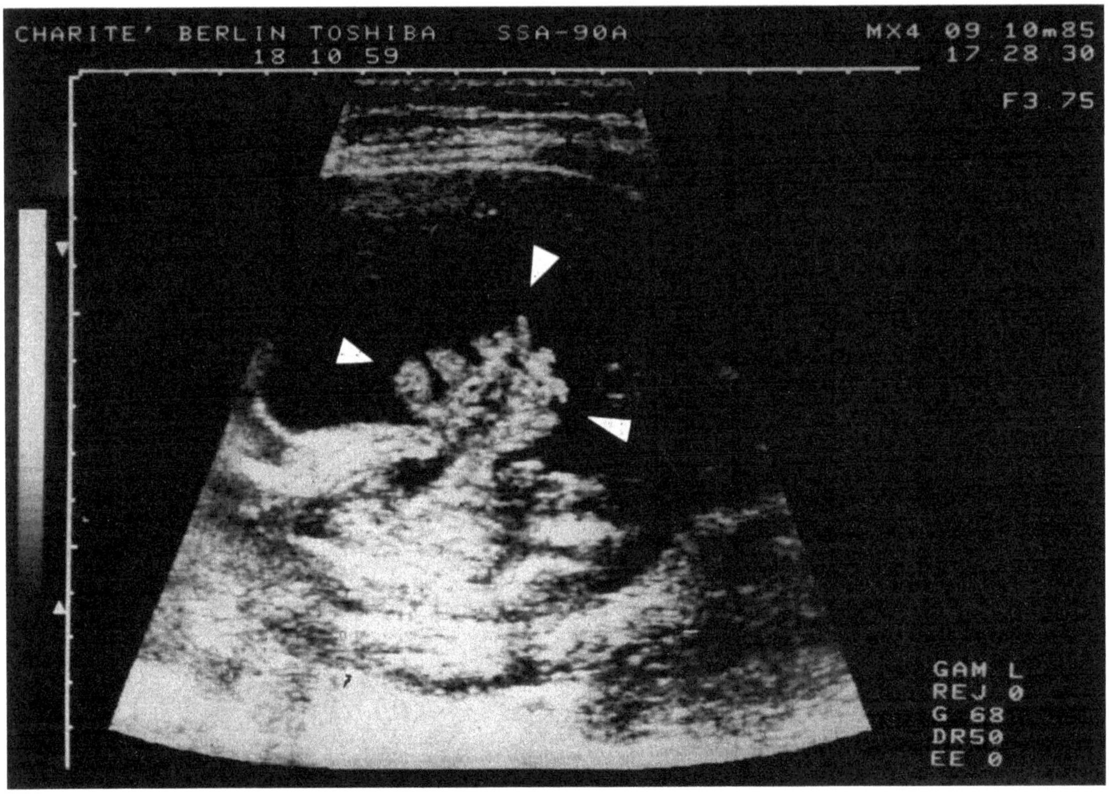

**Indication for AFG:** Verification of sonographic suspicious diagnosis; search for additional malformations.
**AFG findings** (Fig. 43: foetogram 24 hours from injection): Sex of foetus not determinable; breech presentation; lateral bending of trunk (A; arrows); loops of small intestine and colon at abdominal wall (B).

Case 24

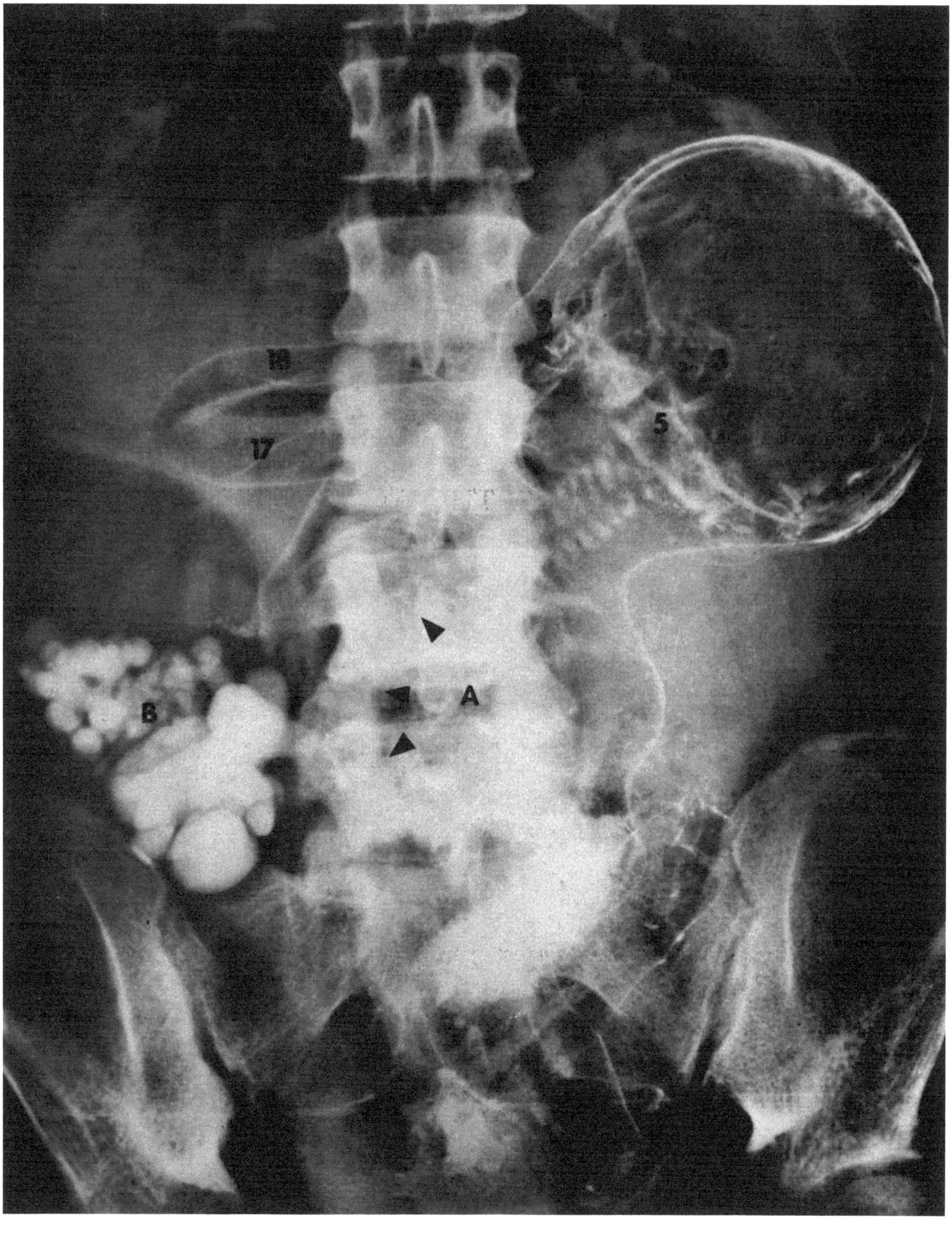


Fig. 43

Case 24 **Prenatal summary diagnosis:** Large omphalocele.
**Clinical course:** Spontaneous labour in 35th week of pregnancy; female foetus; 1,300 g, 40 cm; intrapartum death.
**Radiogram** (Fig. 44) and **post-mortem findings:** Rectangular flexion of vertebral column; omphalocele with liver, spleen, pancreas, stomach, small intestine, and colon; aplasia of left kidney; bilateral club-foot postures. ◁

Fig. 44

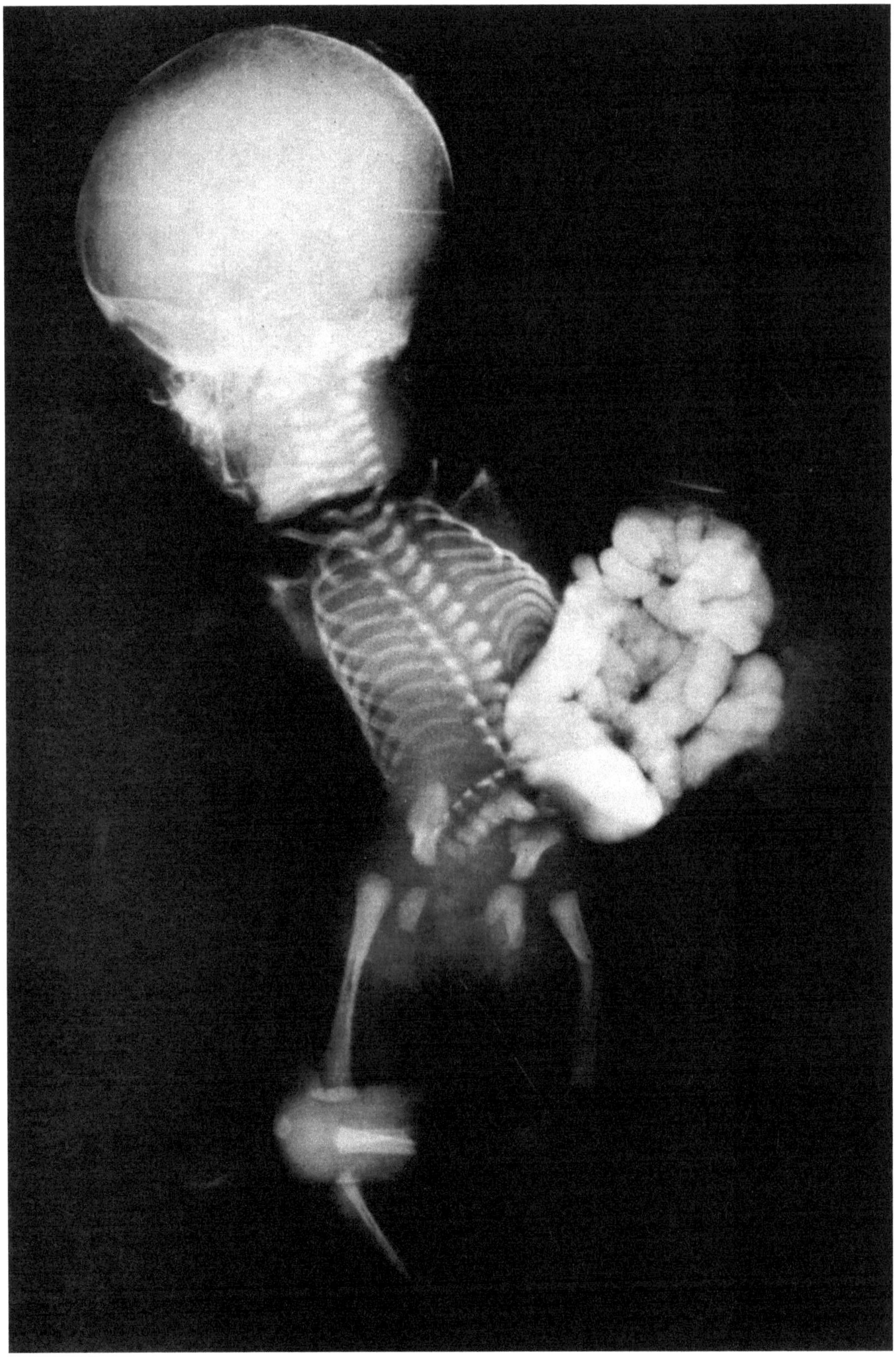

**Patient T.U./85,** 24 years, first gravidity.
**Clinical findings:** 35th week of pregnancy; no contributory findings.
**Ultrasonic findings** (Fig. 45a, b): Loops of small intestine and colon with thickened walls floating freely in amniotic fluid; no additional malformations detectable.
**Indication for AFG:** Search for additional malformations.
**AFG findings** (Fig. 46: foetogram 24 hours from injection): Female foetus; cephalic presentation; time-adequate passage of contrast medium through gastro-intestinal tract; enlarged

**Case 25**

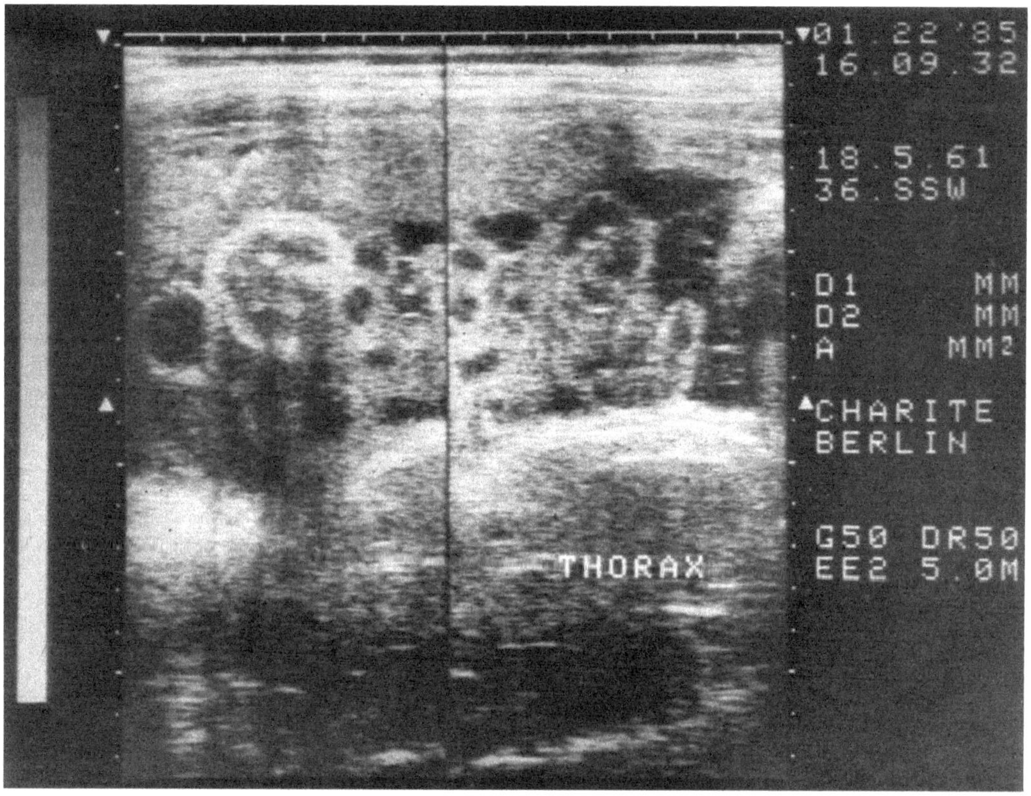


Fig. 45a

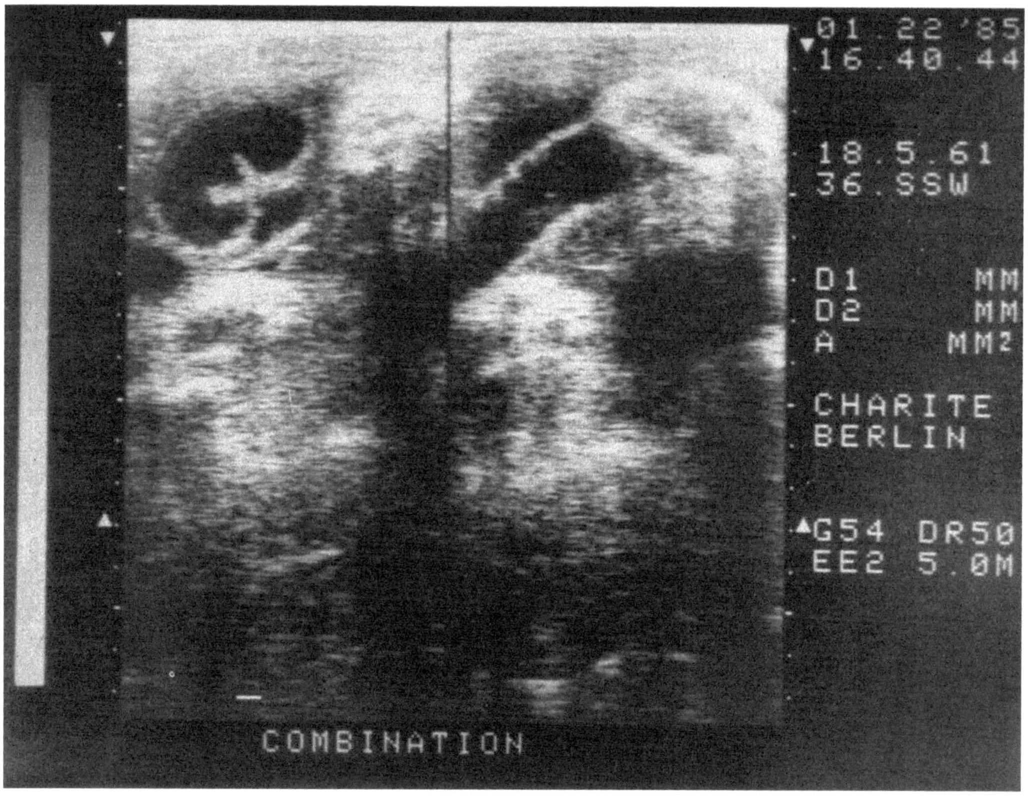


Fig. 45b

Case 25 loops of small intestine and colon ventral from abdominal wall and between legs (A; arrows); no additional malformation detectable.

**Prenatal summary diagnosis:** Gastroschisis (Omphalocele without a sac).

Intestinal loops, different from omphalocele, not localised in delimited space but ventral from abdominal wall in a fetus with gastroschisis; their lumen being enlarged because of unphysiological contact with amniotic fluid.

**Clinical course:** Delivery by caesarean section in 36th week of pregnancy; 2,560 g, 47 cm; surgical treatment of gastroschisis immediately after birth; no postnatal complications. ◁

Fig. 46

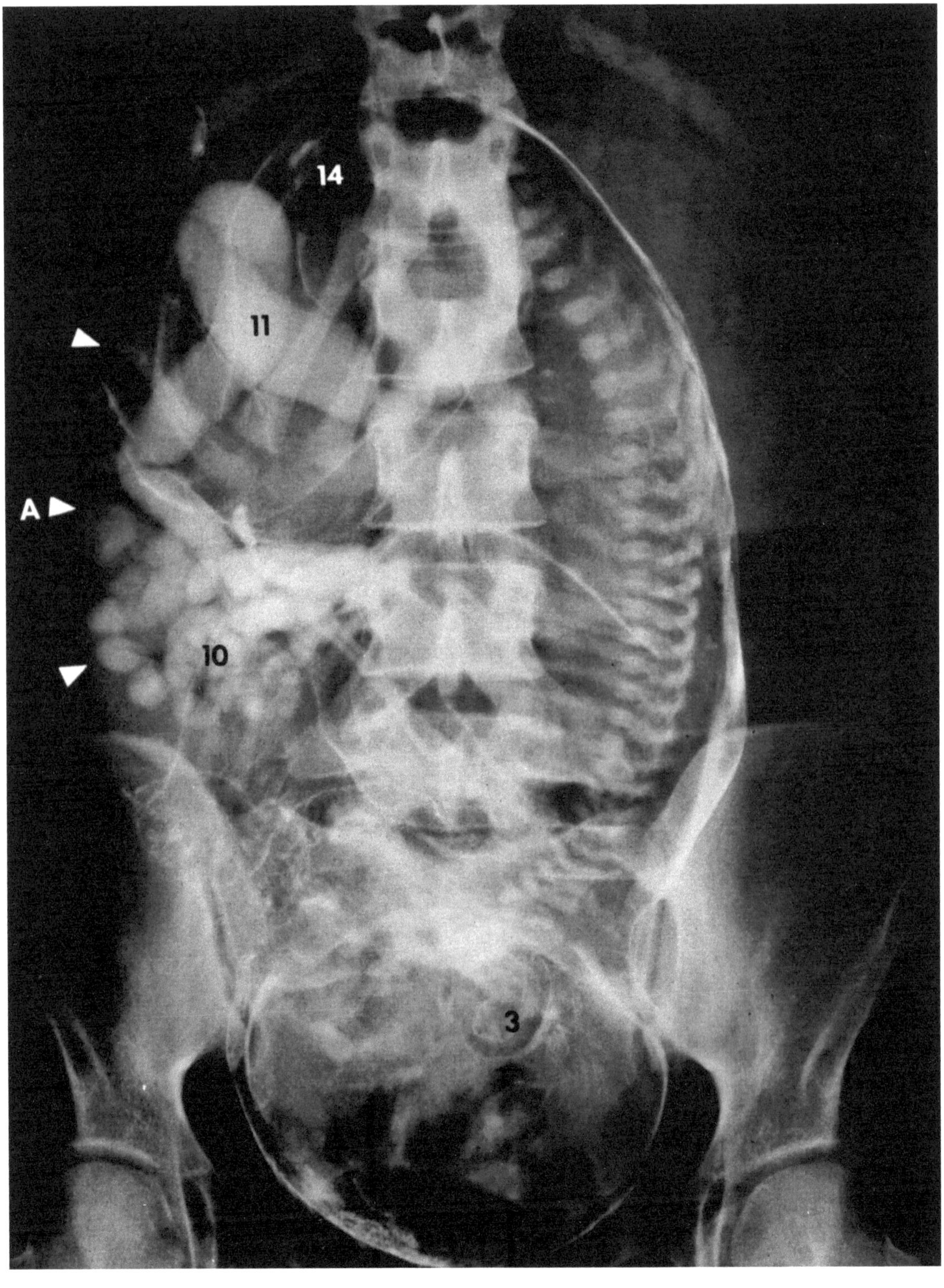

**Patient B.G./84,** 30 years, third gravidity, one parturition.
**Record:** One live-born child, death nine hours postpartum for malformation of lung; one interruption.
**Clinical findings:** 30th week of pregnancy; polyhydramnion.
**Ultrasonic findings** (Fig. 47 a): Polyhydramnion; no detectable malformation. Normal diaphragma (arrows; REN = kidney)
**Indication for AFG:** Polyhydramnion; search for malformations.
**AFG findings** (Fig. 47 b: foetogram 24 hours from injection). Female foetus; cephalic presentation; complete contrast

**Case 26**

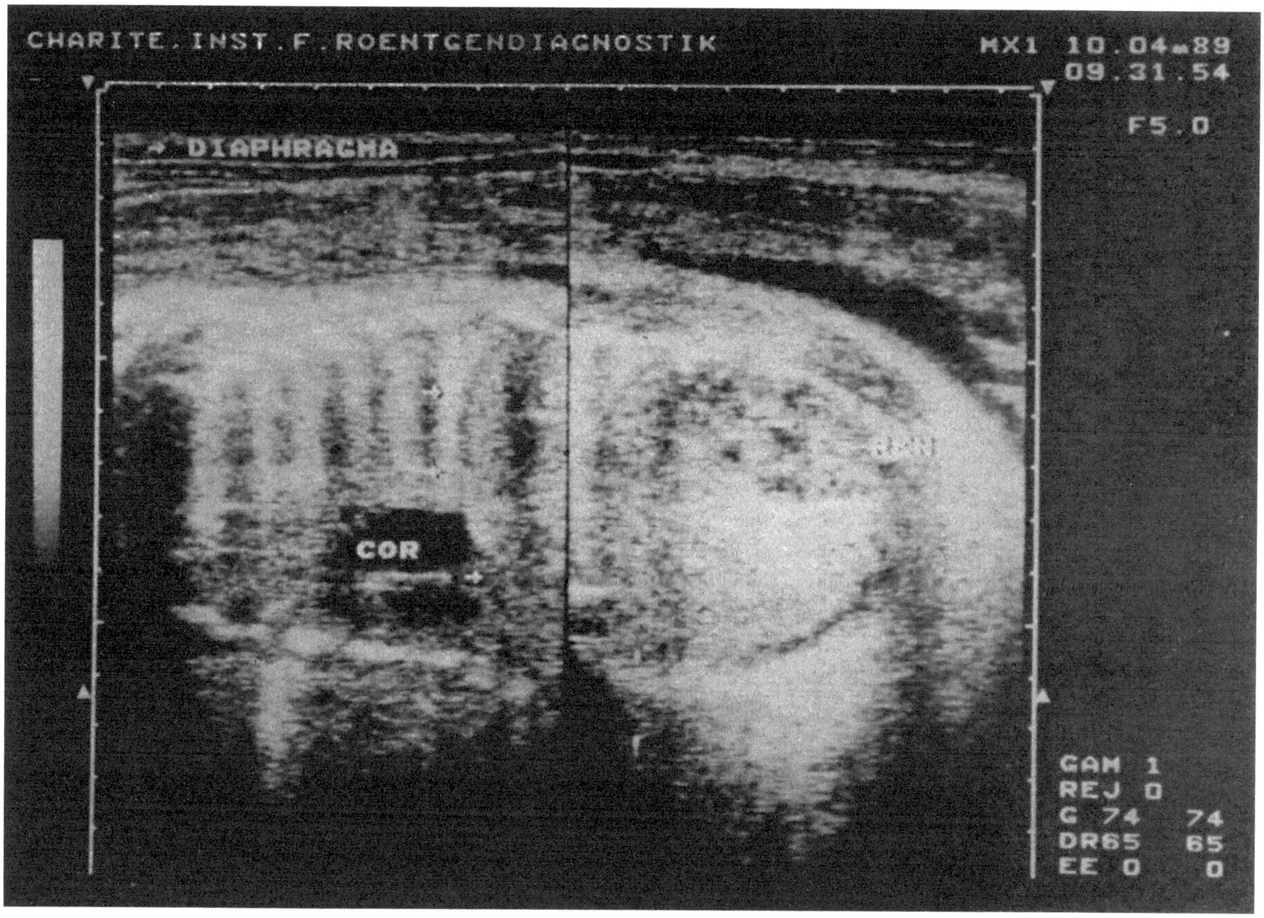


Fig. 47 a

Case 26 image of gastro-intestinal tract; no signs indicative of malmations.

**Prenatal summary diagnosis:** No detection of malformations.

**Clinical course:** Spontaneous labour in 35th week of pregnancy; 3,250 g, 50 cm; death nine hours postpartum of respiratory distress syndrome and right-side diaphragmatic defect with intrathoracic displacement of liver.

**Post-mortem findings.:** Right-side diaphragmatic defect with herniation of liver and pulmonary hypoplasia (right); no additional organic malformations. ◁

Fig. 47 b

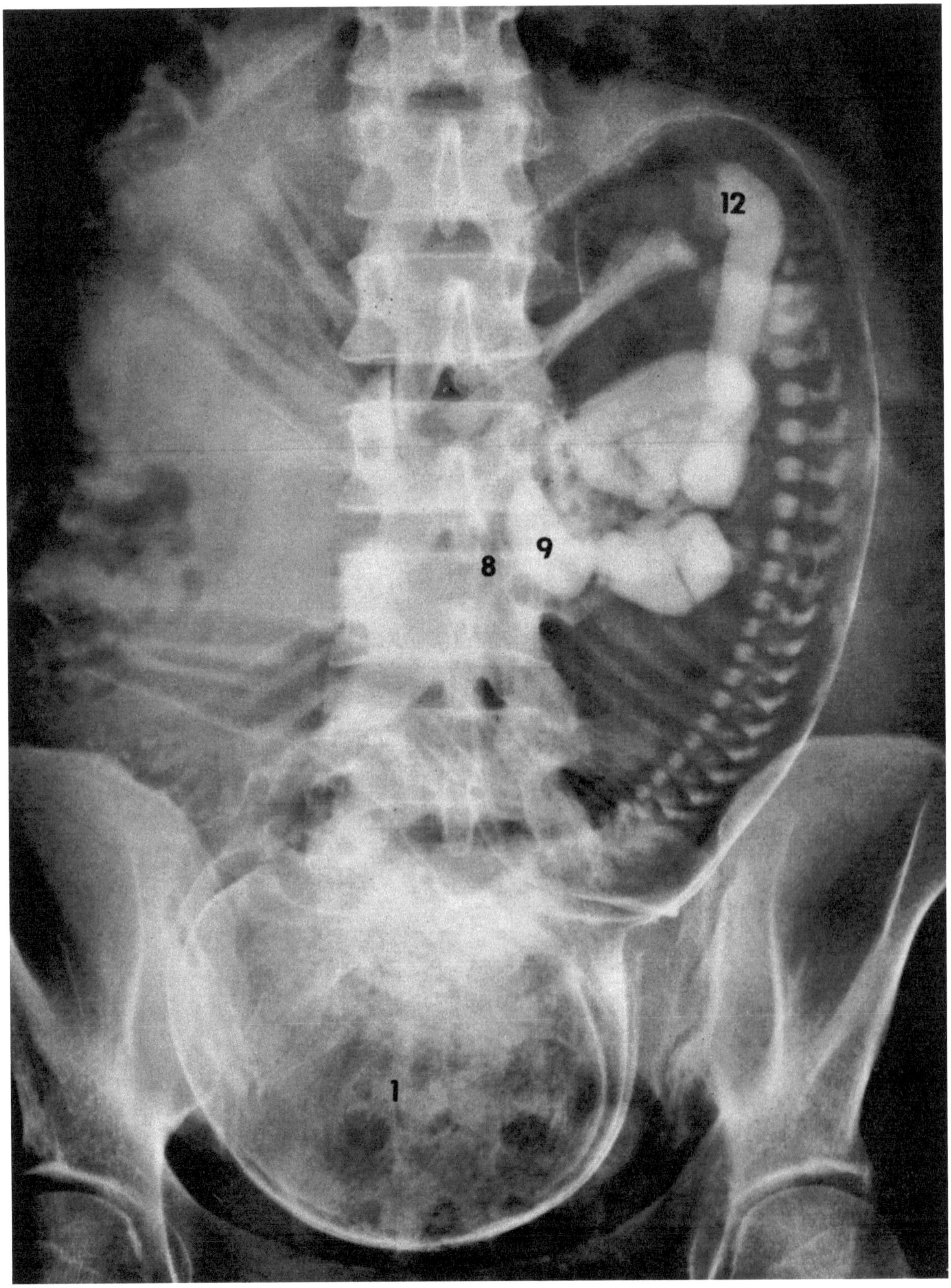

**Case 27**

**Patient W.A./84,** 26 years, second gravidity, one parturition.
**Record:** Polyhydramnion of unelucidated genesis in first gravidity; normal birth; clinically intact child.
**Clinical findings:** 35th week of pregnancy; polyhydramnion.
**Ultrasonic findings** (Fig. 48a, b): Polyhydramnion; moderate dermal oedema; ascites (MD); enlarged small intestine loops (D) of rigid appearance with clearly thickened walls.
(LE = liver)
**Indication for AFG:** Assessment of gastro-intestinal canal; search for malformations.

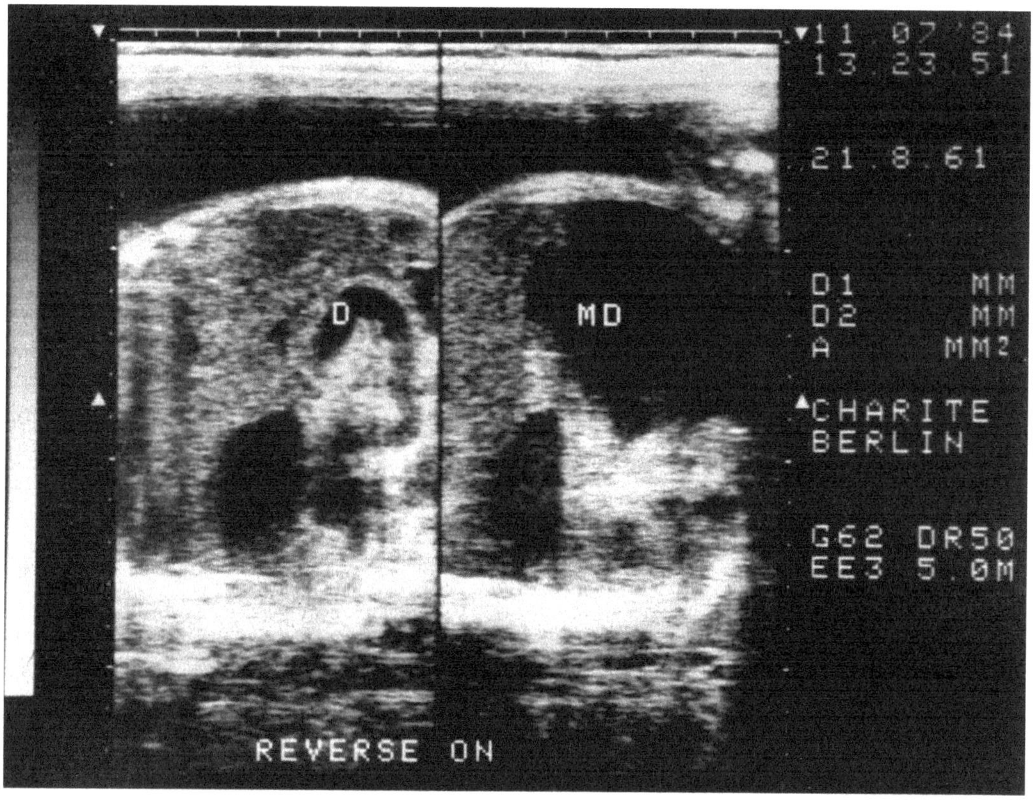


Fig. 48a

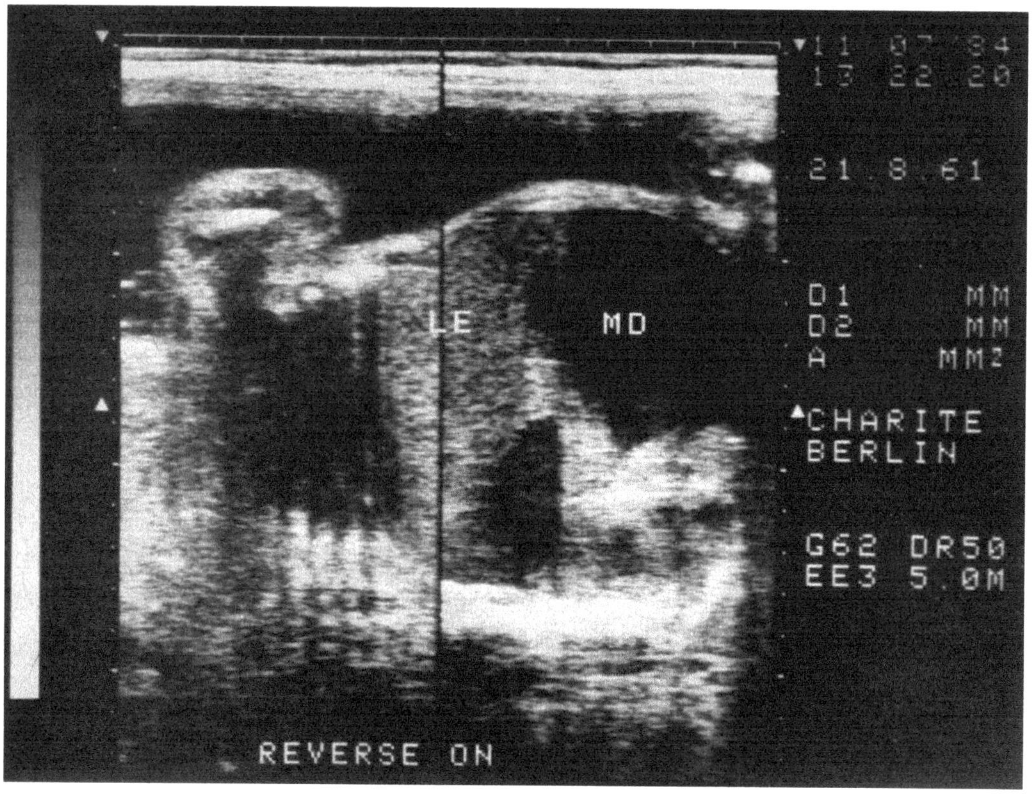


Fig. 48b

Case 27 **AFG findings** (Fig. 49: foetogram 24 hours from injection): Male foetus; cephalic presentation; protrusion of abdominal region (A; arrows); no contrast medium detectable in gastro-intestinal tract.

**Prenatal summary diagnosis:** Suspicion of atresia in gastro-intestinal tract.

**Clinical course:** Spontaneous labour in 35th week of pregnancy; child with moderate hydrops, 2,620 g, 47 cm; laparotomy immediately after birth shows atresia of small intestine, volvulus, perforation of small intestine, meconium peritonitis; no postoperative complications. ◁

Fig. 49

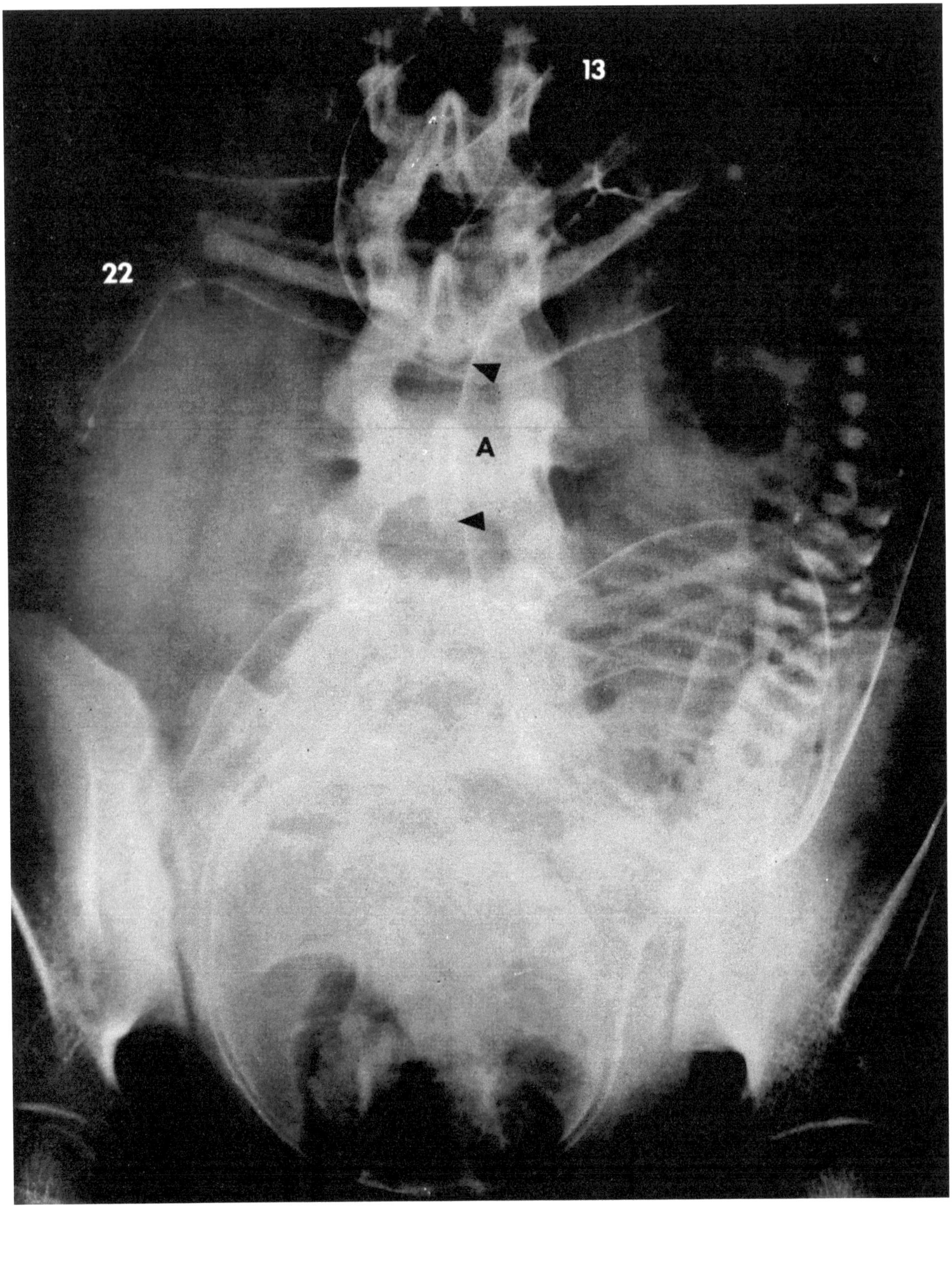

Case 28

**Patient K.K./86,** 25 years, second gravidity, one parturition.
**Record:** One clinically intact child.
**Clinical findings:** 30th week of pregnancy; polyhydramnion; treatment initiated for fresh toxoplasmosis infection in 24th week of pregnancy.

**Ultrasonic findings:** Polyhydramnion; no detectable malformation.
**Indication for AFG:** Polyhydramnion; search for malformations.
**AFG findings** (Fig. 50a: foetogram 24 hours from injection;

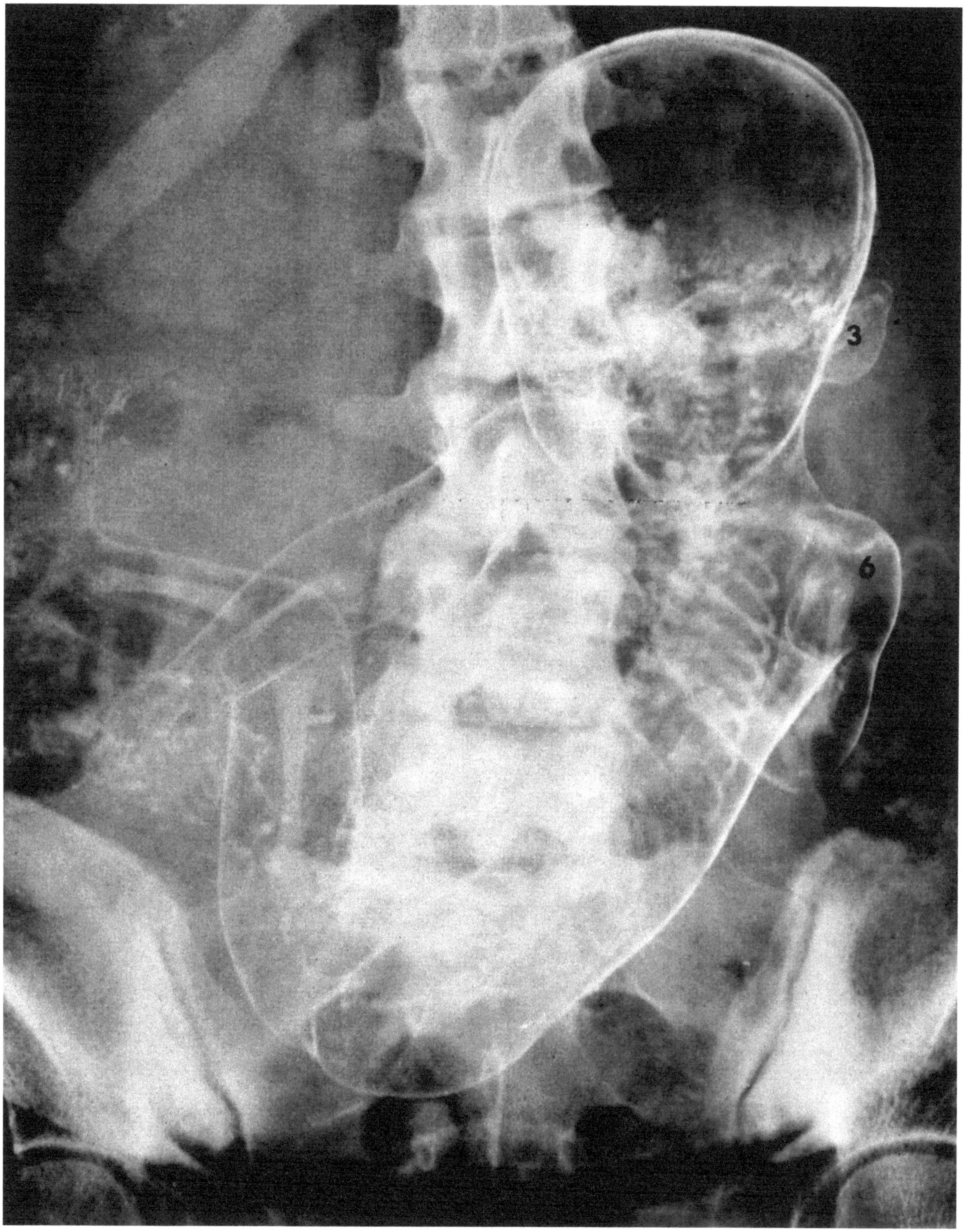


Fig. 50a

Case 28 Fig. 50b: foetogram 48 hours from injection): Male foetus; breech presentation; inconspicuous Lipiodol marking of foetal skin surface; skeleton without signs of pathological alterations; normal contrast image of gastro-intestinal tract with contrast medium not obtainable; deposition of contrast medium visible below foetal chest after 24 and 48 hours; fluoroscopic image (Fig. 50b) suggests that contrast medium is probably in foetal stomach (A).

Fig. 50b

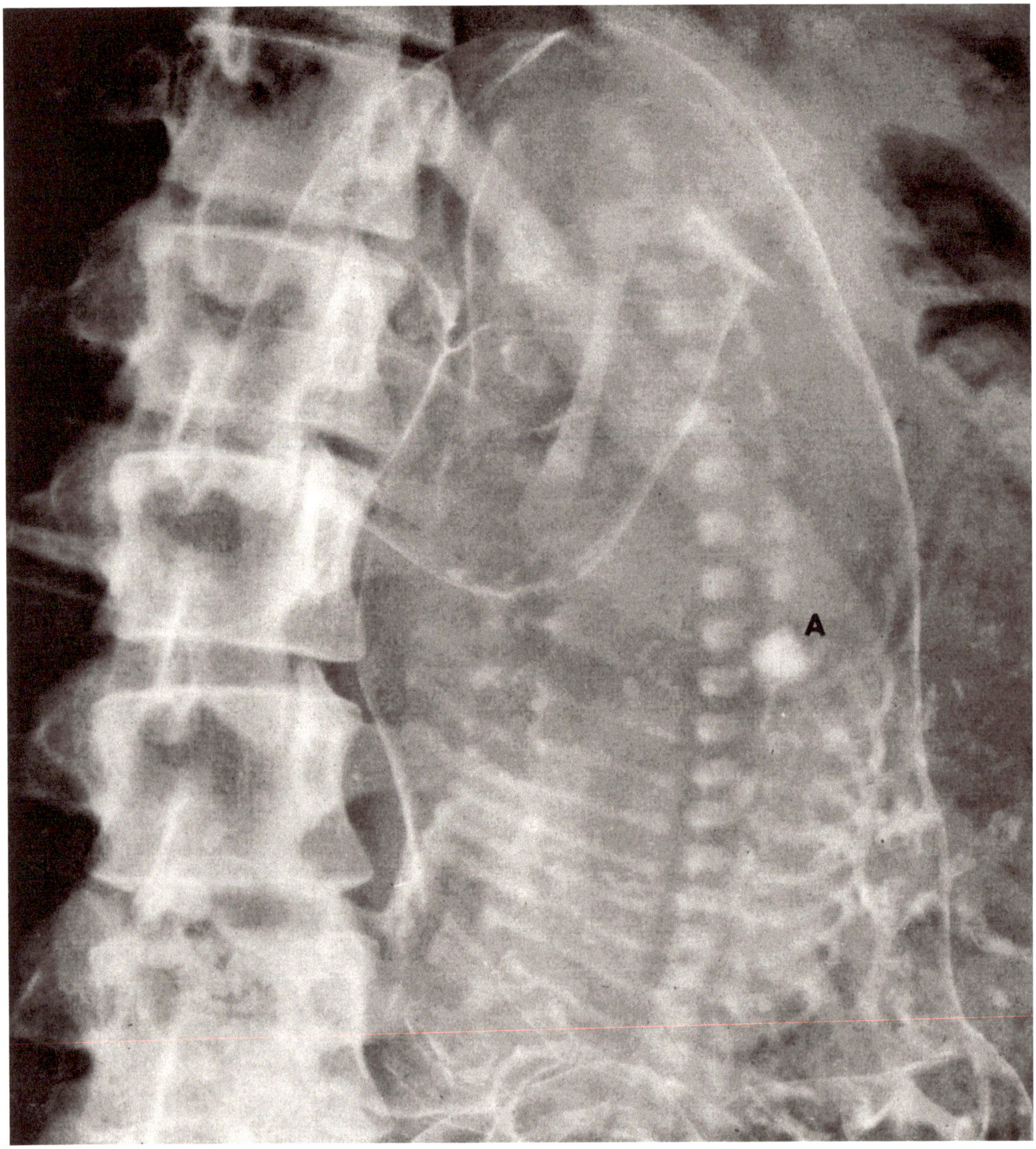

**Additional ultrasonographic follow-up checks** showed typical image of "double bubble" or "hour-glass" (Fig. 51 a, b, arrows); intravenous application of Cerucal® (metoclopramide hydrochloride, 0.01 g) to mother was followed by detectable contractions of foetal intestine but failed to produce contraction of stomach (MA).
**Genetic findings:** Trisomy 21 (Down's syndrome).
**Prenatal summary diagnosis:** Suspicion of severe duodenal

Fig. 50 b

Case 28 stenosis and trisomy 21 (Down's syndrome).

**Clinical course:** Spontaneous labour in 38th week of pregnancy; 2,530 g, 49 cm; operation on second day of age for clinically and radiologically established duodenal stenosis and annular pancreas; death on tenth postoperative day of diffuse peritonitis. ◁

Fig. 51a

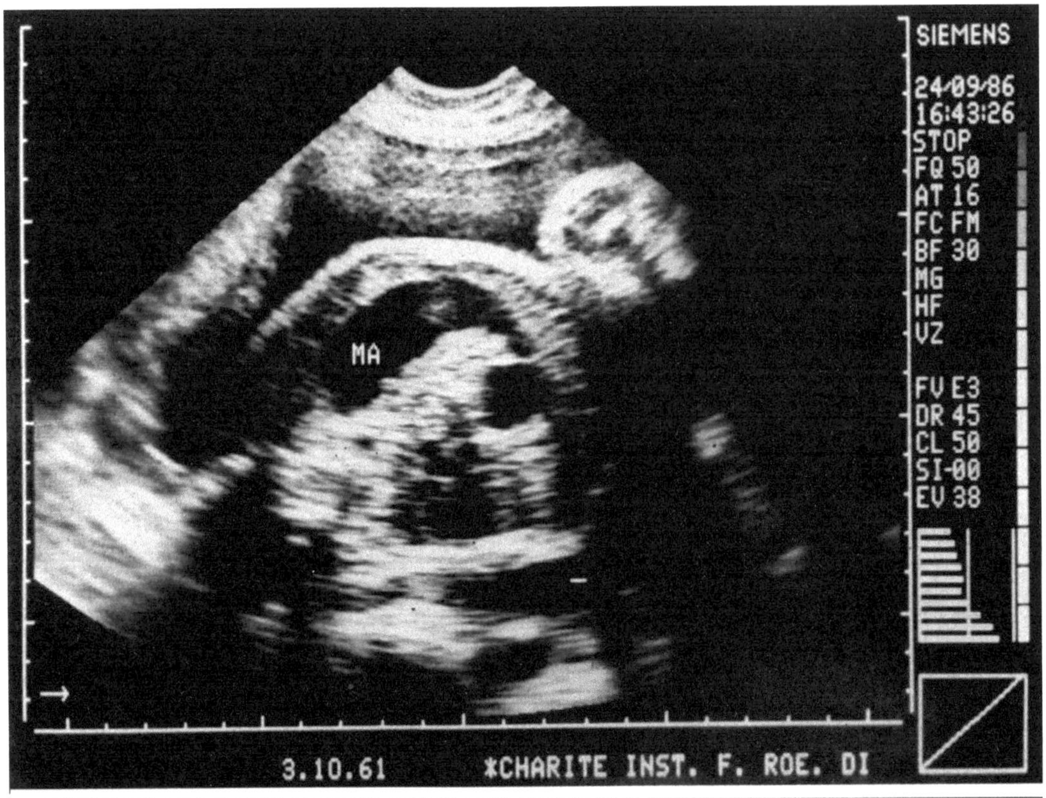


Fig. 51b

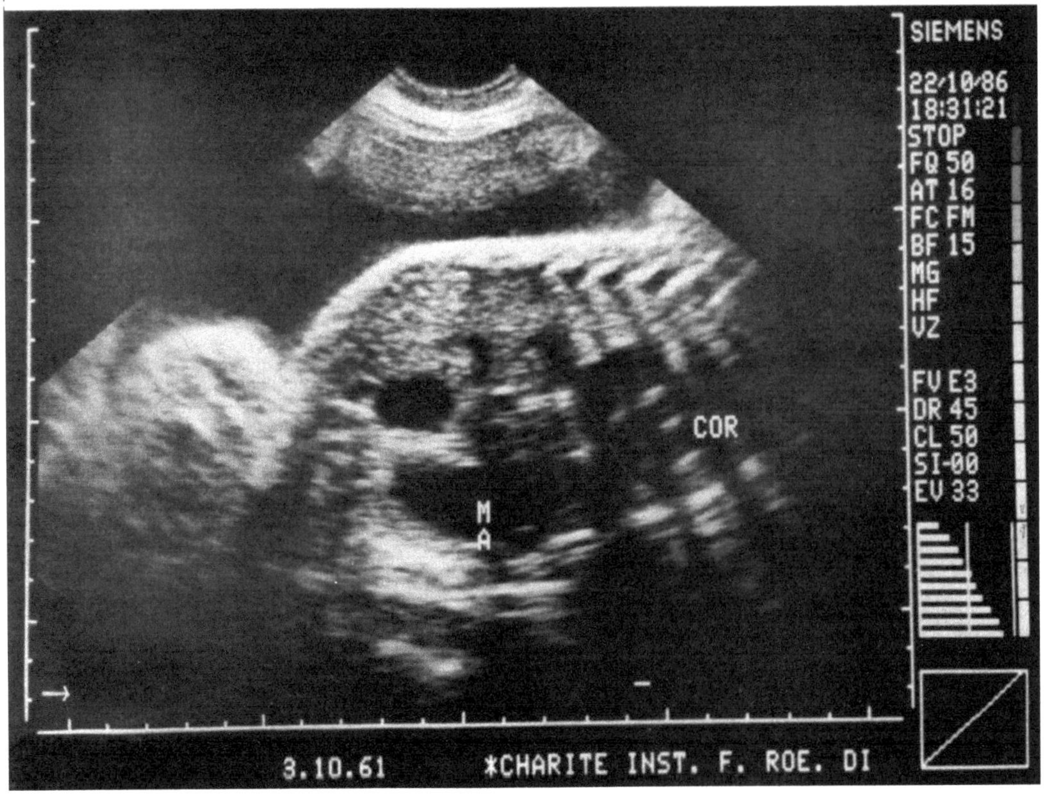

**Case 29**

**Patient H.M./83,** 23 years, second gravidity, one parturition.
**Record:** One clinically intact child.
**Clinical findings:** 30th week of pregnancy; polyhydramnion.
**Ultrasonic findings:** Polyhydramnion; foetal ascites; no detectable malformation.
**Indication for AFG:** Search for malformations.
**AFG findings:** (Fig. 52a: foetogram 21.5 hours from injection; Fig. 52b: peritoneography 18 days from injection and 30 minutes from puncture of ascites): Foetogram (Fig. 52a), shows male foetus; cephalic presentation; polyhydramnion; protrusion of abdominal region (A; arrows); somewhat retarded passage of contrast medium through gastro-intestinal tract (image of stomach, incomplete colon contrast); narrow colonic lumen (B); dilated colonic frame; dorsal and caudal displacement of gastro-intestinal tract.
Puncture of ascites for relief and infection diagnosis and

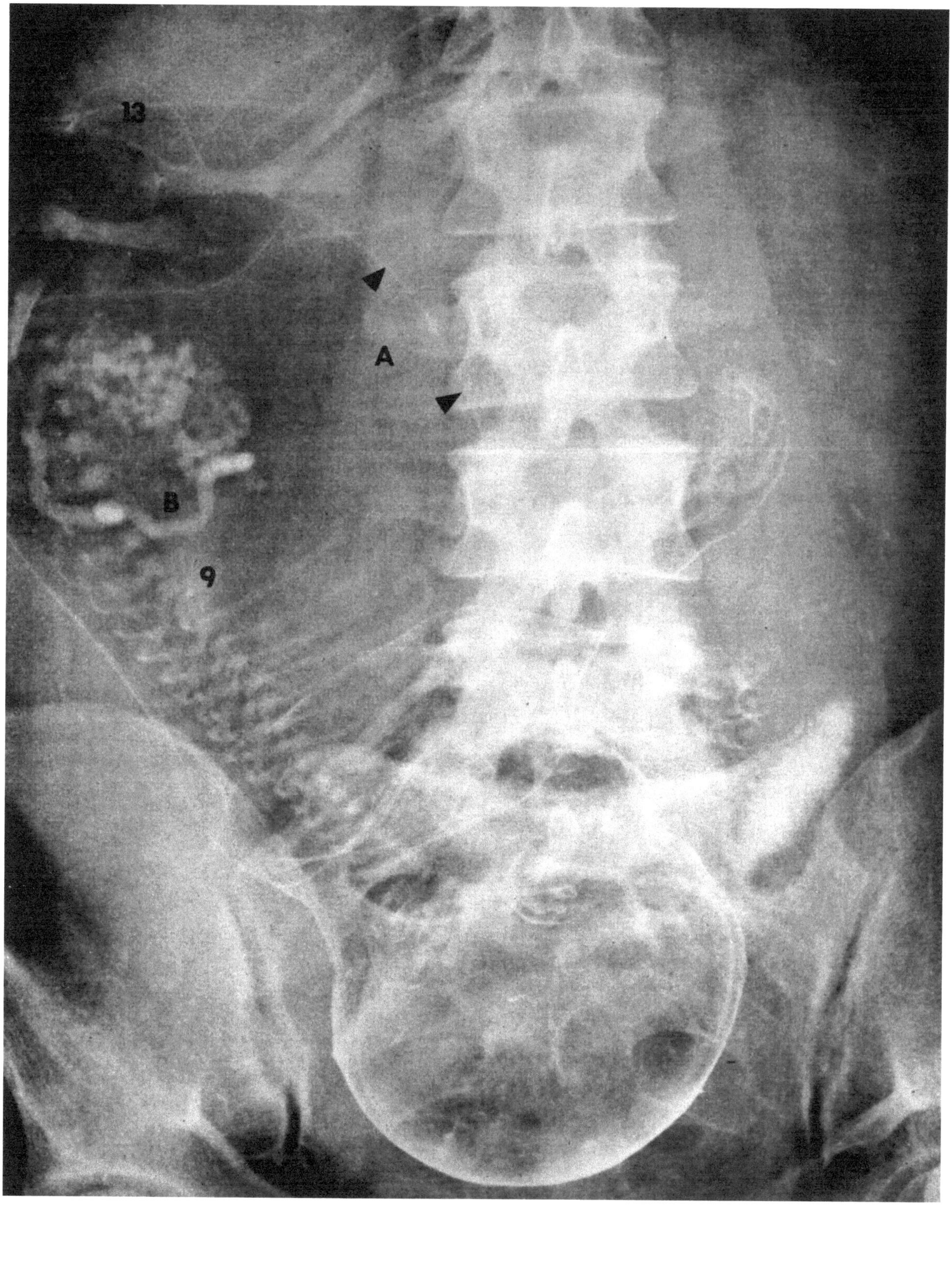


Fig. 52a

Case 29 peritoneography (Fig. 52b) for assessment of liver and spleen sizes, three weeks after AFG, because of progressing ascites; hepatosplenomegaly (C; arrows); intestinal loops visible in negative contrast; contrast medium has disappeared from intestinal lumen; signs indicative of intra-uterine discharge of meconium for foetal hypoxia.

No intra-uterine infection verified by microbiological and serological diagnosis.

**Prenatal summary diagnosis:** Polyhydramnion and foetal ascites of obscure genesis.

**Clinical course:** Spontaneous labour in 37th week of pregnancy; 3,210 g, 49 cm; postnatal ultrasonographic follow-up shows continuous regression of both ascites and hepatosplenomegaly. ◁

Fig. 52b

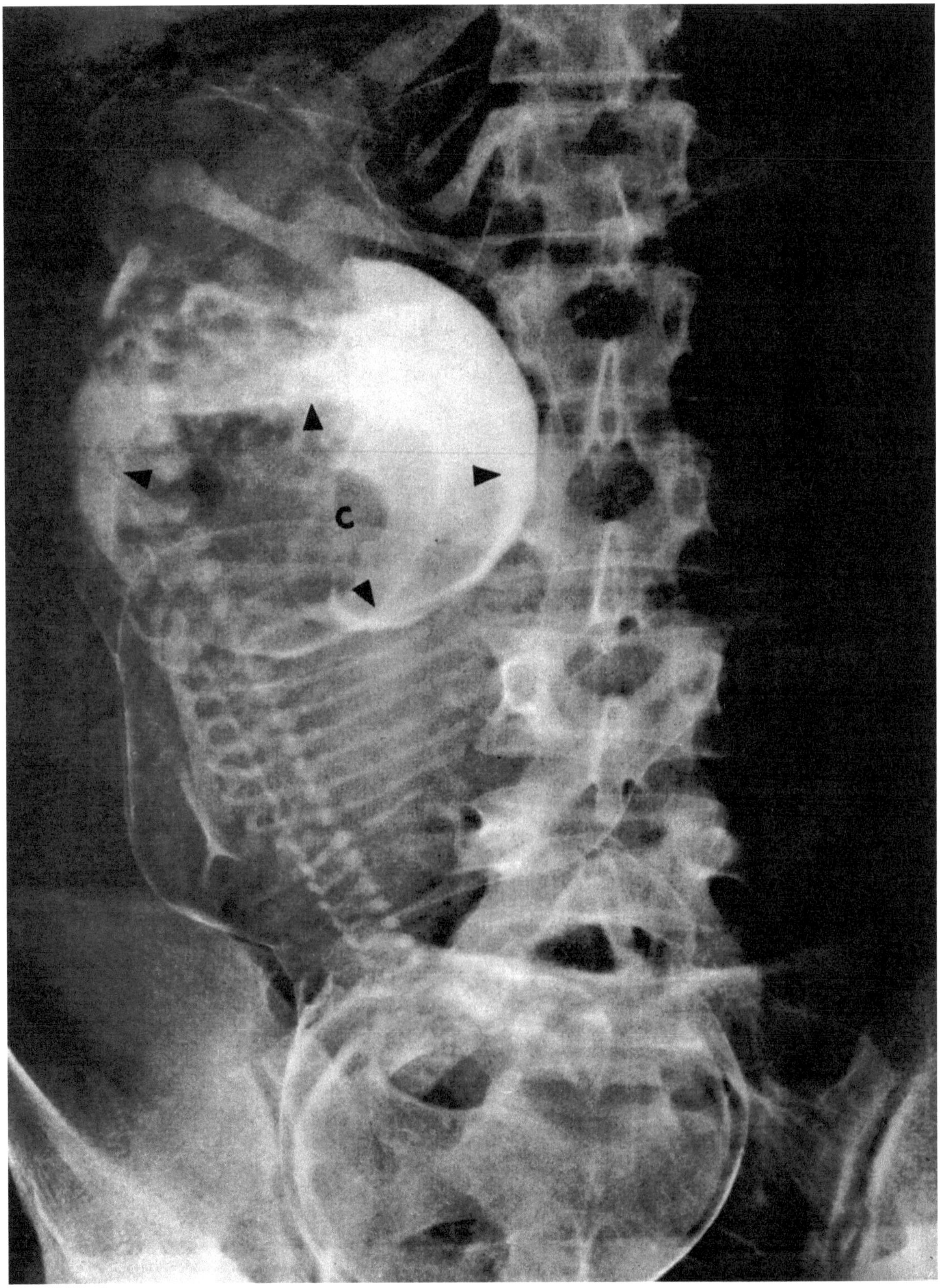

**Patient G.M./84,** 30 years, second gravidity, one parturition.
**Record:** One clinically intact child.
**Clinical findings:** 25th week of pregnancy; oligohydramnion.
**Ultrasonic findings** (Fig. 53 a, b): Oligohydramnion; kidneys and urinary bladder not detectable, but sonographic visibility was limited because of oligohydramnion.

Instillation into amniotic cavity of 80 ml glucose, 40 ml watersoluble contrast medium, and 4 ml Lipiodol UF (arrows).
**Indication for AFG:** Oligohydramnion; signs indicative of additional malformations.
**AFG findings** (Fig. 53 c: amniogram 30 minutes from injec-

**Case 30**

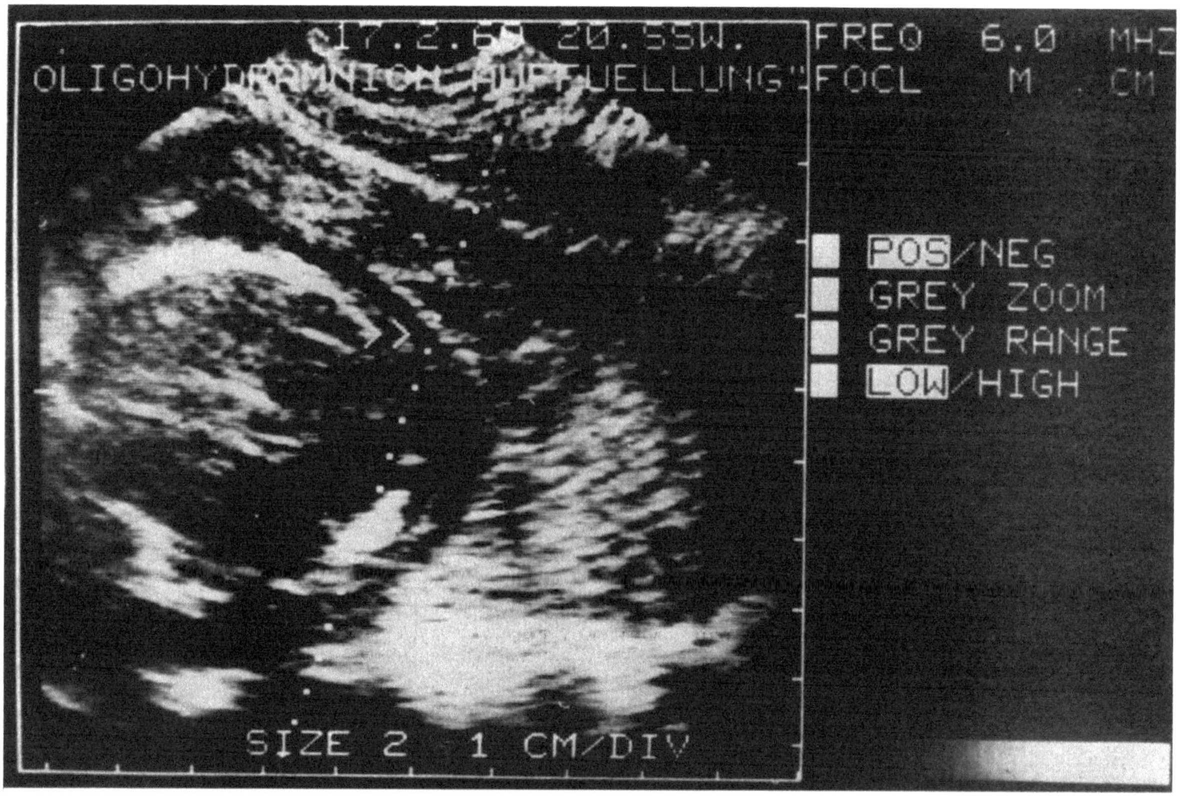


Fig. 53 a

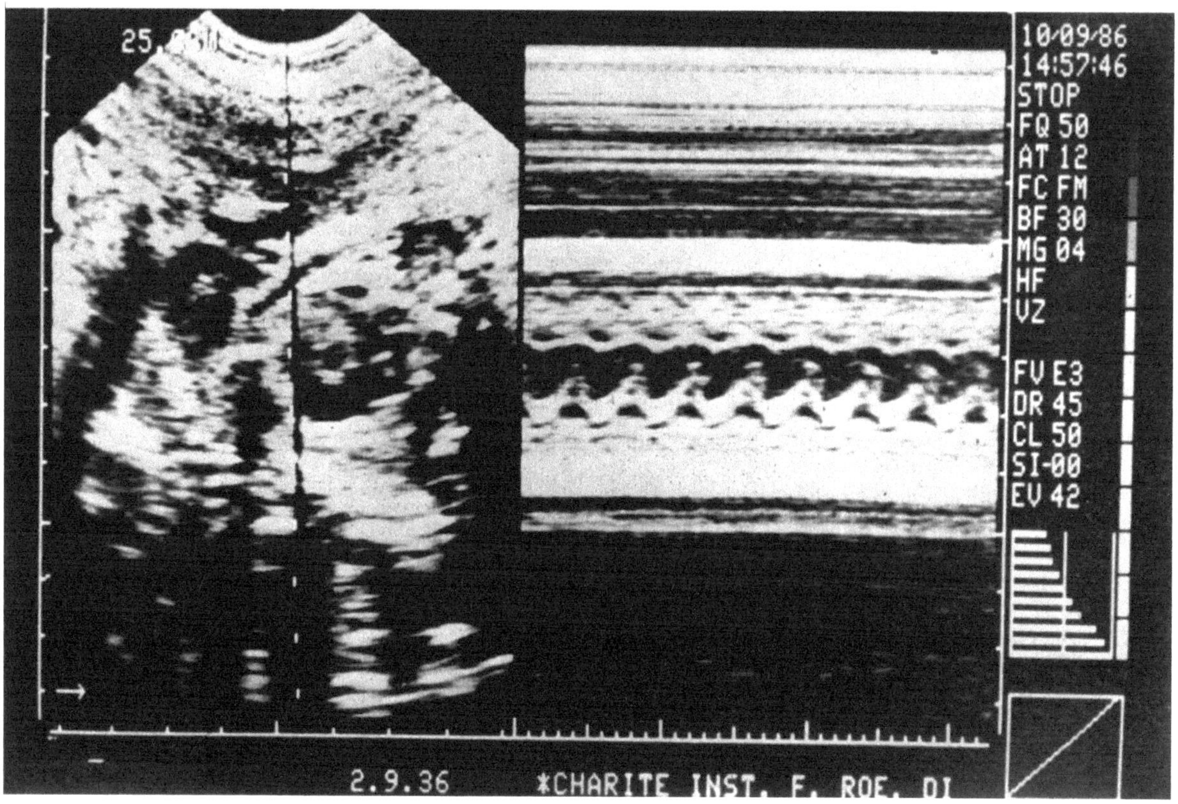


Fig. 53 b

Case 30 tion): Sex of foetus not safely determinable; breech presentation; oligohydramnion (A); time-adequate visualisation of small intestine and stomach; no detectable malformation; contrast medium recesses in left cornu of uterus due to umbilical cord; additional sideline findings from maternal excretory urogram.

**Prenatal summary diagnosis:** Suspicion of Potter syndrome.
**Clinical course.** Spontaneous labour in 37th week of pregnancy; girl, 2,250 g, 45 cm; child died immediately after birth.
**Post-mortem findings:** Bilateral renal agenesis (Potter-I syndrome). ◁

Fig. 53 c

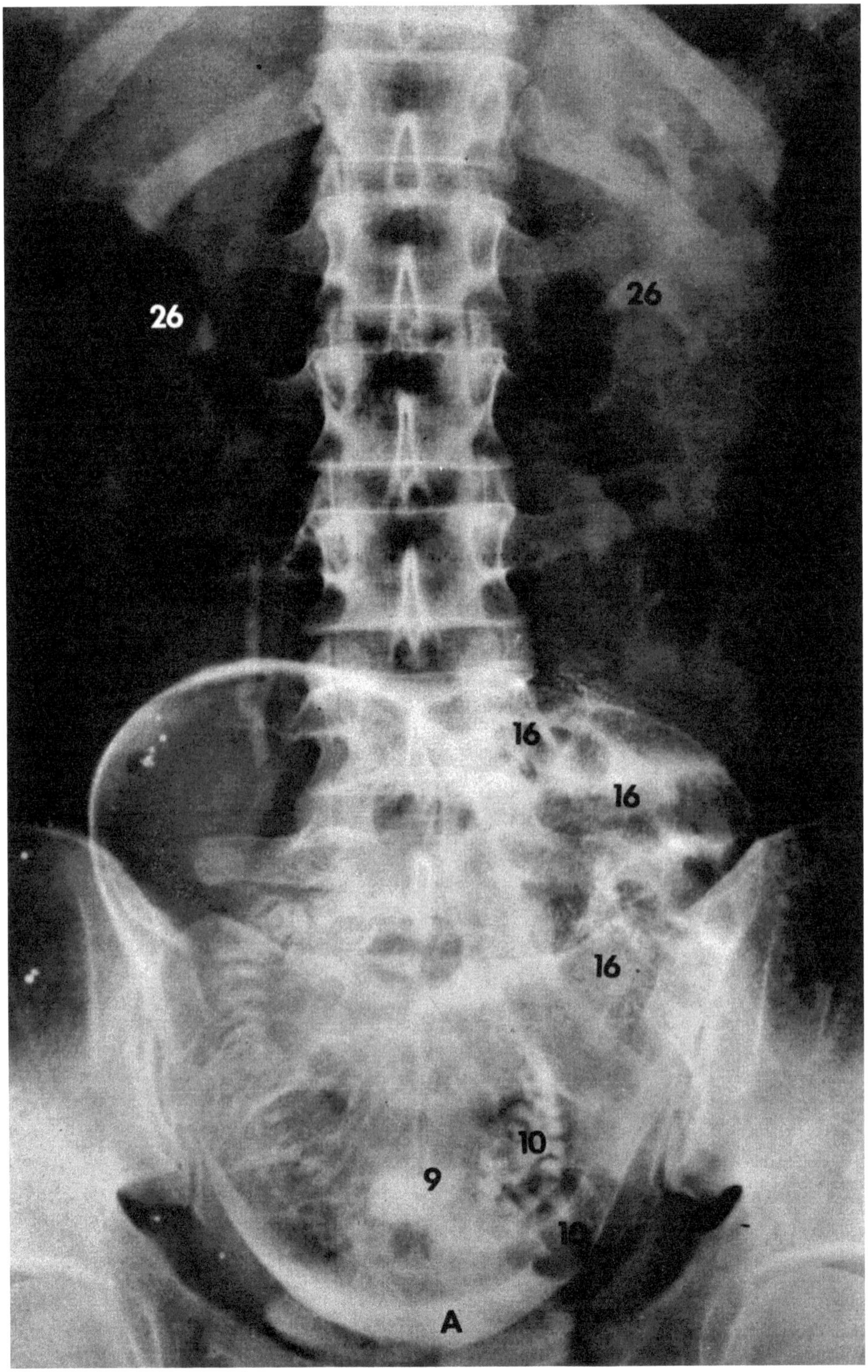

**Case 31**

**Patient A.U./84,** 22 years, second gravidity, first parturition.
**Record:** One child with Potter-2 syndrome, Type I; death one week after birth.
**Clinical findings:** 34th week of pregnancy; oligohydramnion.
**Ultrasonic findings** (Fig. 54): Oligohydramnion; large hyperechoic kidneys on both sides, 6.5 cm (arrows); renal pelvis hardly delimitable; no safe detection of urinary bladder.
**Indication for AFG:** Detection of additional malformations.
**AFG findings** (Fig. 55: foetogram 24 hours from injection): Male foetus; breech presentation; apparent microcephalus (A); short nape (B); lowered ear insertion (C); elevated

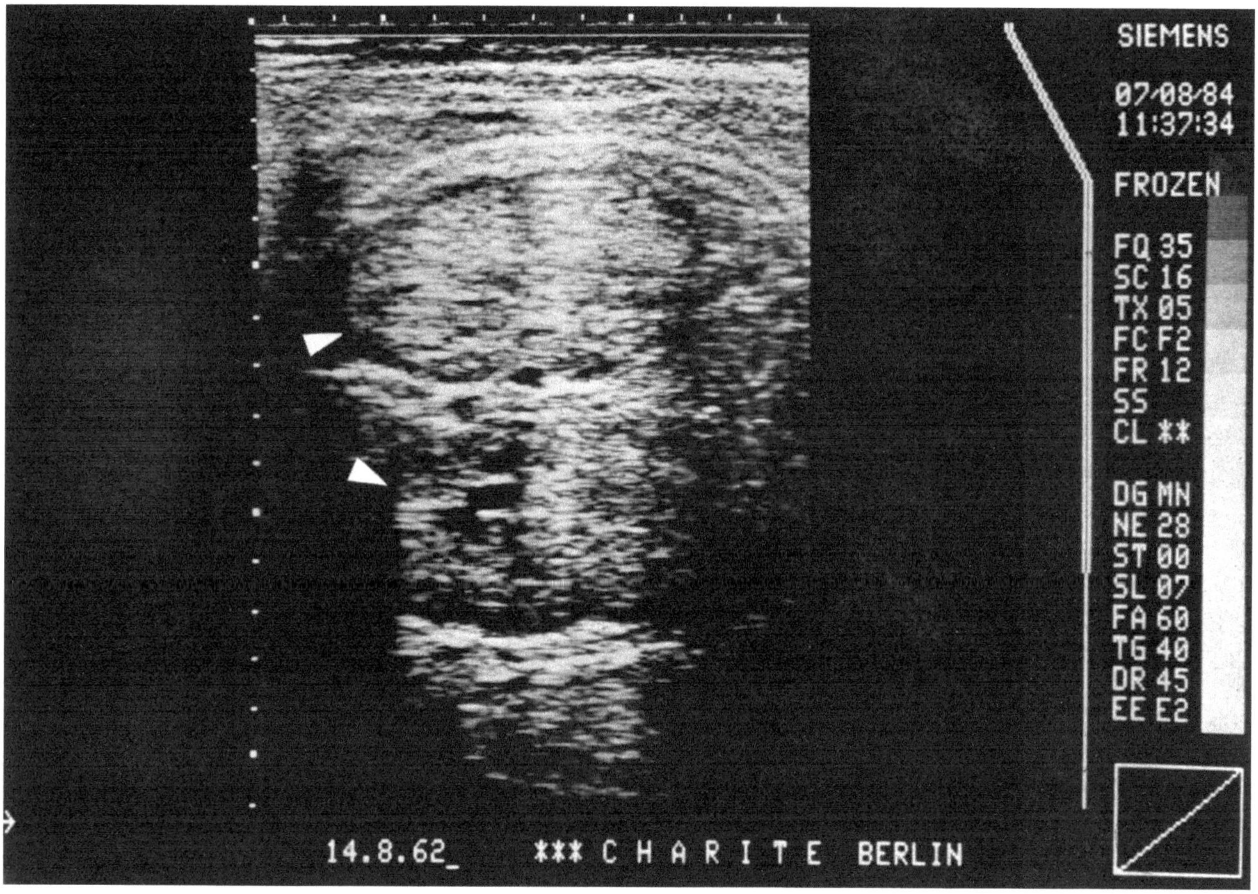


Fig. 54

Case 31 shoulders; marked protrusion of abdominal region (D; arrows); poor gastro-intestinal passage of contrast medium; constrained posture of hands and feet; no skeletal abnormality.

**Prenatal summary diagnosis:** Potter syndrome.

**Clinical course:** Spontaneous labour in 35th week of pregnancy; 3,500 g; death of newborn two hours after birth; hydrops; collateral tumours in abdominal flanks; ungainly hands; lowered ears.

**Post-mortem diagnosis:** Potter-2 syndrome, type I; hypoplastic lungs; bile duct dysplasia; moderate anasarca. ◁

Fig. 55

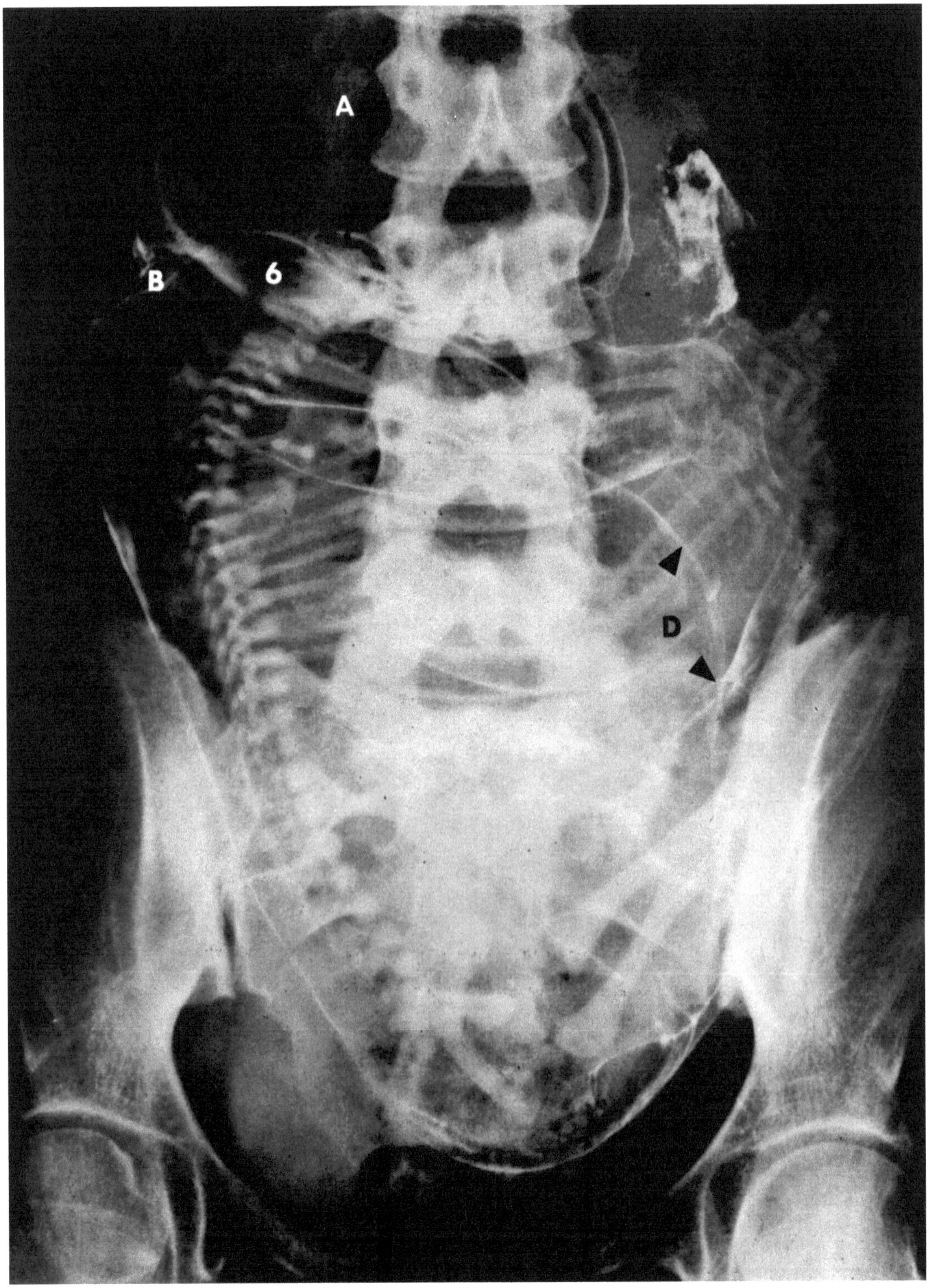

**Patient B.L./83,** 18 years, first gravidity.
**Record:** Patient's sister gave birth to child with hydrocephalus.
**Clinical findings:** 21st week of pregnancy; oligohydramnion.
**Ultrasonic findings:** Oligohydramnion; large expansive cysts in abdominal region but not clearly attributable to specific organs; puncture of cystic tumour and instillation of water-soluble contrast medium; bell-shaped deformation of thorax.
**Radiological findings:** Breech presentation; oligohydramnion; forced posture of foetus; large intra-abdominal expansive growth filled with contrast medium and with dorsal outlet; unambiguous interpretation impossible; check-up was repeated in 31st week of pregnancy to clear up ultrasonic and radiological findings.

**Case 32**

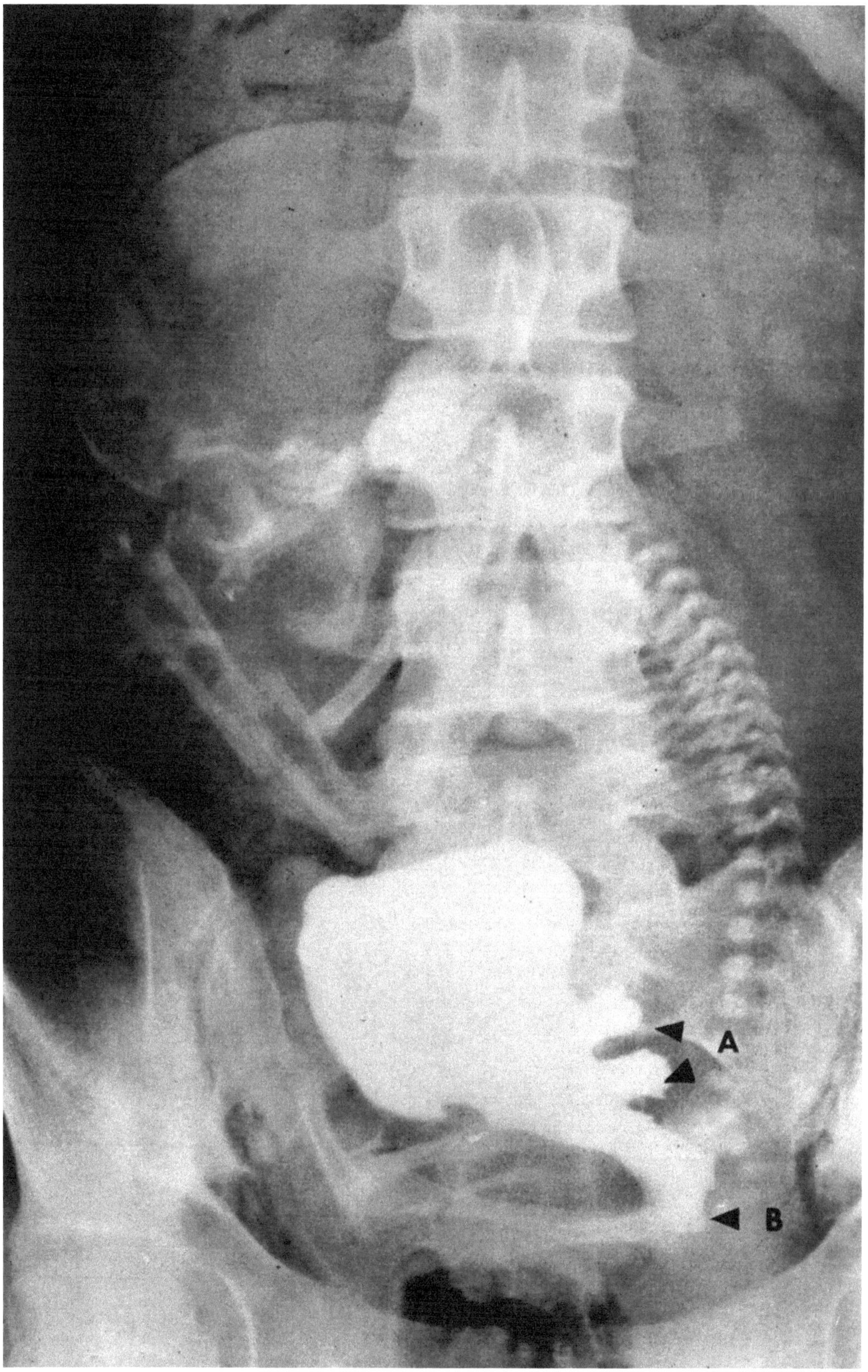


Fig. 56

Case 32 **Radiological findings** (Fig. 56): Cystic growth with three dorsal runners; two cranial processi are distal sections of ureter (A; arrows); broader caudal processus represents enlarged urethra with distal stenosis (B; arrow).
**Prenatal summary diagnosis:** Complex malformation of urinary tract according to prune-belly syndrome.
**Clinical course:** Spontaneous labour after induction; newborn died at birth.
**Radiographic** (Fig. 57) and **post-mortem findings:** Prune-belly syndrome with multiple stenosis of hydro-ureters; bilateral macrocystic dysplasia of kidneys; distal occlusion of urethra; mesenterium ilio-colicum communis; microcephalus; lowered ears. ◁

Fig. 57

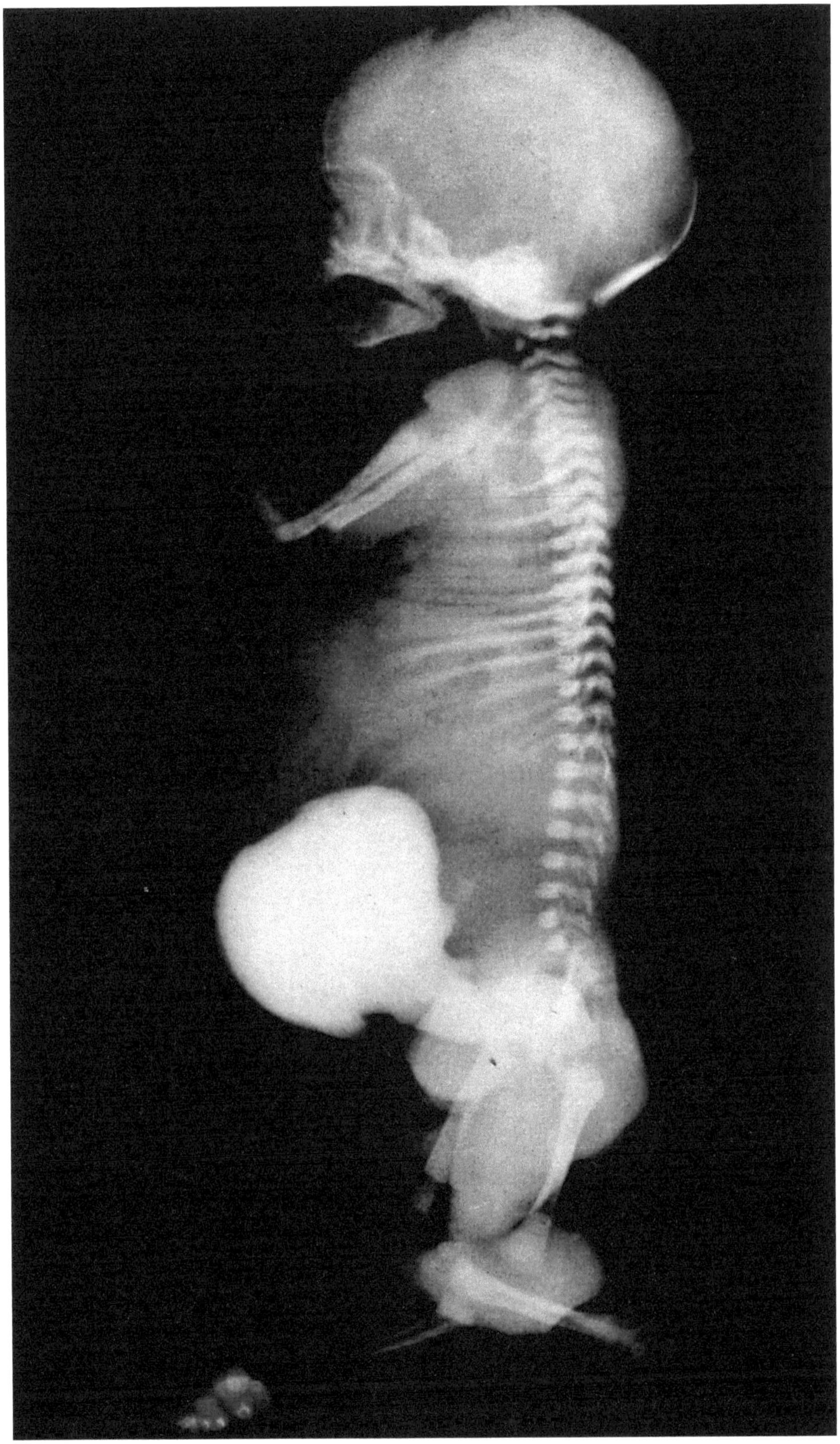

Patient E.C./84, 31 years, fifth gravidity, two parturitions. **Record:** One live born child with brain damage, died in sixth year of age; one clinically intact child; two abortions. **Clinical findings:** 33rd week of pregnancy; no contributory findings.
**Ultrasonic findings** (Fig. 58a, b): Accurate delimitation of left kidney with multiple cystic areas; right kidney not delimitable; multiple cystic structures stretching from latter zone; in differential diagnosis, due to clearly pronounced findings, no distinction between hydronephrosis and cystorenal dysplasia (R = rigth, L = left).
Amniofoetography and puncture of cystic area with instillation of water-soluble contrast medium to clear up condition.
**Indication for AFG:** Verification of ultrasonic findings; infa-

**Case 33**

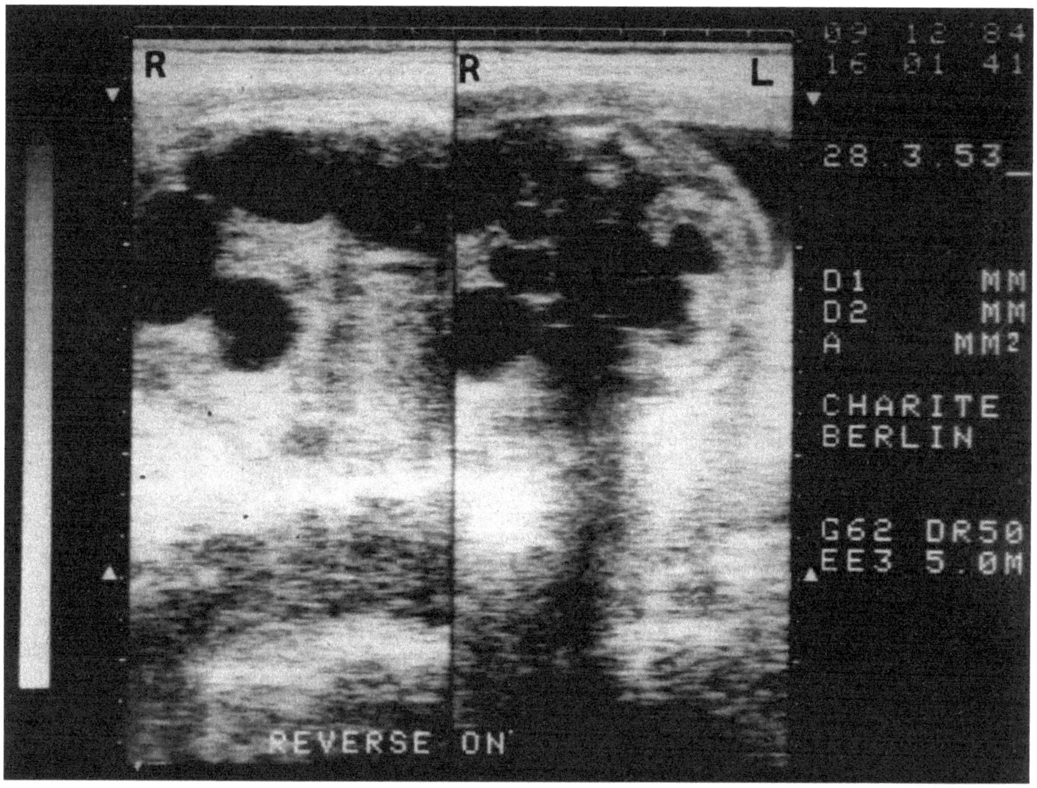


Fig. 58a

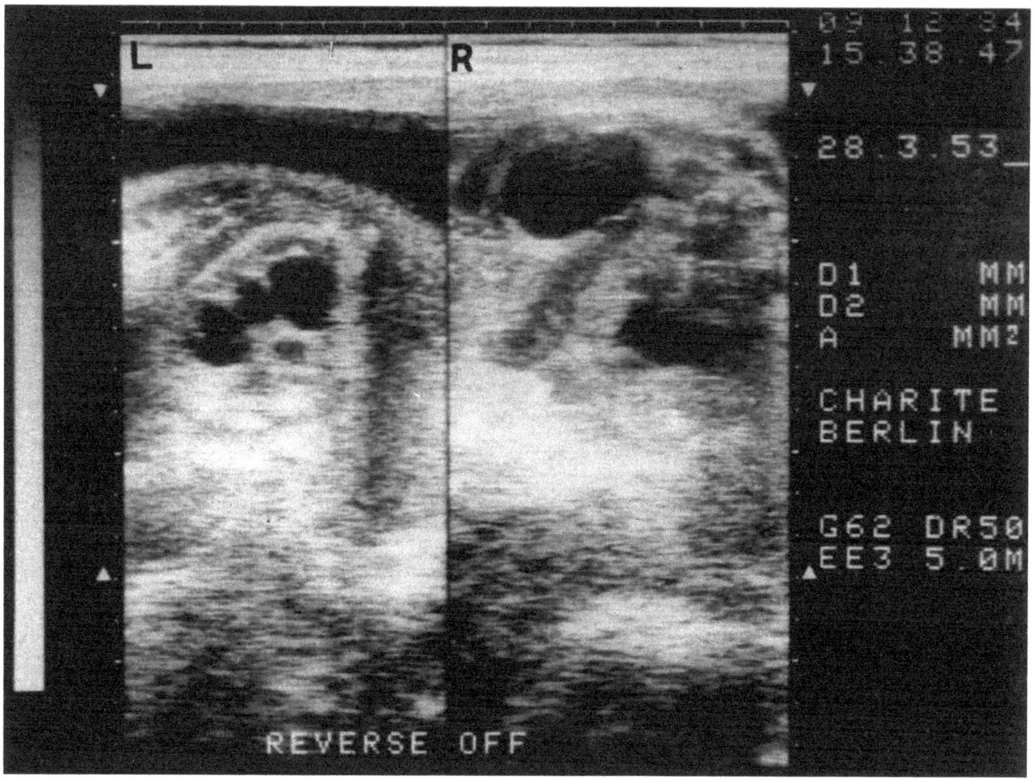


Fig. 58b

Case 33 vourable record; signs indicative of additional malformations.
**AFG findings** (Fig. 59: foetogram 24 hours from injection): Sex not safely determinable; cephalic presentation; bilateral distension of flanks, right more than left; cyst filled up with contrast medium on right side in abdominal cavity (A); no additional malformation.
**Prenatal summary diagnosis:** Large cystic dysplasia of right kidney; left-side findings continued to be hard to interpret.
**Clinical course:** Spontaneous labour in 37th week of pregnancy; male child; 3,790 g, 54 cm; postnatal urological X-ray examination failed to depict right kidney and showed moderate left-side hydronephrosis; polycystic renal dysplasia revealed by right-side nephrectomy. ◁

Fig. 59

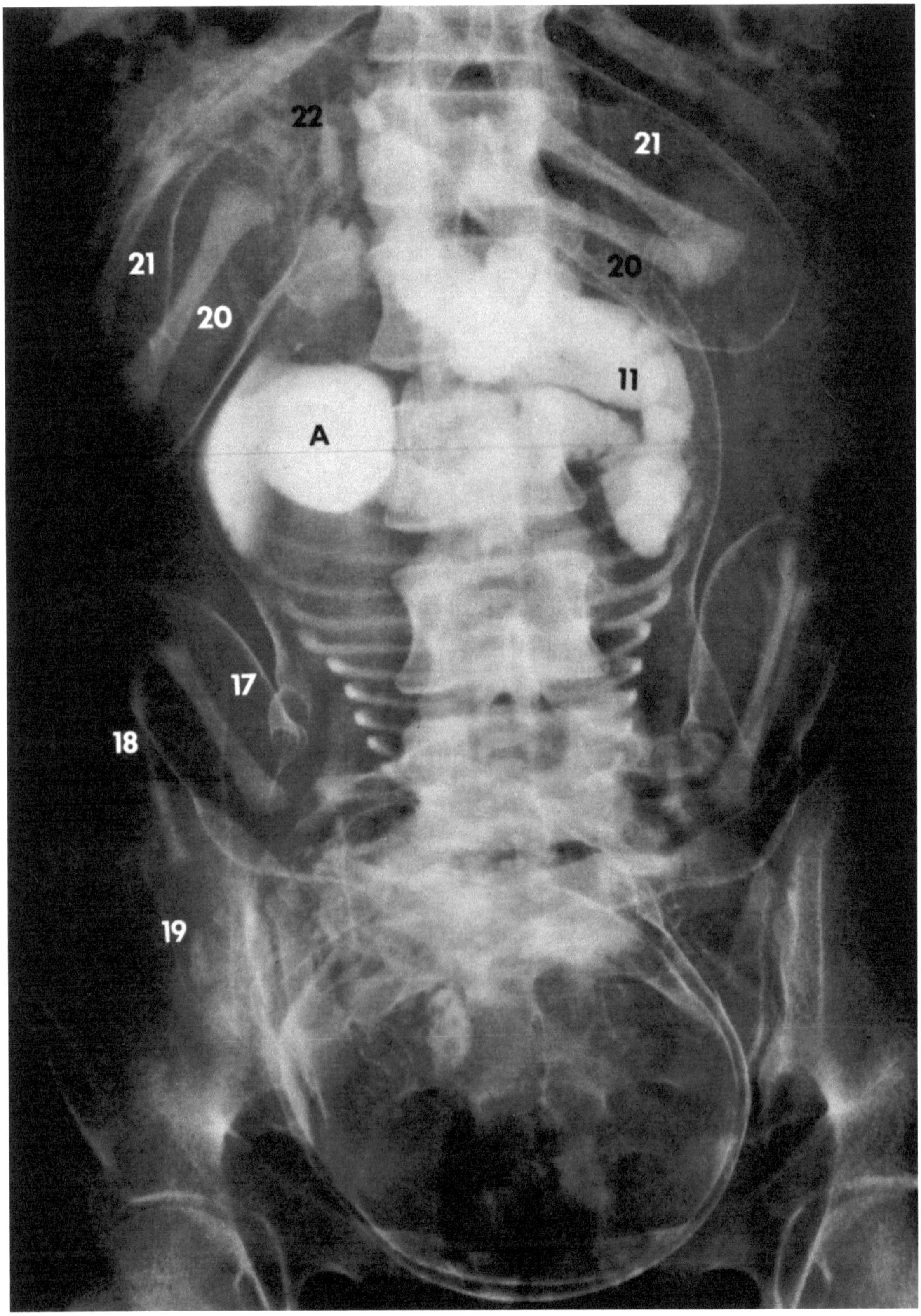

**Patient K.K./85,** 20 years, first gravidity.
**Clinical findings:** 30th week of pregnancy; no contributory findings.
**Ultrasonic findings** (Fig. 60): Bilateral urinary stasis (REN); multiply convoluted hydro-ureters (UR); urinary bladder visible; no signs of additional malformations.
**Indication for AFG:** Search for additional malformations.
**AFG findings** (Fig. 61: foetogram 23 hours from injection): Female foetus; cephalic presentation; slight protrusion of abdominal region (A; arrows); time-adequate gastro-intesti-

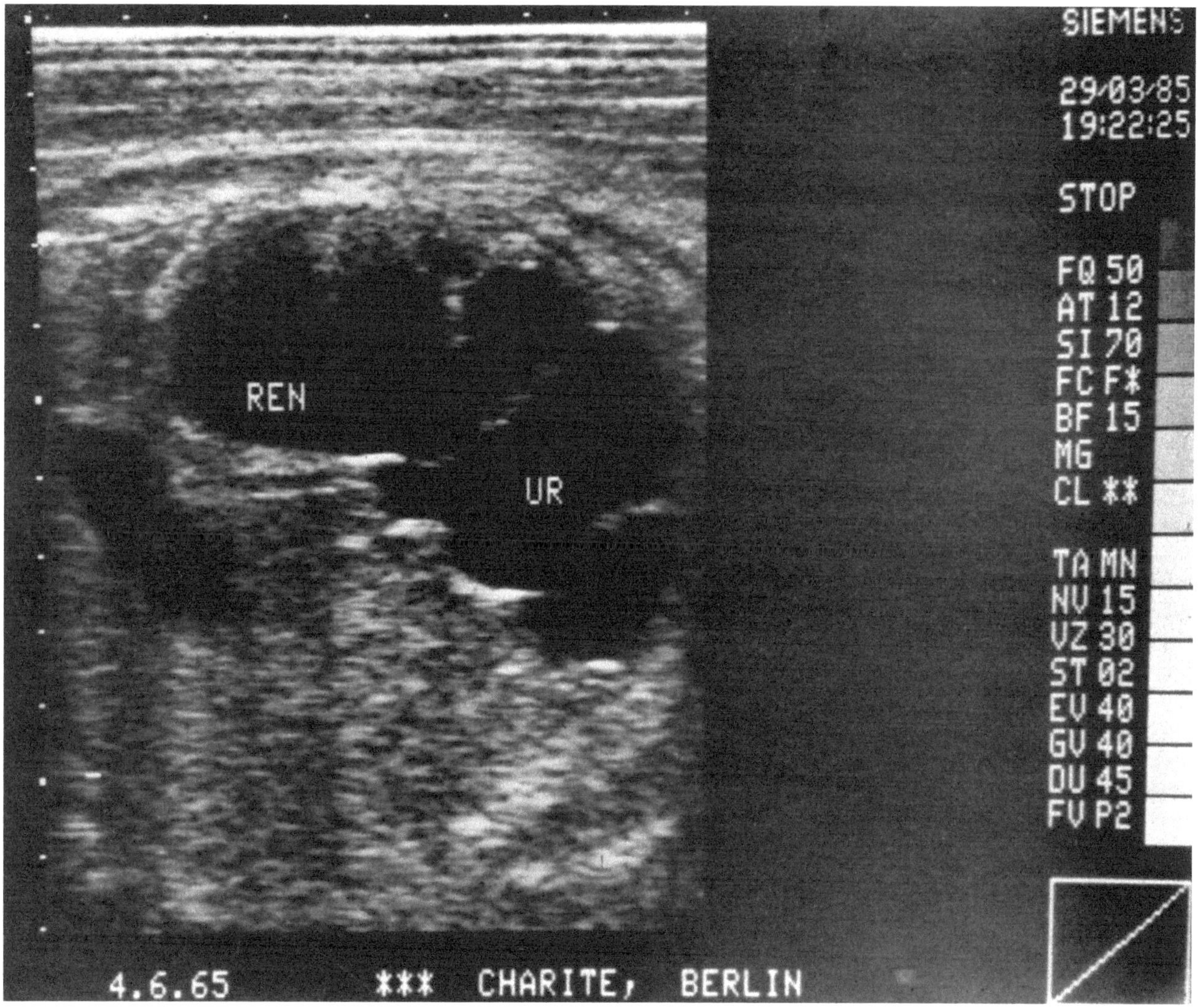


Fig. 60

Case 34 nal passage of contrast medium; ventral displacement of ascending or descending colon (B; arrows); no detectable malformation; maternal ureter in contrast at L 1/2 level.
**Prenatal summary diagnosis.** Clearly pronounced bilateral hydronephrosis and hydro-ureters.

**Clinical course.** No progression of bilateral hydronephrosis detected by weekly ultrasonographic checks; hence, premature induction of labour only in 37th week of pregnancy; 3,250 g, 52 cm; prenatal findings confirmed by postnatal diagnosis and surgery. ◁

Fig. 61

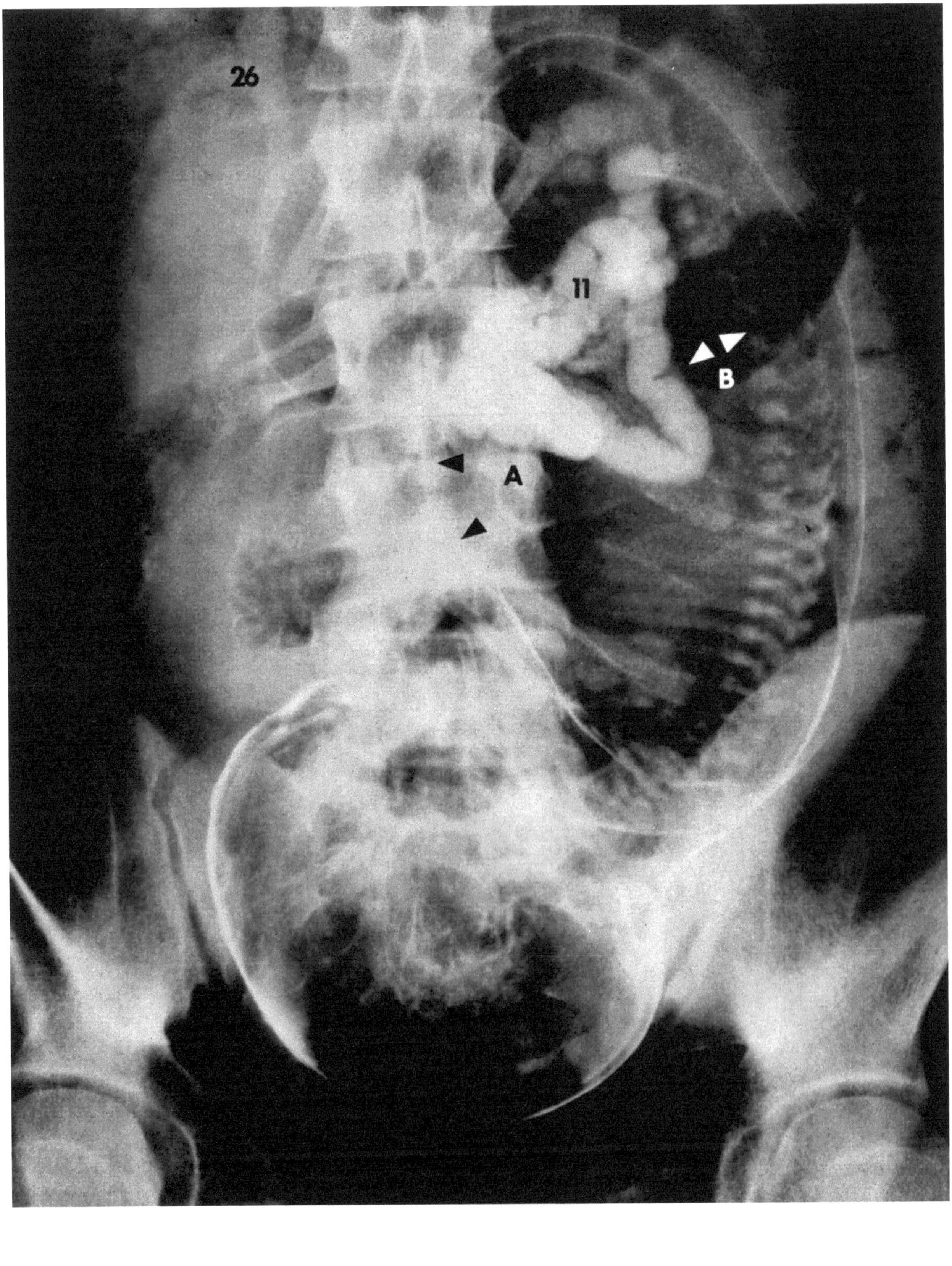

Case 35

**Patient M.C./85,** 23 years, second gravidity, one parturition.
**Record.** One clinically intact child.
**Clinical findings.** 34th week of pregnancy; no contributory findings.
**Ultrasonic findings** (Fig. 62a, b): Bilateral enlargement of renal cavity system with hydro-ureters; lumen growing in caudal direction; hyperperistalsis; large cystic areas in left part of abdominal region; suspicion of expanded colon; (Fig. 62b: LE  liver, kidney).
**Indication for AFG.** To clear up ultrasonic findings; search for additional malformations.
**AFG findings** (Fig. 63: foetogram 24 hours from injection):

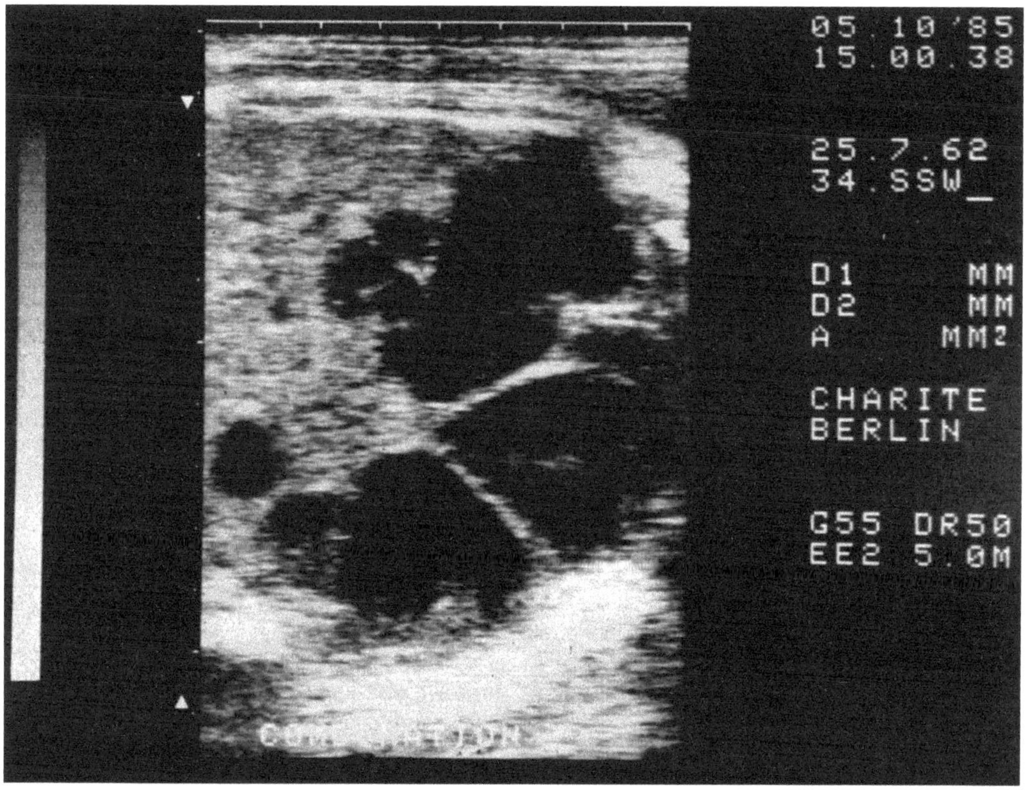


Fig. 62a

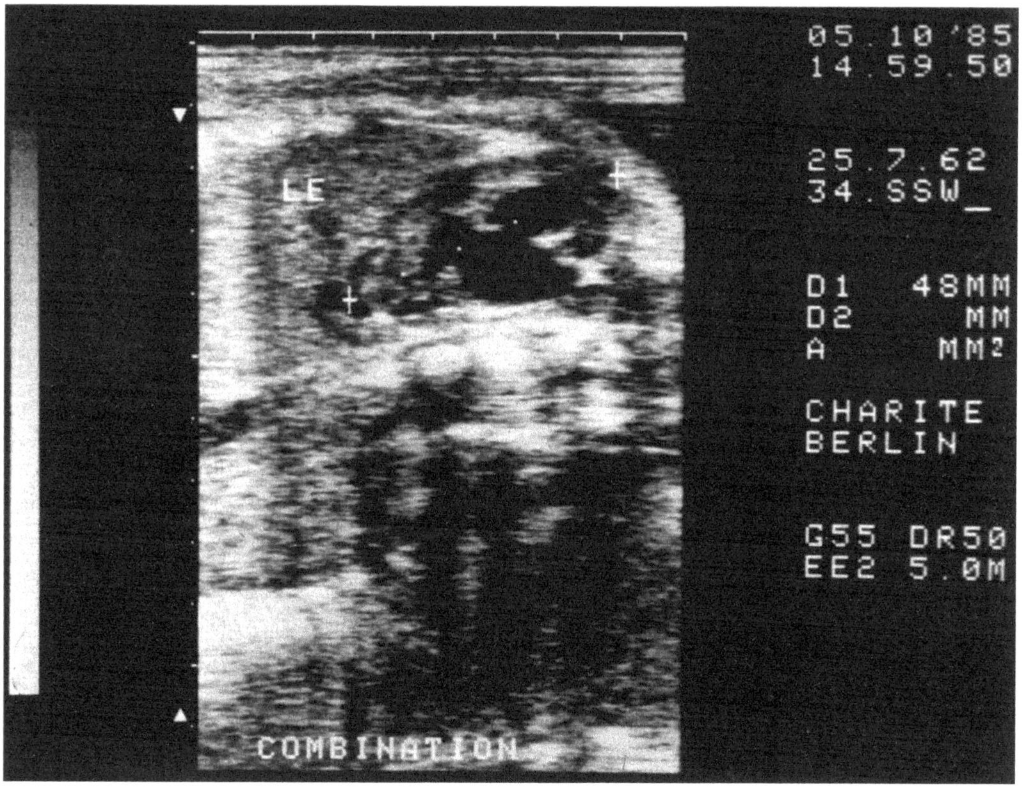


Fig. 62b

Case 35 Male foetus; cephalic presentation; protrusion of abdominal region (A; arrows); time-adequate gastro-intestinal passage of contrast medium up to rectal ampulla; no expanded colonic sections detectable; dorsal-to-cranial pressure effect of upper sigmoid (B; arrow); no malformation.

**Prenatal summary diagnosis.** Bilateral hydronephrosis and bilateral hydro-ureters causing sigmoid pressure effect.

**Clinical course.** Spontaneous labour after premature induction in 38th week; 3,500 g, 51 cm; hydronephrosis and hydro-ureters with subvesical obstruction (urethral valve) confirmed by postnatal diagnosis and surgery; bilateral Sober plasty. ◁

Fig. 63

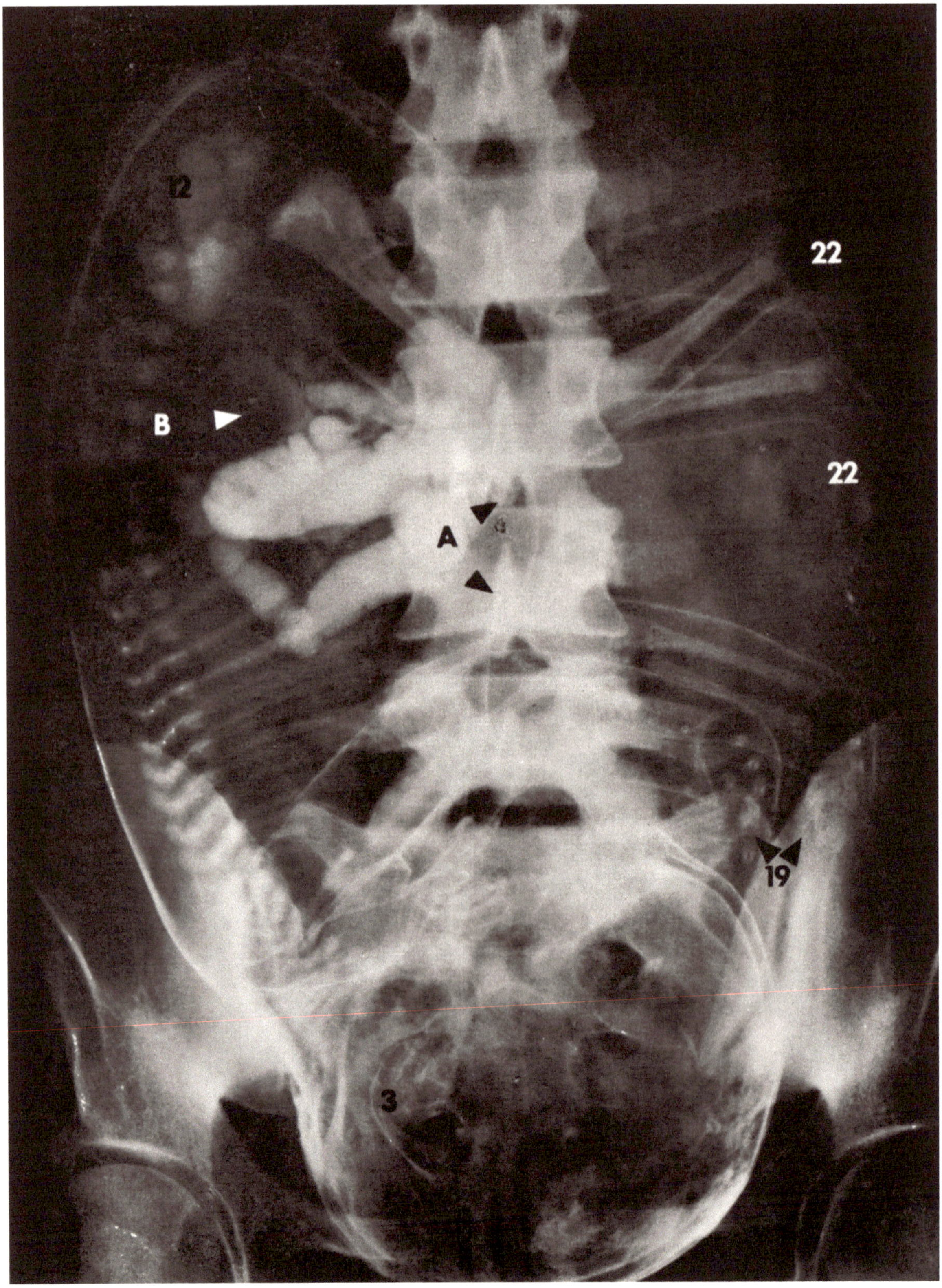

Case 36

**Patient K.K./85,** 23 years, first gravidity.
**Clinical findings.** 35th week of pregnancy; no contributory findings.
**Ultrasonic findings** (Fig. 64): Left-side hydronephrosis; ureter not detectable; transitory enlargement of cavity system of right kidney; strong motility detectable of renal pelvis and ureter; presence of urinary bladder; (Fig. 64: LI = left; RE = right; WS = vertebral column).
**Indication for AFG.** Search for additional malformations.
**AFG findings** (Fig. 65: foetogram 20 hours from injection): Female foetus; cephalic presentation; protrusion of abdominal region (A; arrow); time-adequate gastro-intestinal

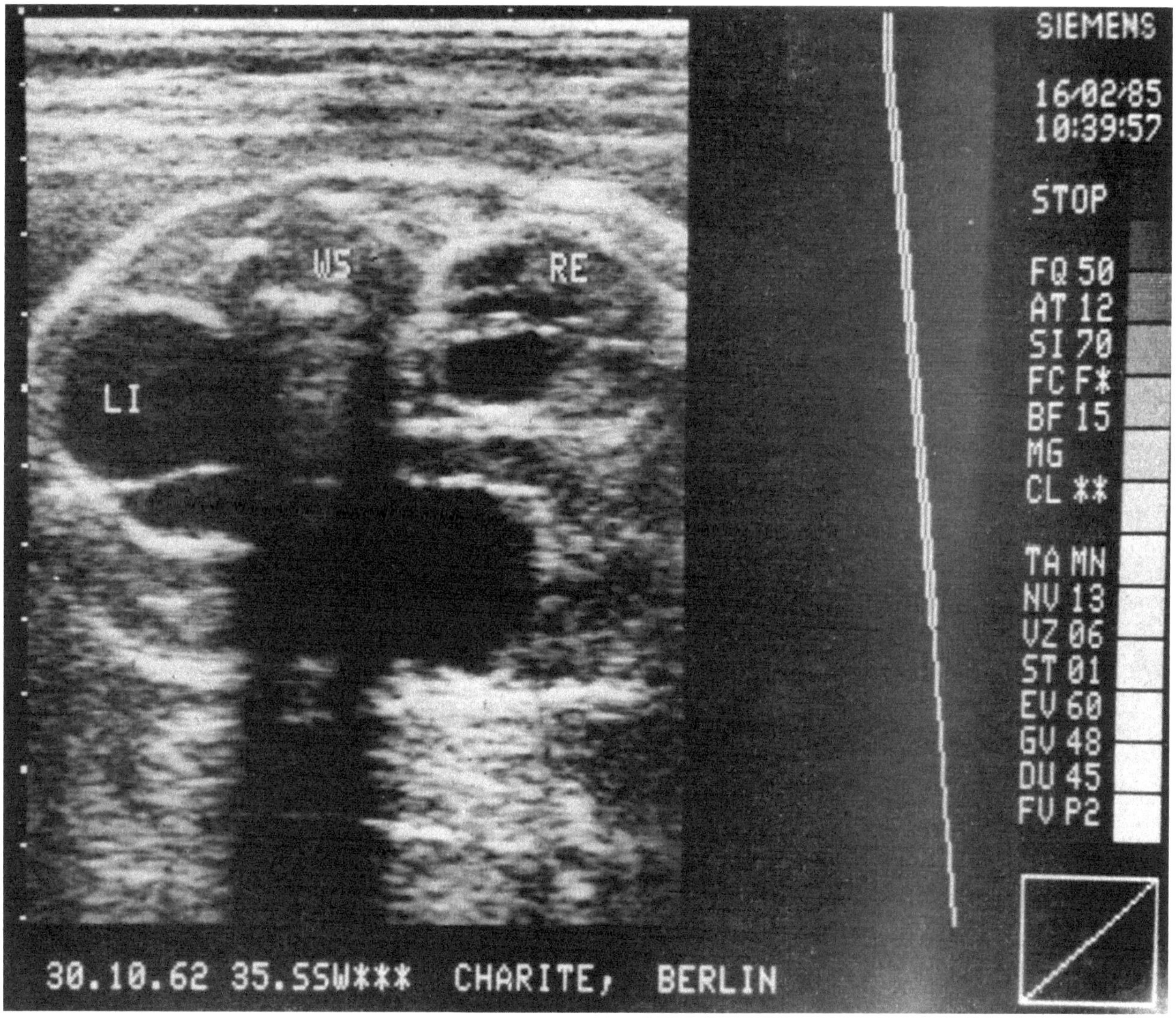


Fig. 64

Case 36 passage of contrast medium (11); suspicion of dolichocolon with caudal displacement of transverse colon (B; arrow); no detectable malformation.

**Prenatal summary diagnosis.** Clearly pronounced hydronephrosis due to stenosis of left-side ureter drainage; dubious hydronephrosis on right side; differential diagnosis: vesico-ureteral reflux.

**Clinical course.** Spontaneous labour in 39th week of pregnancy; 3,230 g, 50 cm; postnatal diagnosis and surgery revealed bilateral dual development of kidneys, one inactive kidney on the left along with ureteral stenosis and moderate right-side hydronephrosis of caudal primordium; no vesico-ureteral reflux detectable; nephrectomy on the left. ◁

Fig. 65

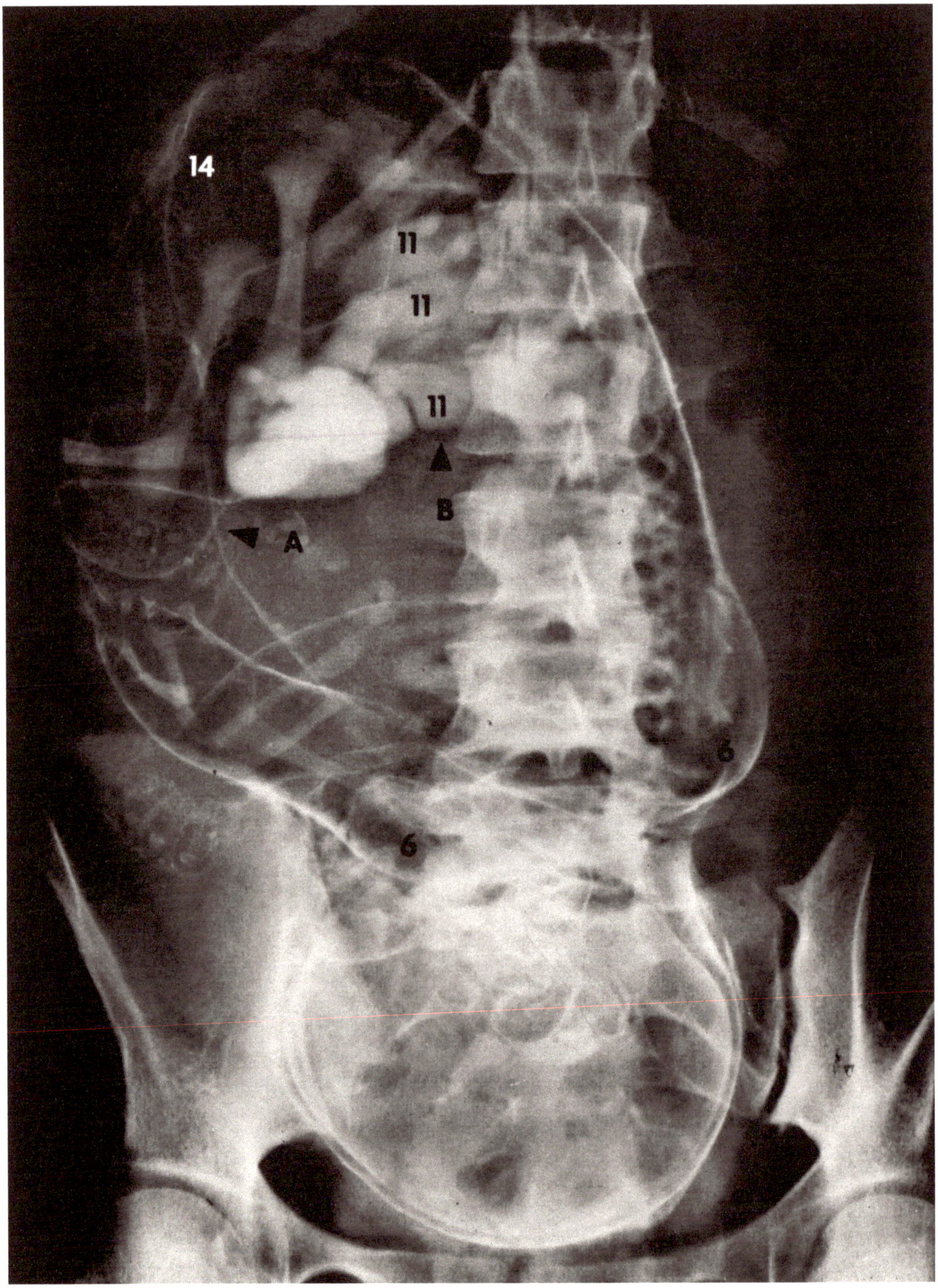

**Case 37**

**Patient R.S./86,** 22 years, first gravidity.
**Clinical findings:** 34th week of pregnancy; no contributory findings.
**Ultrasonic findings** (Fig. 66): Multicystic areas, 7 cm in diameter, in either renal bed; both kidneys delimitable; parenchymal configurations of conspicuous inhomogeneity; systems of renal pelvis moderately enlarged; bilateral enlargement of ureters and convolution traceable to urinary bladder; no enlargement of urinary bladder; normal rhythm of bladder filling and voiding established by repetitive tests; moderate perihepatic ascites; bilateral elevation of diaphragm; cardiac arrhythmia. (Fig. 66: VC = vertebral column).
**Indication for AFG:** Cystic area punctured on the right, since sonographic findings were typical neither of polycystic kidneys nor of urinary stasis in isolation; purpose of puncture was collection of fluid for chemical laboratory analysis;

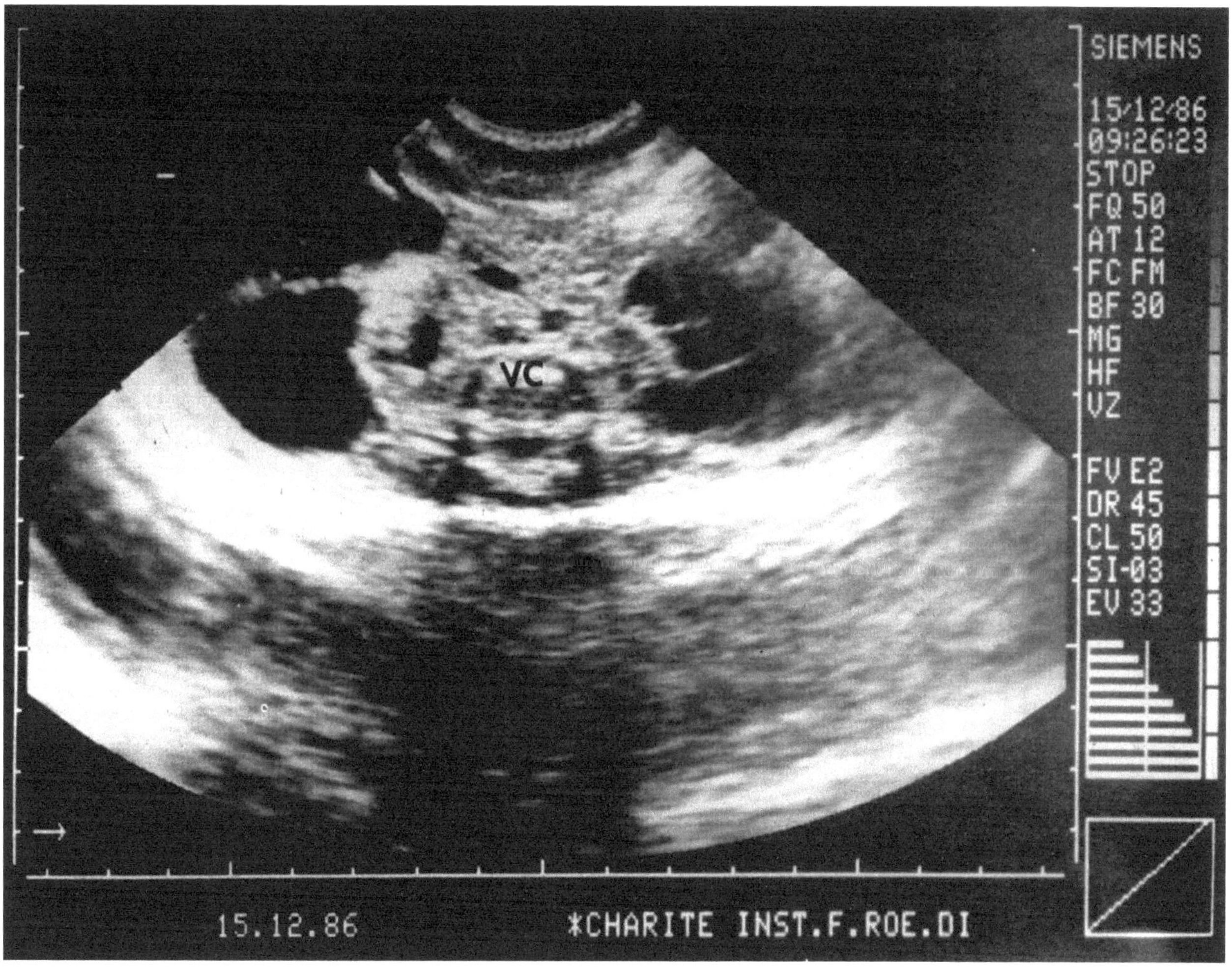


Fig. 66

Case 37 visualisation by contrast medium for additional information on genesis.

**AFG findings** (Fig. 67: foetogram 5 hours from injection): Male foetus; cephalic presentation; ventriculated cystic expansion, 5 cm, in epigastrium (A); convolution of small intestine in contrast; no additional malformation detectable.

**Chemical laboratory analysis** of punctured matter revealed foetal urine.

**Prenatal summary diagnosis:** Bilateral urinoma with hydronephrosis, depending on reflux (?).

**Clinical course:** Spontaneous labour in 36th week of pregnancy; 2,900 g, 48 cm; postnatal ultrasonographic checkup revealed continuous enlargement of urinomas; puncture of urinoma and complete drainage on eighth day of age; no recurrence; micturating cystoureterography showed urethral valve and bilateral 5 vesico-ureteral reflux with flow of contrast medium into renal parenchyma. ◁

Fig. 67

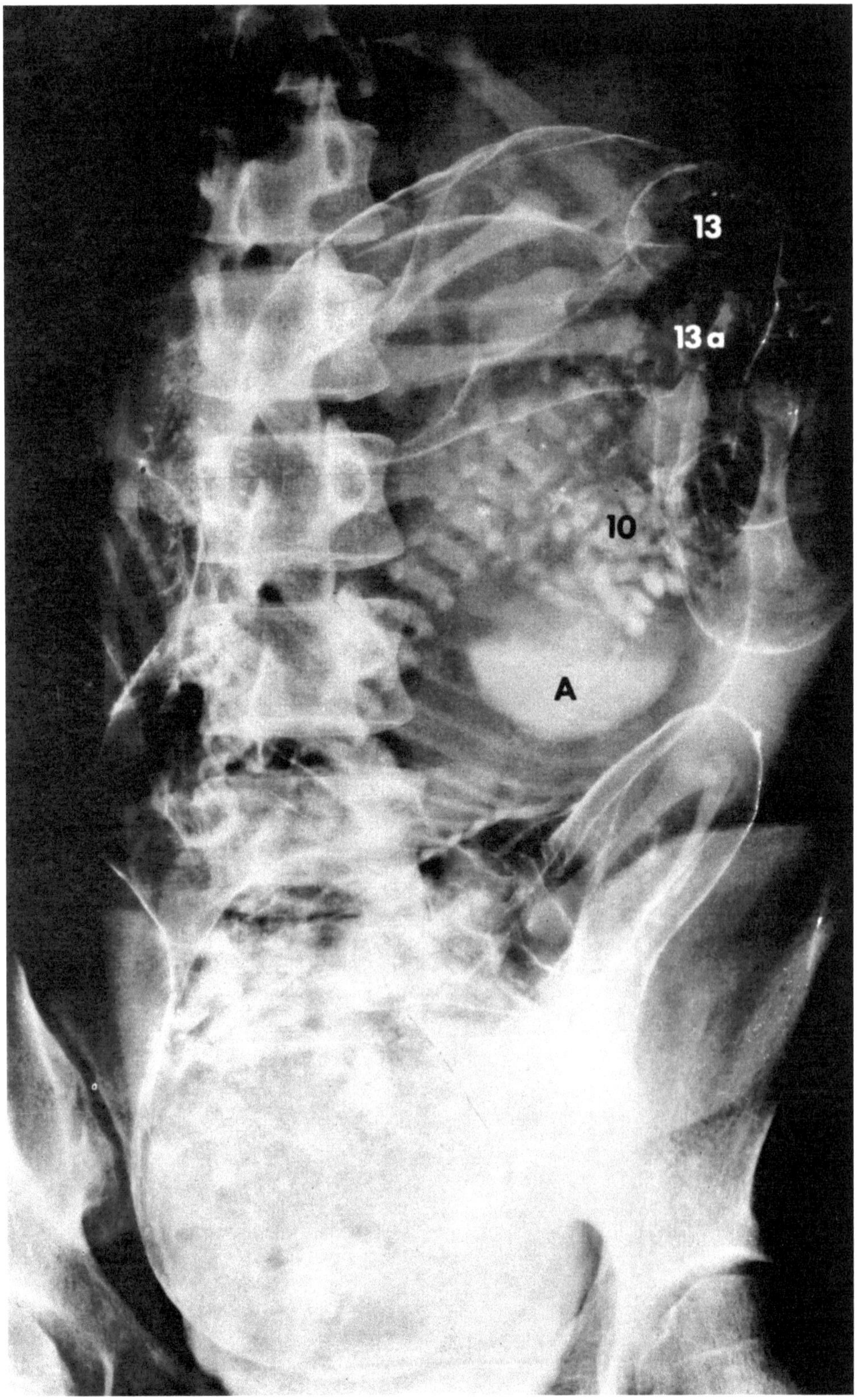

**Patient B.S./86,** 23 years, first gravidity.
**Clinical findings:** 35th week of pregnancy; no contributory findings.
**Ultrasonic findings** (Fig. 68 a): 8-cm cystic expansion in centre-right abdominal region; finely structured matter in lumen; strong reflection of wall.
**Indication for AFG:** Complementary information in addition to ultrasonic findings.
**AFG findings** (Fig. 68 b: foetogram 24 hours from injection): Female foetus; cephalic presentation; no signs indicative of

**Case 38**

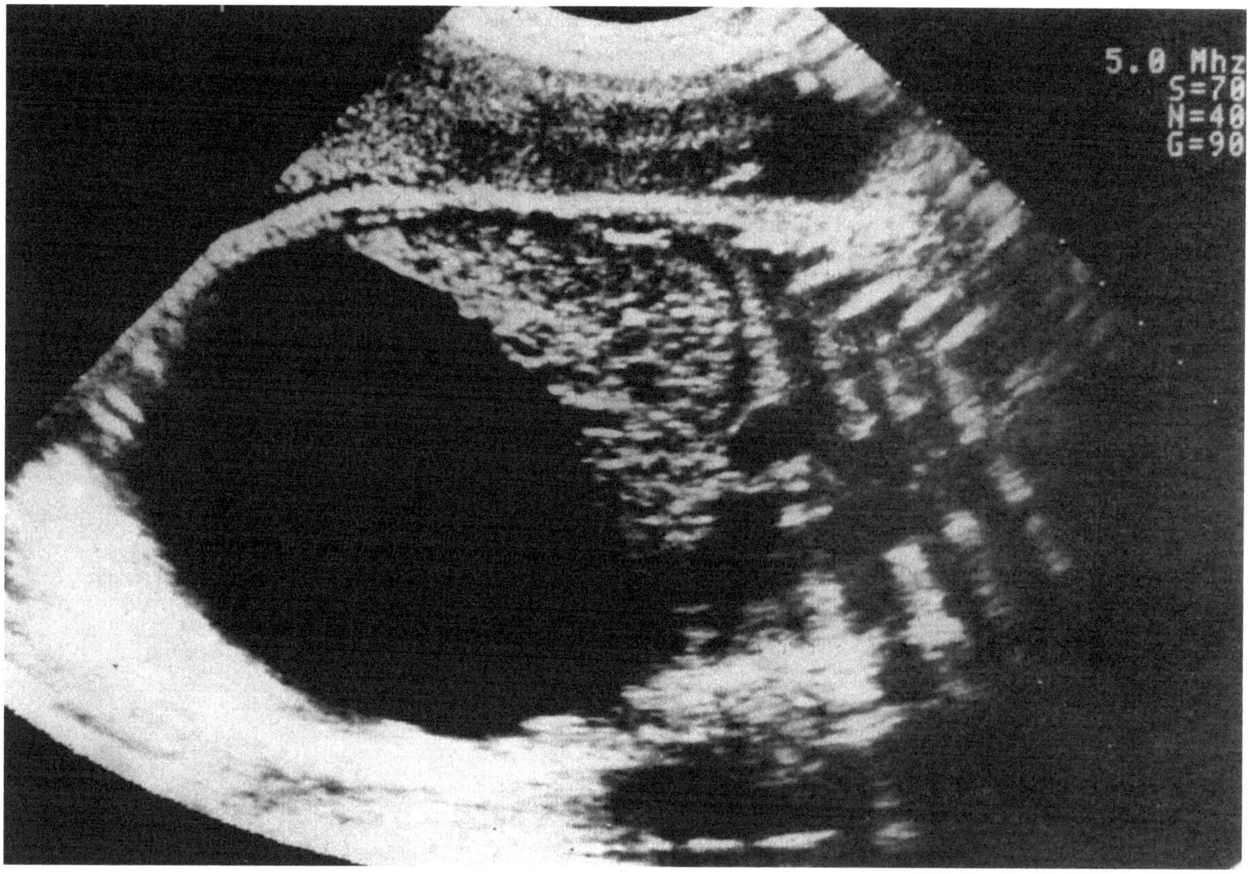


Fig. 68 a

Case 38 malformations; contrast image of intestinal tract from stomach to rectal ampulla.

**Prenatal summary diagnosis:** Cystic expansion in abdominal region not clearly attributable to specific organ; suspicion of inflammatory genesis.

**Clinical course:** Spontaneous labour in 37th week of pregnancy; unchanged postnatal ultrasonic findings; laparotomy on fifth day of age shows ovarian cyst with haemorrhagic infarction; no postoperative complications. ◁

Fig. 68 b

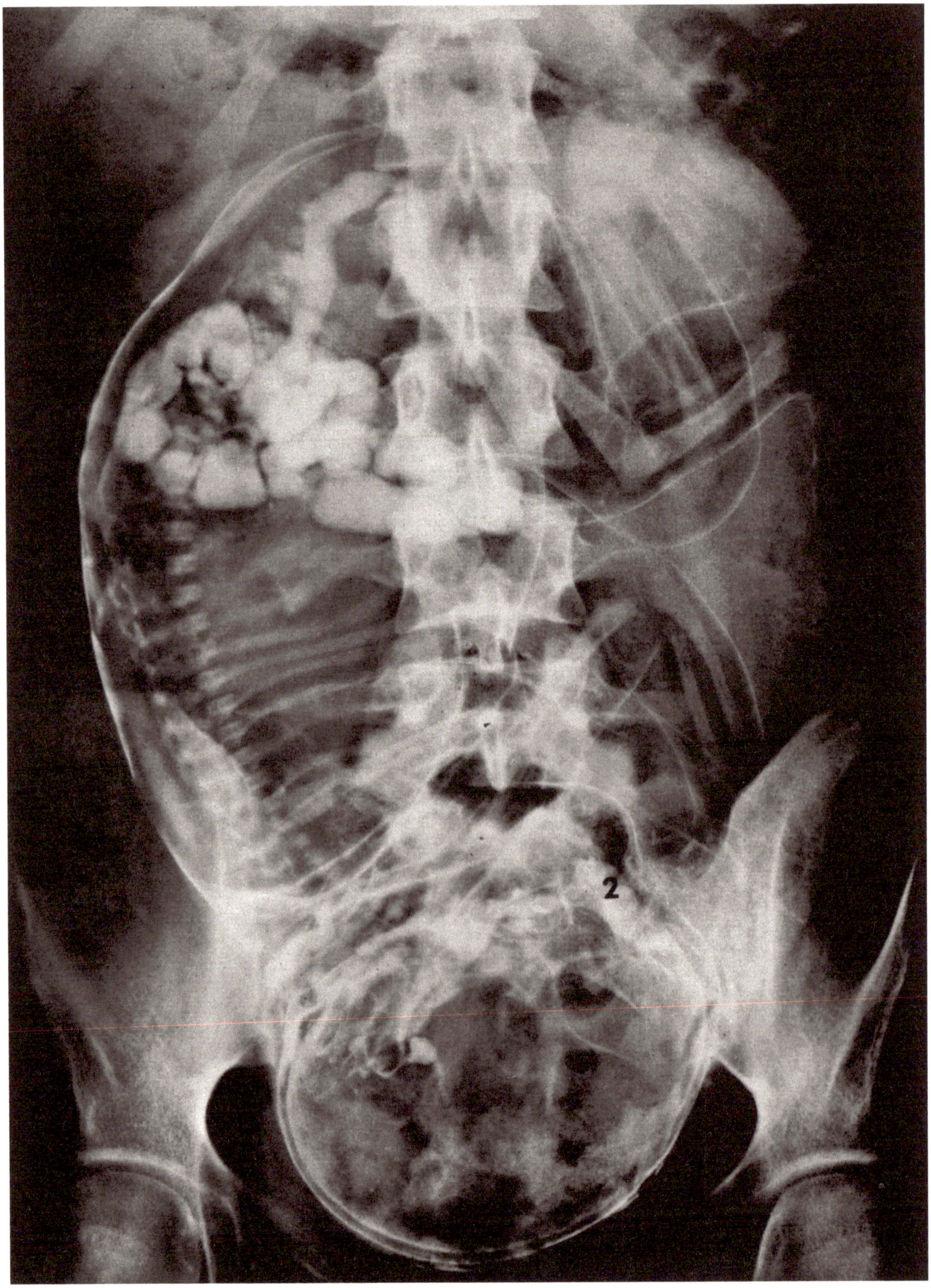

**Patient D.M./76,** 26 years, second gravidity, one parturition.
**Record:** One clinically intact child.
**Clinical findings:** 35th week of pregnancy; acute polyhydramnion.
**Ultrasonic findings:** Polyhydramnion; double contour of soft tissues of head and trunk; no detectable malformations.
**Indication for AFG:** Information indicative of malformations.
**AFG findings** (Fig. 69a: amniogram 30 minutes from injection; Fig. 69b: foetogram 16 hours from injection): Male foetus; cephalic presentation; enlargement of soft tissue of

**Case 39**

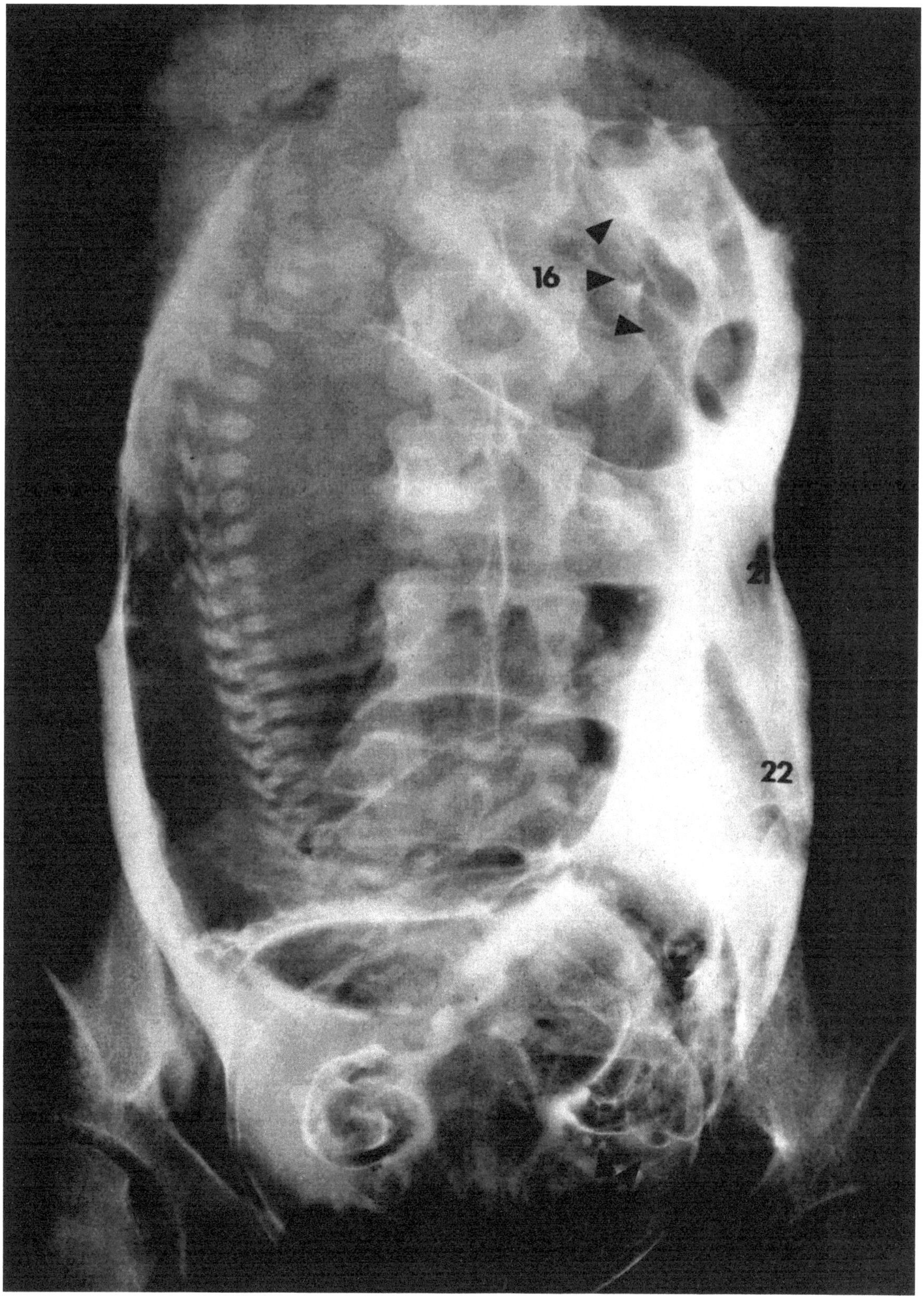


Fig. 69a

Case 39 trunk (A; arrows); protrusion of abdominal region (B; arrow); homogeneous contrast of small intestine and colon; rectal ampulla unfilled; constant foetal presentation; no detectable malformation.

**Prenatal summary diagnosis:** Hydrops fetus universalis.

**Clinical course:** Spontaneous labour after induction in 36th week of pregnancy; newborn died 20 minutes after birth.

**Post-mortem findings:** Hydrops fetus universalis; ascites; no malformation; cytomegalic infection. ◁

Fig. 69b

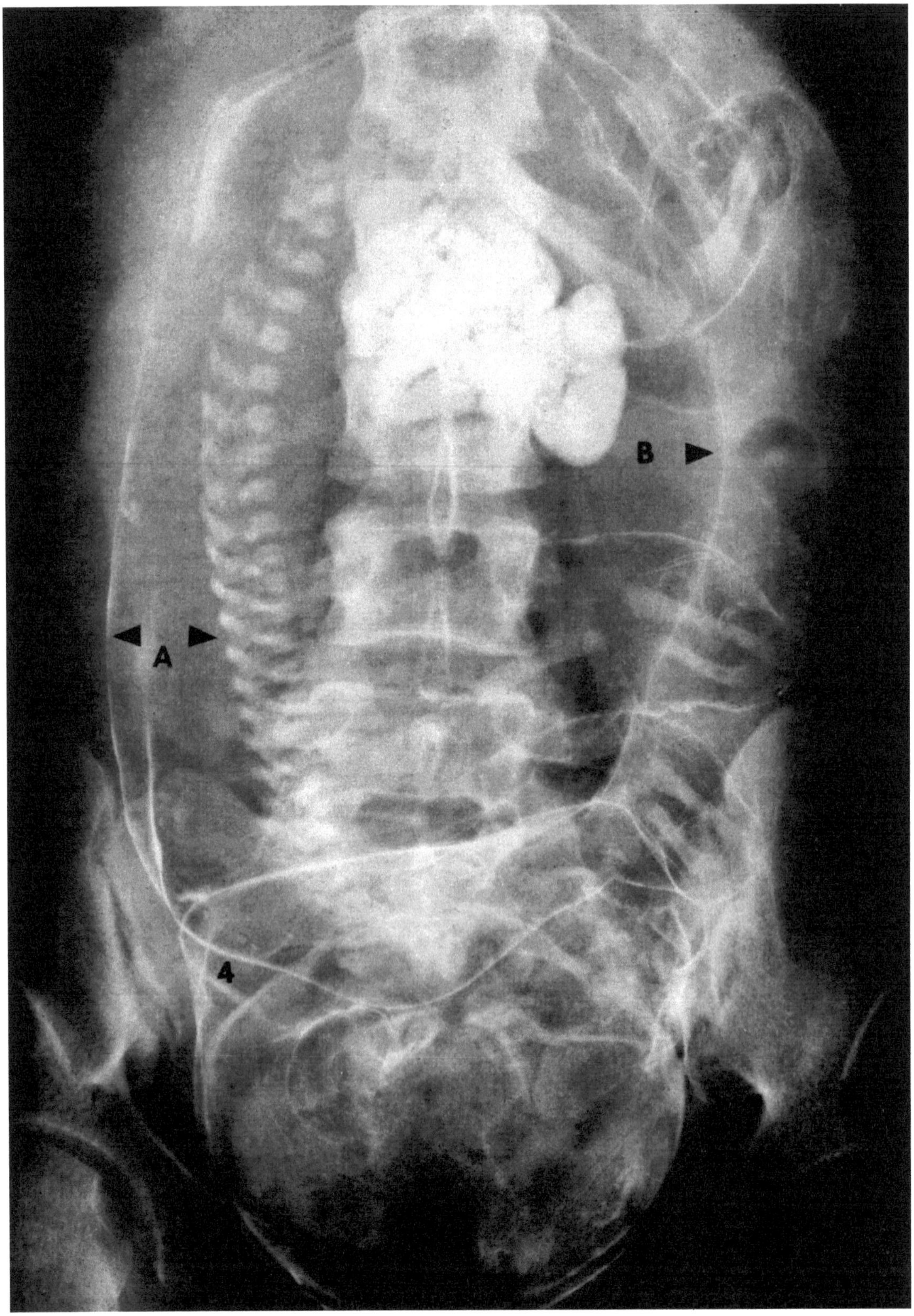

**Patient T.K./83,** 22 years, first gravidity.
**Clinical findings:** 34th week of pregnancy; no contributory findings.
**Ultrasonic findings:** Subcutaneous accumulation of fluid, 2 cm in average width and circular in craniocervical region; no detectable malformation.
**Computed tomography** (Fig. 70a, b): Skull cap surrounded by liquid rim (arrows); no additional findings.

**Case 40**

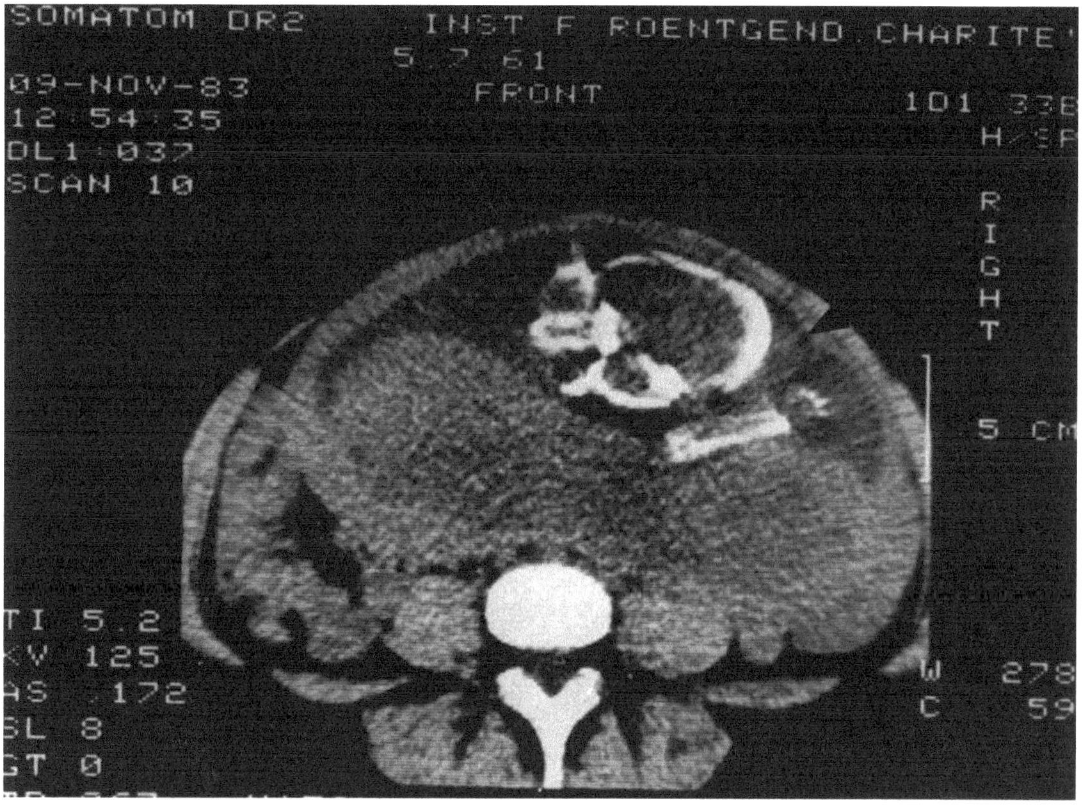


Fig. 70a

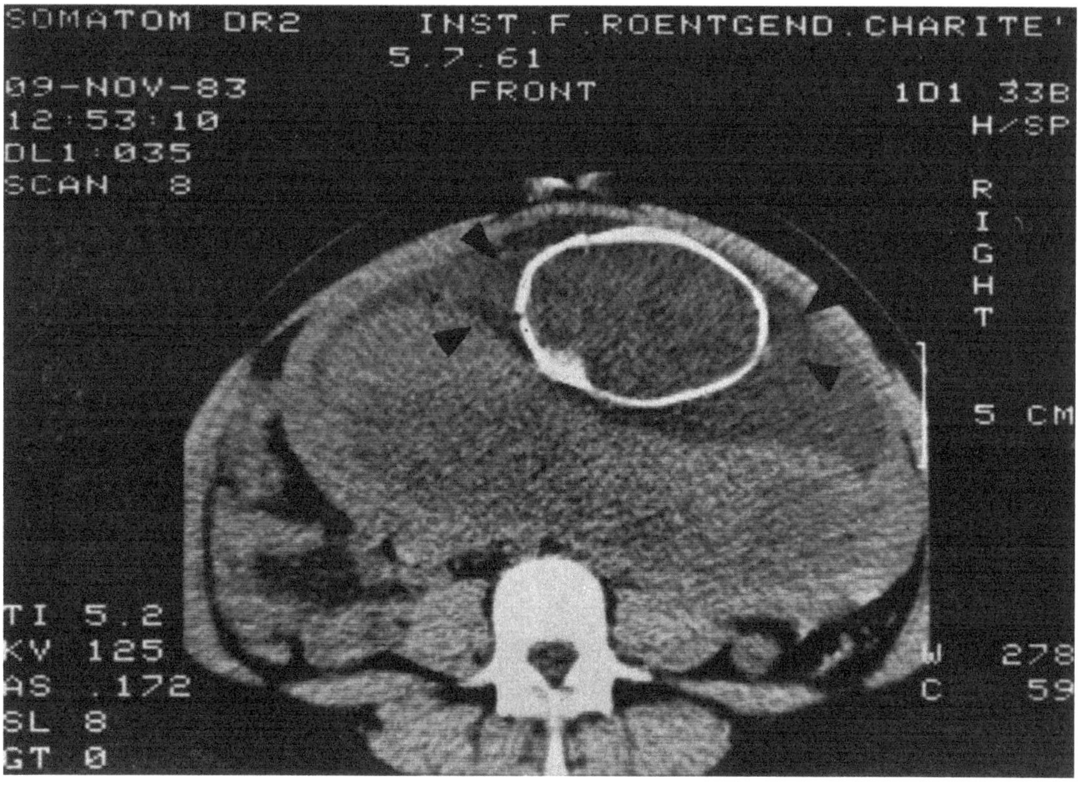


Fig. 70b

Case 40 **Indication for AFG:** Attempt to clearing up ultrasonic and CT findings; search for malformations.

**AFG findings** (Fig. 71: amniogram 60 minutes from injection): Female foetus; breech presentation; circumscribed hydrops in craniocervical region (A); contrast medium not detectable yet in gastro-intestinal tract; retardation.

**Prenatal summary diagnosis.** Scalp edema (circumscribed hydrops of obscure genesis in craniocervical region); retar-

Fig. 71

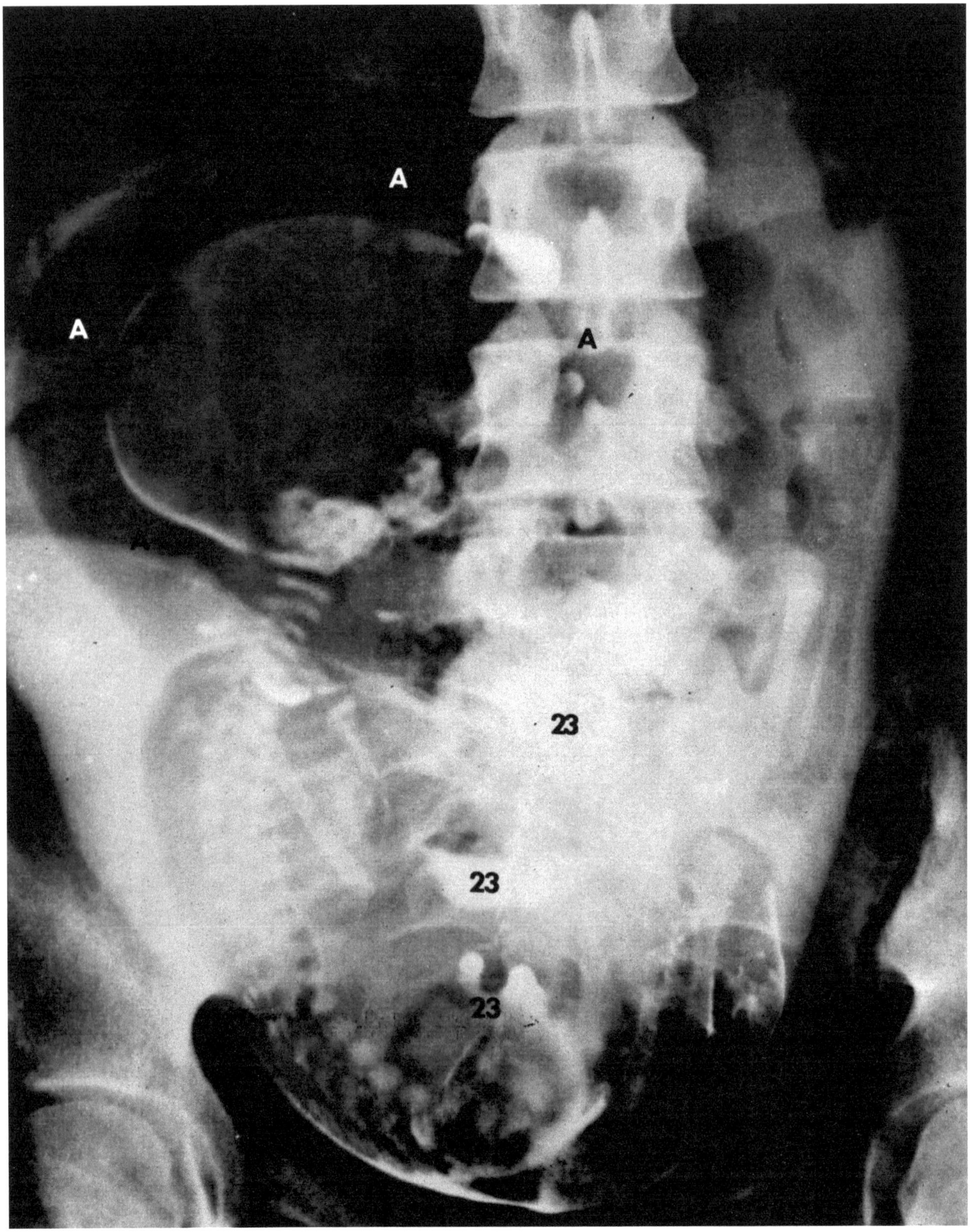

dation; decelerated passage of contrast medium through gastro-intestinal tract (amniogram, Fig. 71).
**Clinical course:** Spontaneous stillbirth in 34th week of pregnancy; 1,650 g, 41 cm.

**Radiogram** (Fig. 72) and **post-mortem findings:** Gelatinous oedema of epicranium; hypertelorism; hypoplasia of left heart. ◁

Case 40

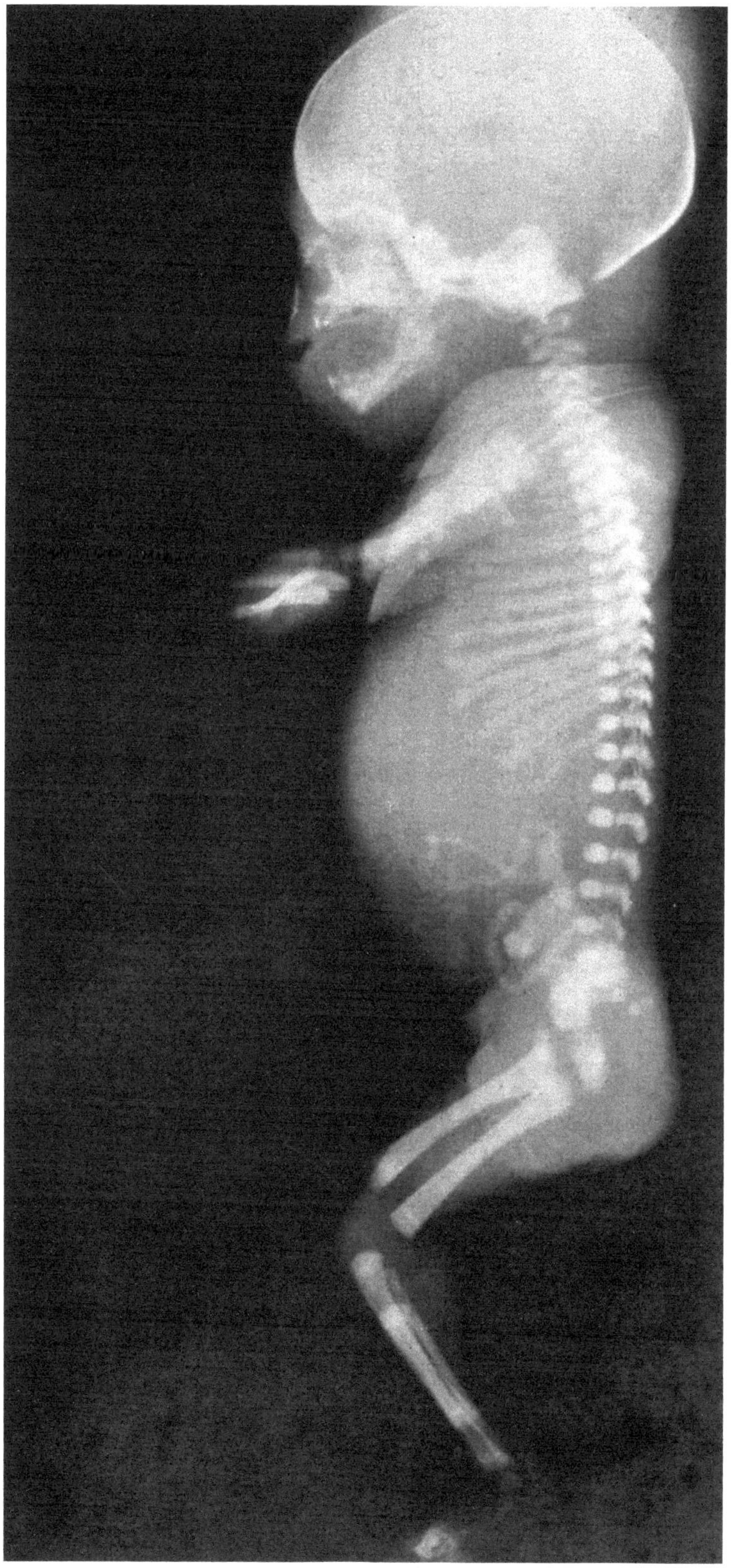

Fig. 72

**Case 41** **Patient L.J./84,** 24 years, first gravidity.

**Clinical findings:** 33rd week of pregnancy; alpha-foeto-protein level twice the normal value.

**Ultrasonic findings** (Fig. 73a, b): No regular cranial echo obtainable; suspicion of malformations of caudal extremities; distension of abdominal region and filled up with undifferentiated tumour mass of homogeneous echo (arrows, VC – vertebral column).

**Indication for AFG:** To clear up ultrasonic findings; search for malformations.

**AFG findings** (Fig. 74: foetogram 23 hours from injection): Female foetus; breech presentation; unround microcephalus (A) with lobular appendages which cause double contours of cerebral cranium (B; arrow); strong distension of abdo-

Fig. 73a

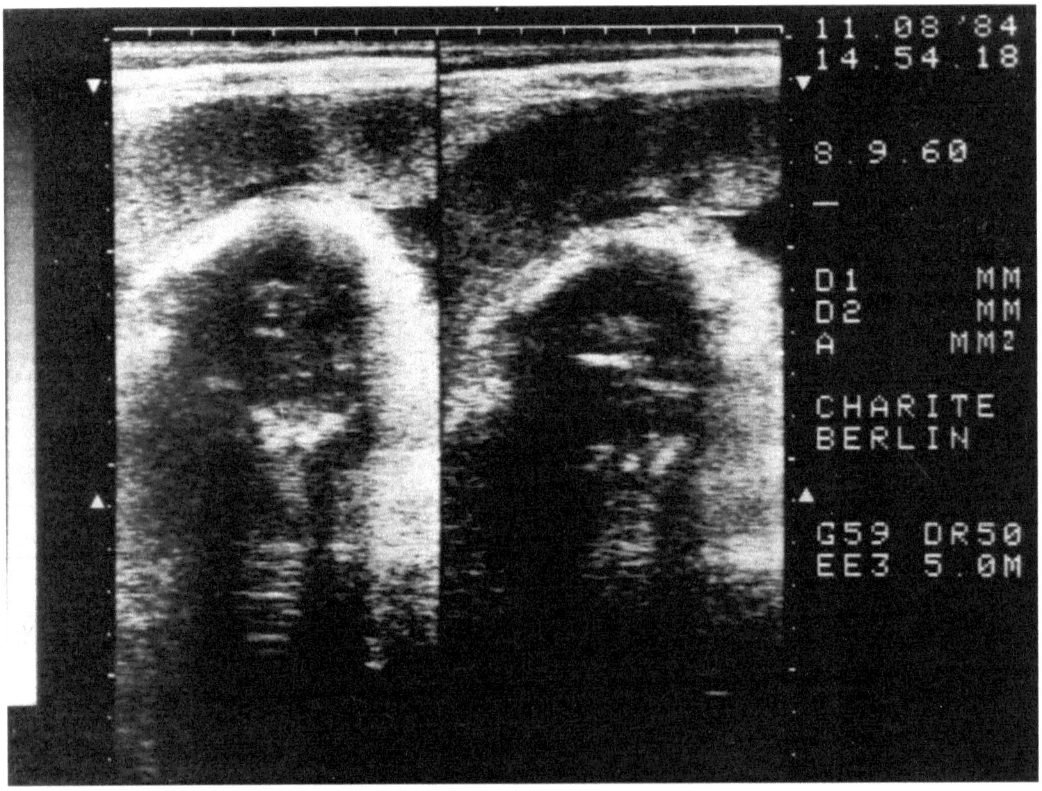


Fig. 73b

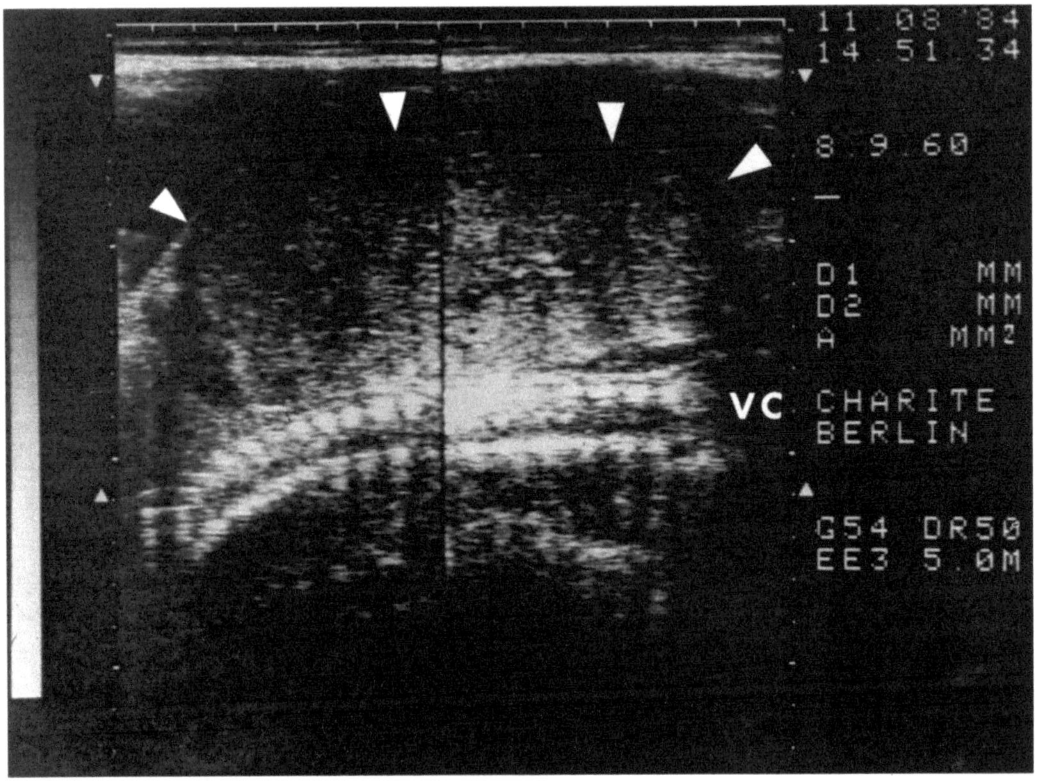

minal region (C); bell-shaped deformation of thorax (D); no contrast medium detectable in gastro-intestinal tract; clump extremities; lower extremities in forced cross-legged position (E).
**Prenatal summary diagnosis:** Multiple malformations of central nervous system, abdominal region, and skeleton.
**Clinical course:** Premature termination of pregnancy in 33rd week; 2,300 g, 42 cm; intrapartum death.
**Post-mortem findings:** Dysplasia of cerebral cranium with cephalocele; dysplastically lowered external ears; palatoschisis; mesenterium ileocolicum commune; microcystic renal degeneration, with size of kidneys being 9 6 3 cm; several hepatocysts up to 10 mm in size; hexadactyly of both hands and feet. ◁

Case 41

Fig. 74

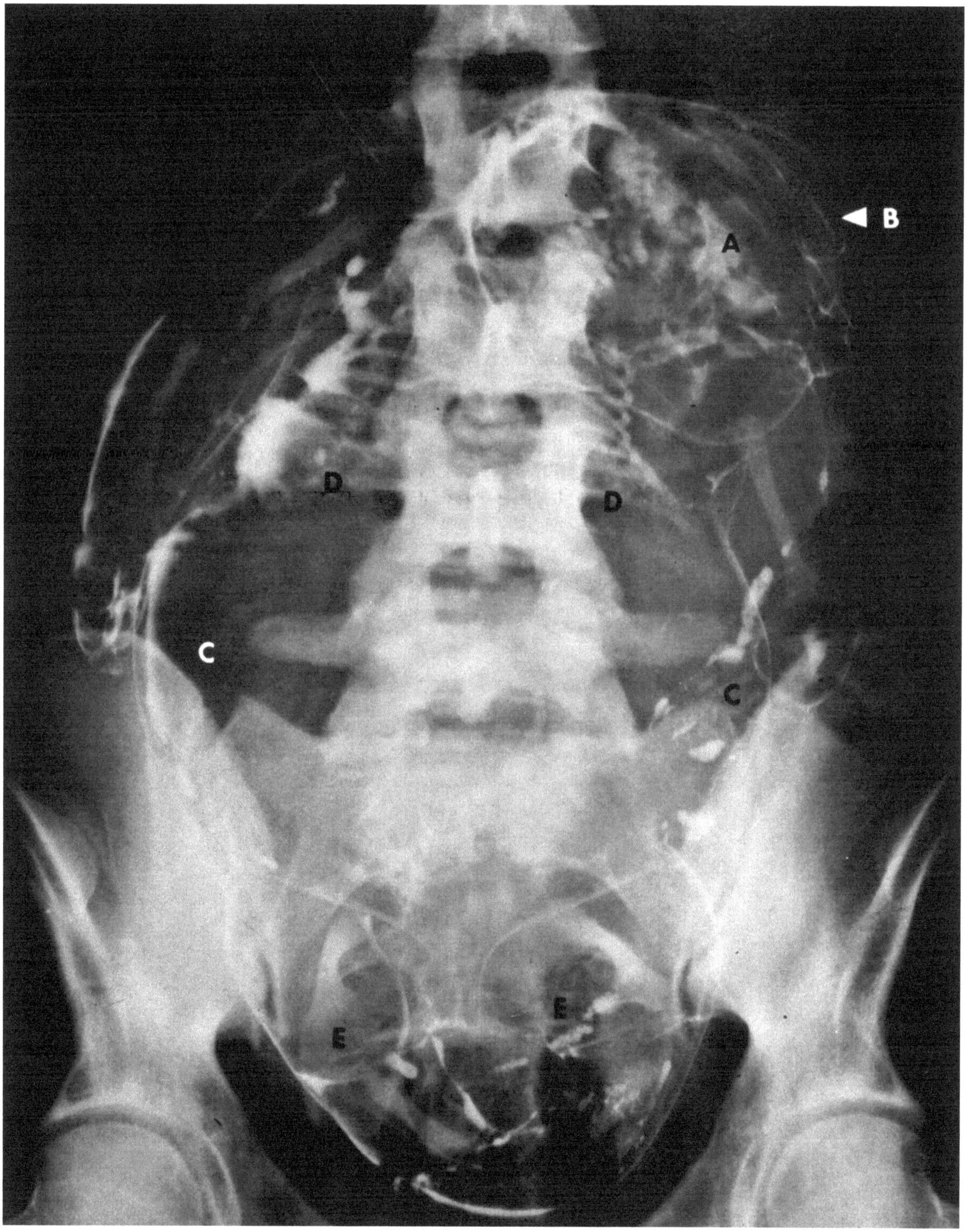

**Case 42** **Patient H.G./82,** 25 years, second gravidity, one parturition.
**Record:** One clinically intact child.
**Clinical findings:** 34th week of pregnancy; no contributory findings.
**Ultrasonic findings:** Suspicion of omphalocele containing fragments of liver and intestine; large cystic areas surrounding both kidneys; more accurate differentiation impossible; no regular kidneys delimitable.
Puncture of one cystic area and instillation of water-soluble contrast medium in conjunction with AFG.

**Indication for AFG:** To clear up ultrasonic findings and search for additional malformations.
**AFG findings** (Fig. 75a: amniogram 30 minutes from injection; Fig. 75b: foetogram 26 hours from injection): Cephalic presentation; sex not safely determinable; amniogram (Fig. 75a): deposition of contrast medium in abdominal region with configuration resembling strongly dilated renal cavity system with distally stenotic hydro-ureter (A); free Lipiodol UF left close to anterior abdominal wall.

Fig. 75a

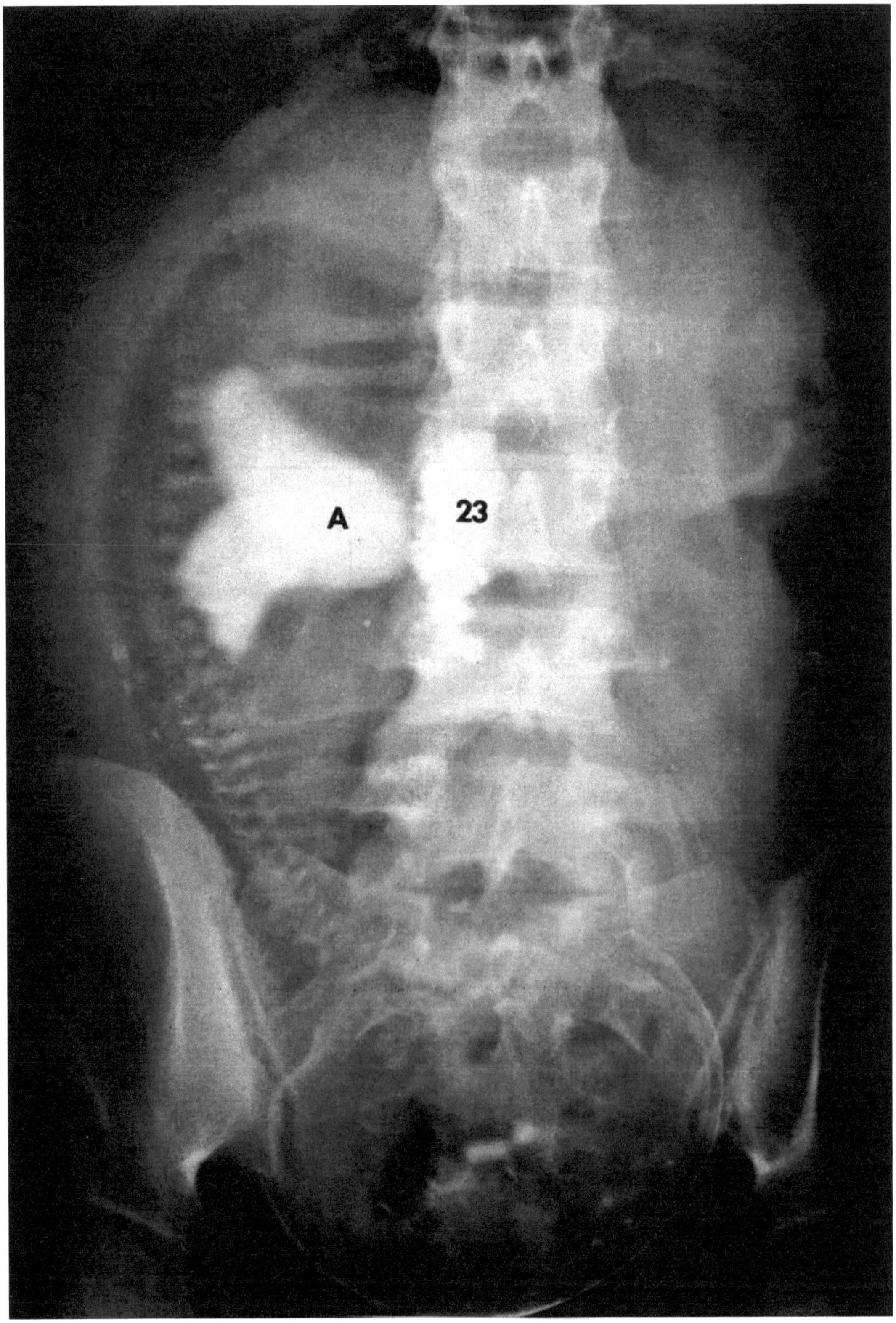

Foetogram (Fig. 75b): sex of foetus not safely determinable; changing presentation of foetus; clear protrusion of abdominal region (B; arrows) with Lipiodol marking only in upper part; no detectable gastro-intestinal passage of contrast mediun; intra-abdominal deposition of contrast medium no longer traceable; drainage of contrast medium from outgoing urinary system with severe ureteral stenosis after 26 hours.

**Prenatal summary diagnosis:** Suspicion of omphalocele with atresia in gastro-intestinal tract; hydronephrosis and hydroureter.

**Clinical course:** Spontaneous labour in 35th week of pregnancy after induction; delivery of girl, 2,400 g, 48 cm; death of child during birth.

**Postmortem diagnosis:** Palatoschisis, oesophageal atresia; large omphalocele with liver and intestine involvement; bilateral hydronephrosis with stenotic hydro-ureters falsely ending in proximal urethra; splenic cysts. ◁

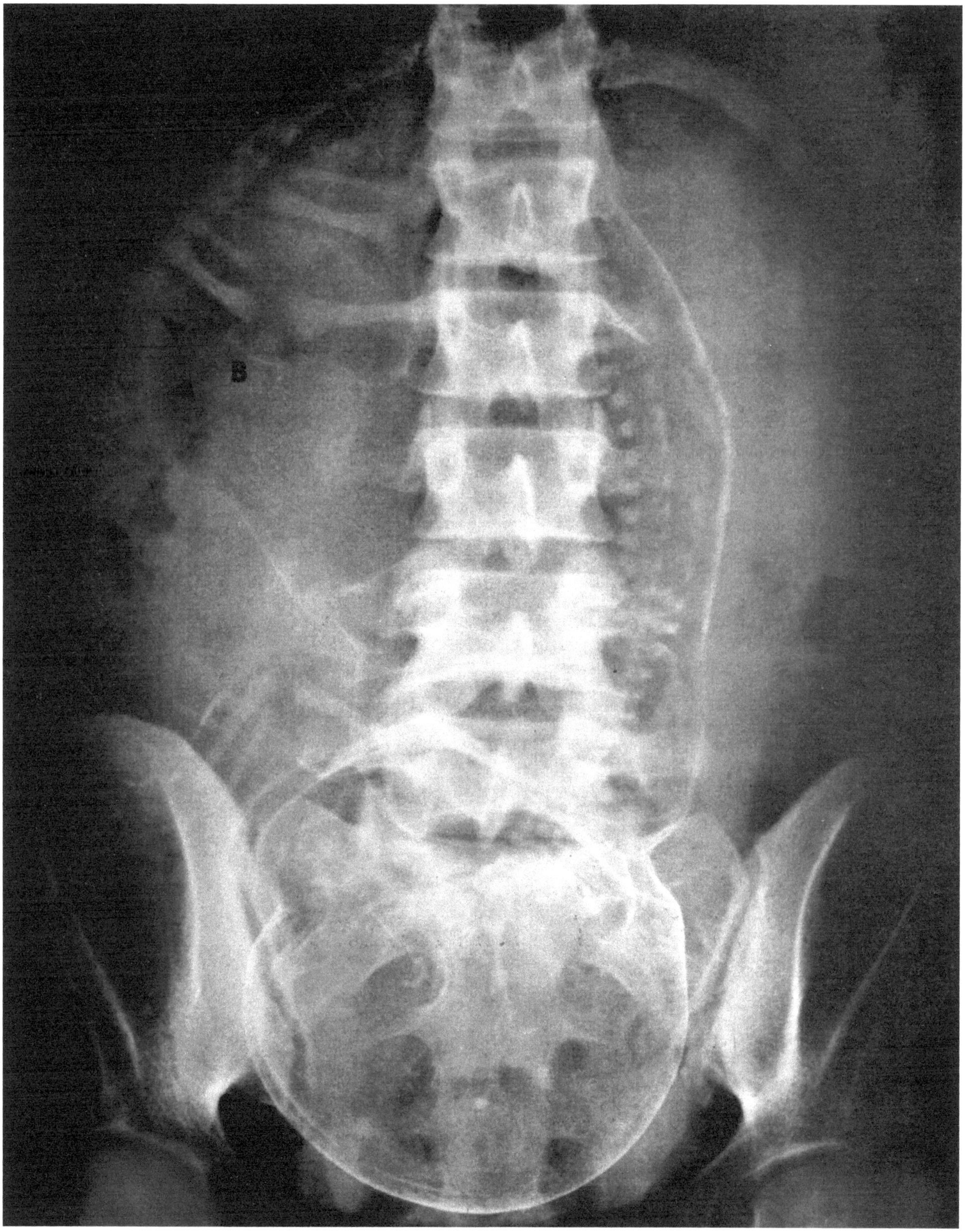


Fig. 75b

**Case 43** **Patient S.T./81**, 23 years, first gravidity.
**Clinical findings:** 30th week of pregnancy; polyhydramnion.
**Ultrasonic findings:** Detection of monstrous omphalocele with fragments of liver and intestine; lumbosacral expansive growth, ca. 8 cm; differential diagnosis: myelomeningocele; coccygeal teratoma.

Fig. 76

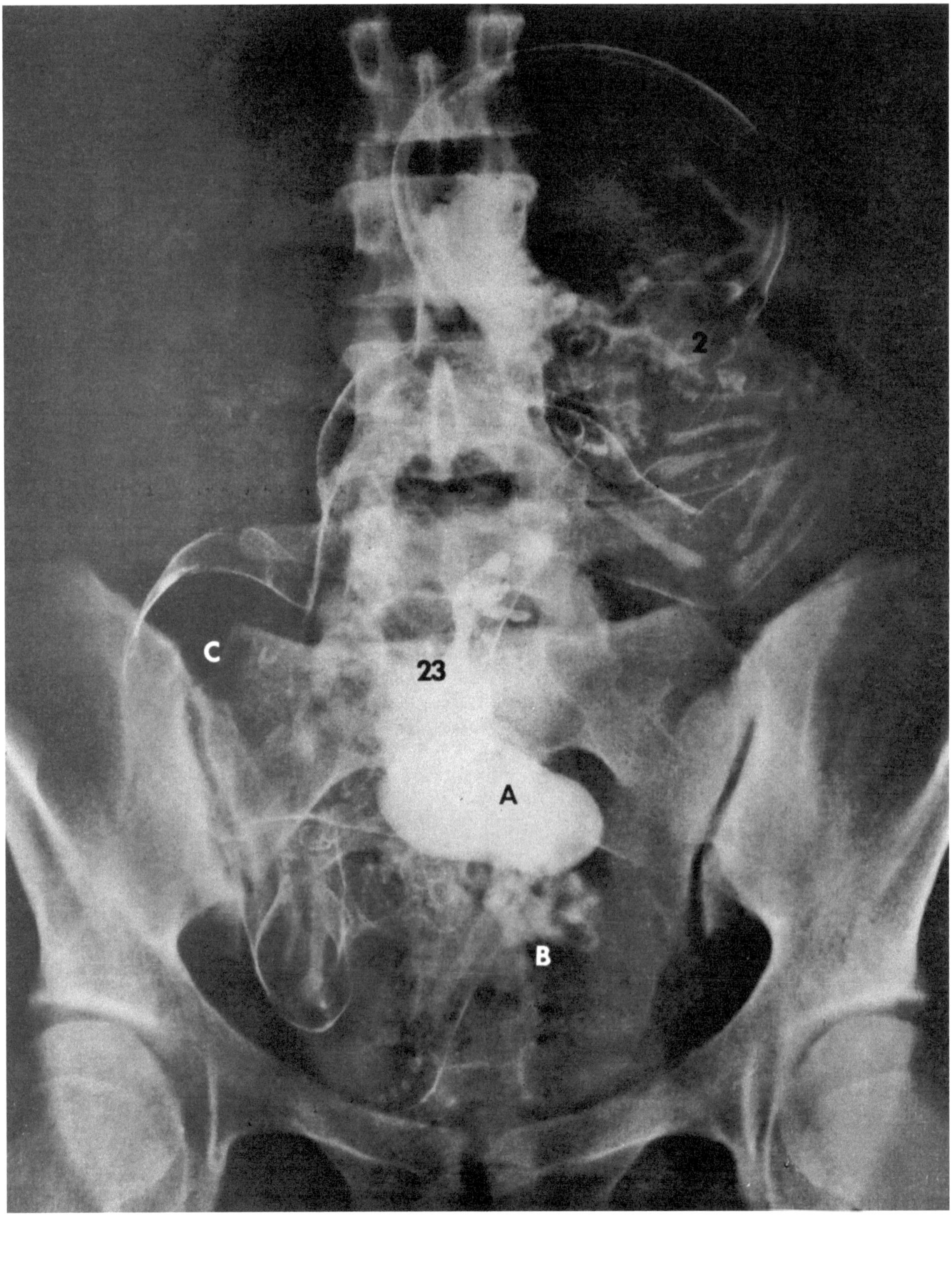

**Indication for AFG:** Verification of ultrasonic findings; search for additional malformations.
**AFG findings** (Fig. 76: foetogram 24 hours from injection): Sex of foetus not determinable; breech presentation; ectatic stomach filled up with contrast medium (A); loops of small intestine ventral from abdominal wall (B); irregular position

Case **43**

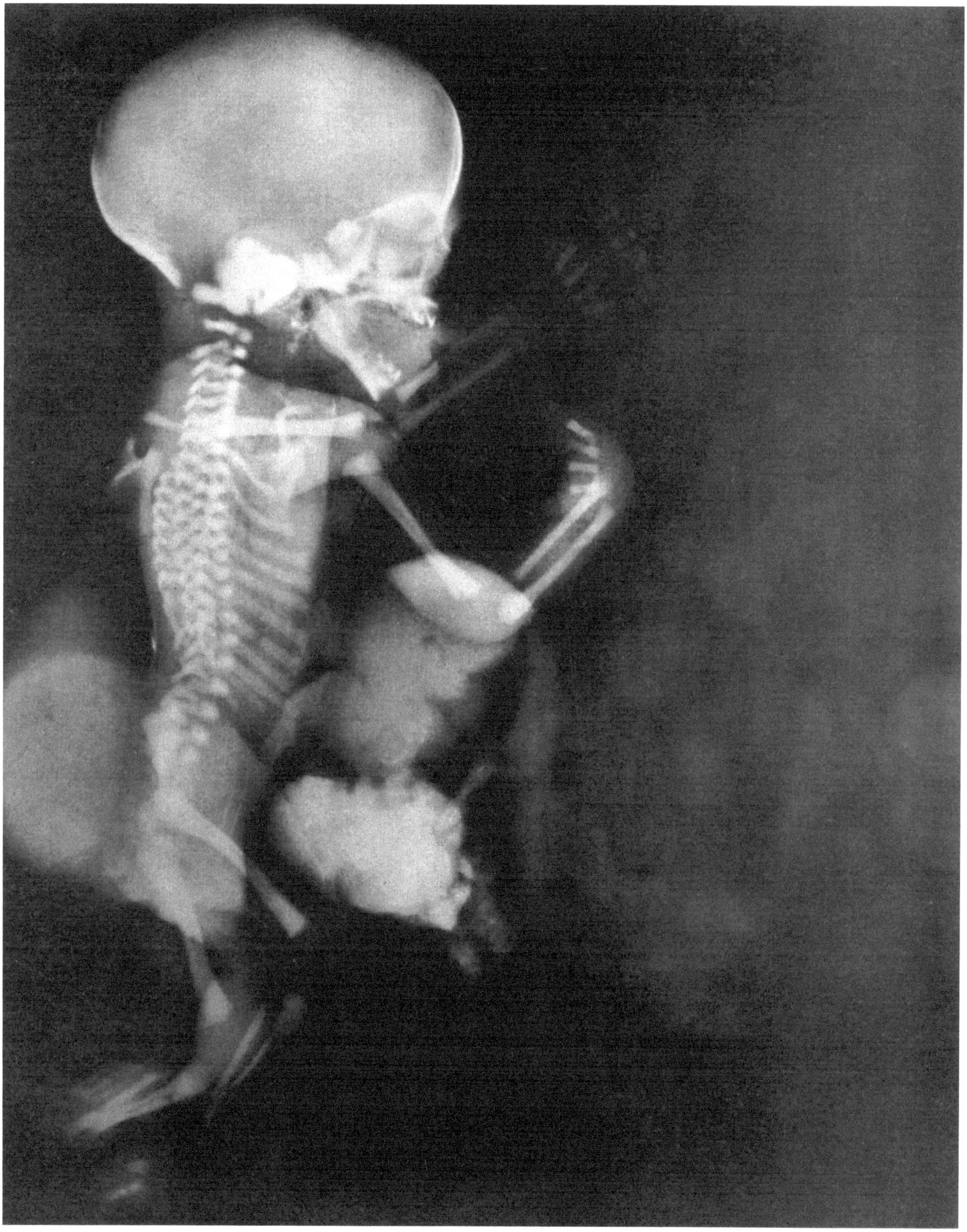

Fig. 77a

Case 43 of lower extremities; large tumour, ca. 8 cm, clearly demarcated in lumbosacral position; high probability of coccygeal teratoma (C); no sign of hydrocephalus.

**Prenatal summary diagnosis:** Omphalocele; coccygeal teratoma.

**Clinical course:** Premature termination of pregnancy in 30th

Fig. 77b

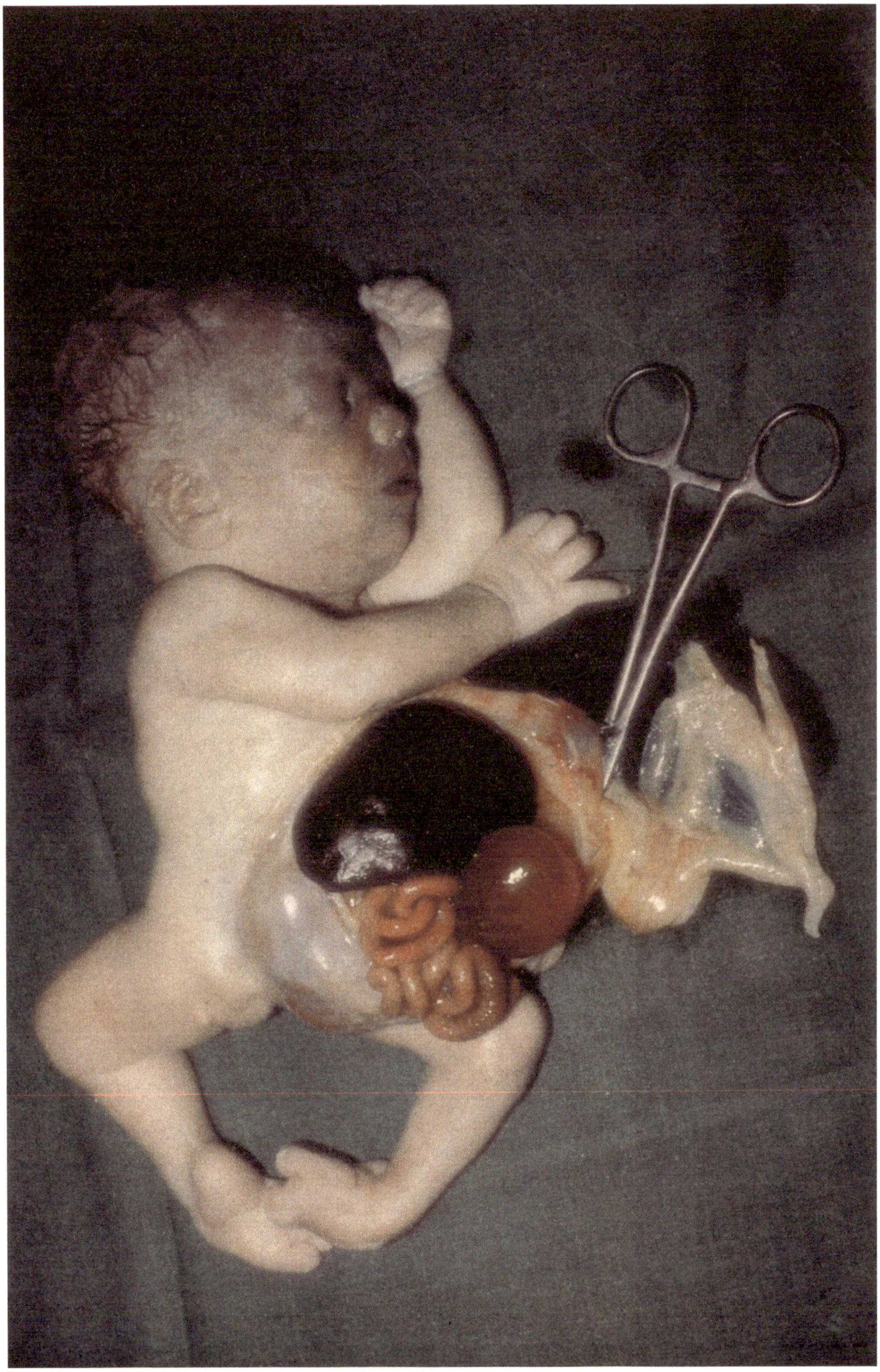

week; male foetus, 1,850 g, 41 cm; death at birth. **Radiogram** (Fig. 77a) and **post-mortem findings:** Coccygeal teratoma; omphalocele with liver, spleen, pancreas, and small intestine; club-hands and club-feet; no hydrocephalus; clinical aspect shows Figures 77b, c. ◁

Case **43**

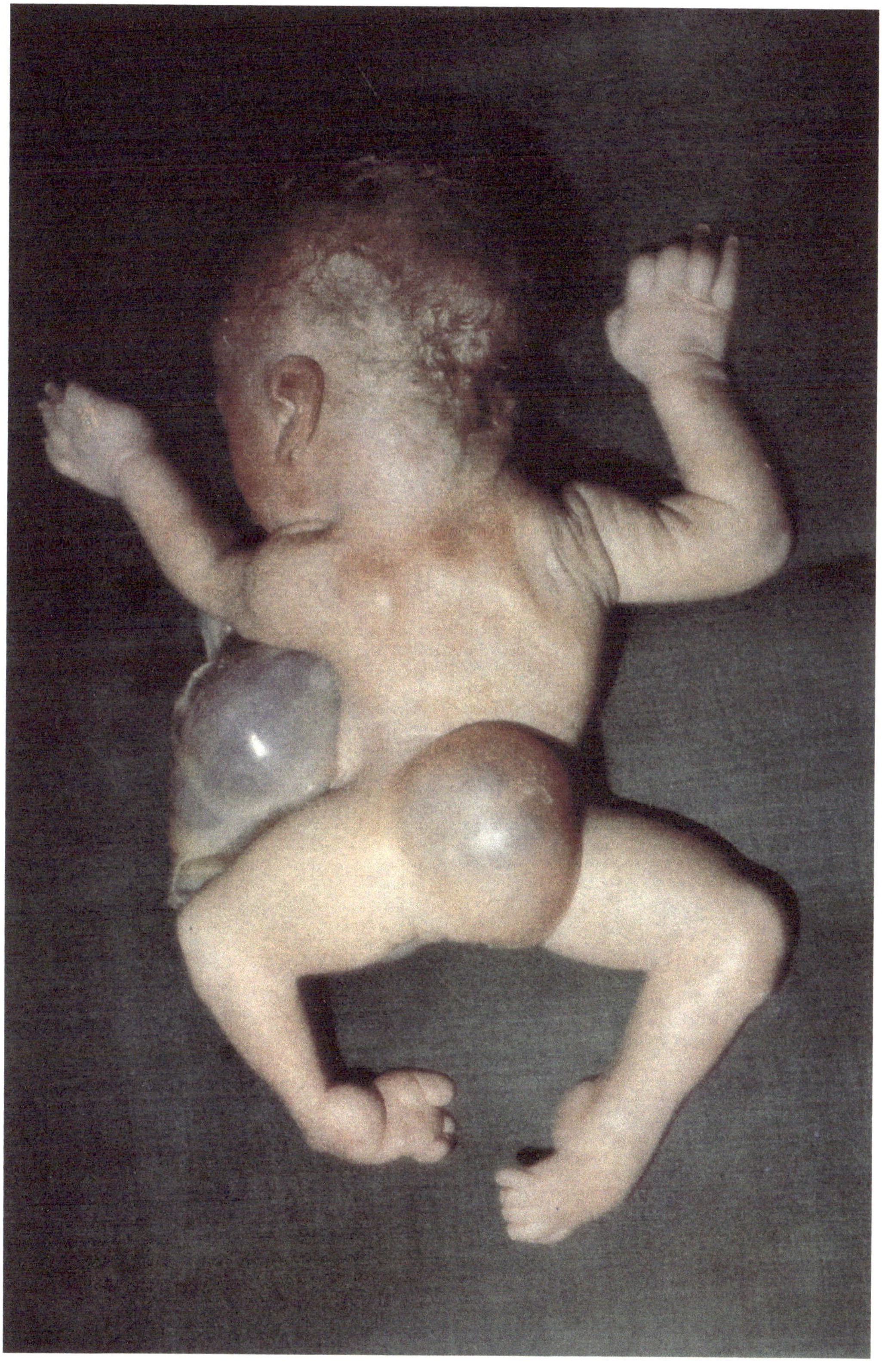

Fig. 77c

**Case 44** **Patient K.S./83,** 33 years, first gravidity.
**Clinical findings:** 36th week of pregnancy; polyhydramnion; alpha-foetoprotein twice the normal value.
**Ultrasonic findings:** Polyhydramnion; internal hydrocephalus; suspicion of thoracolumbar neural tube defect.
**Indication for AFG:** Verification of ultrasonic findings; polyhydramnion; signs indicative of additional malformations.

**AFG findings** (Fig. 78: foetogram 48 hours from injection): Female foetus; cephalic presentation; macrocephalia (A); disruption of dorsal contour at lumbar level (B; arrows) and double contour of thoracic spine (C; arrows); detection of contrast-imaged loops of small intestine and colon in thoracic cavity (D); passage of contrast medium slowed down; 24-hour scan shows contrast medium only in small intestine; no pathological signs of extremities; accurate assessment of

Fig. 78

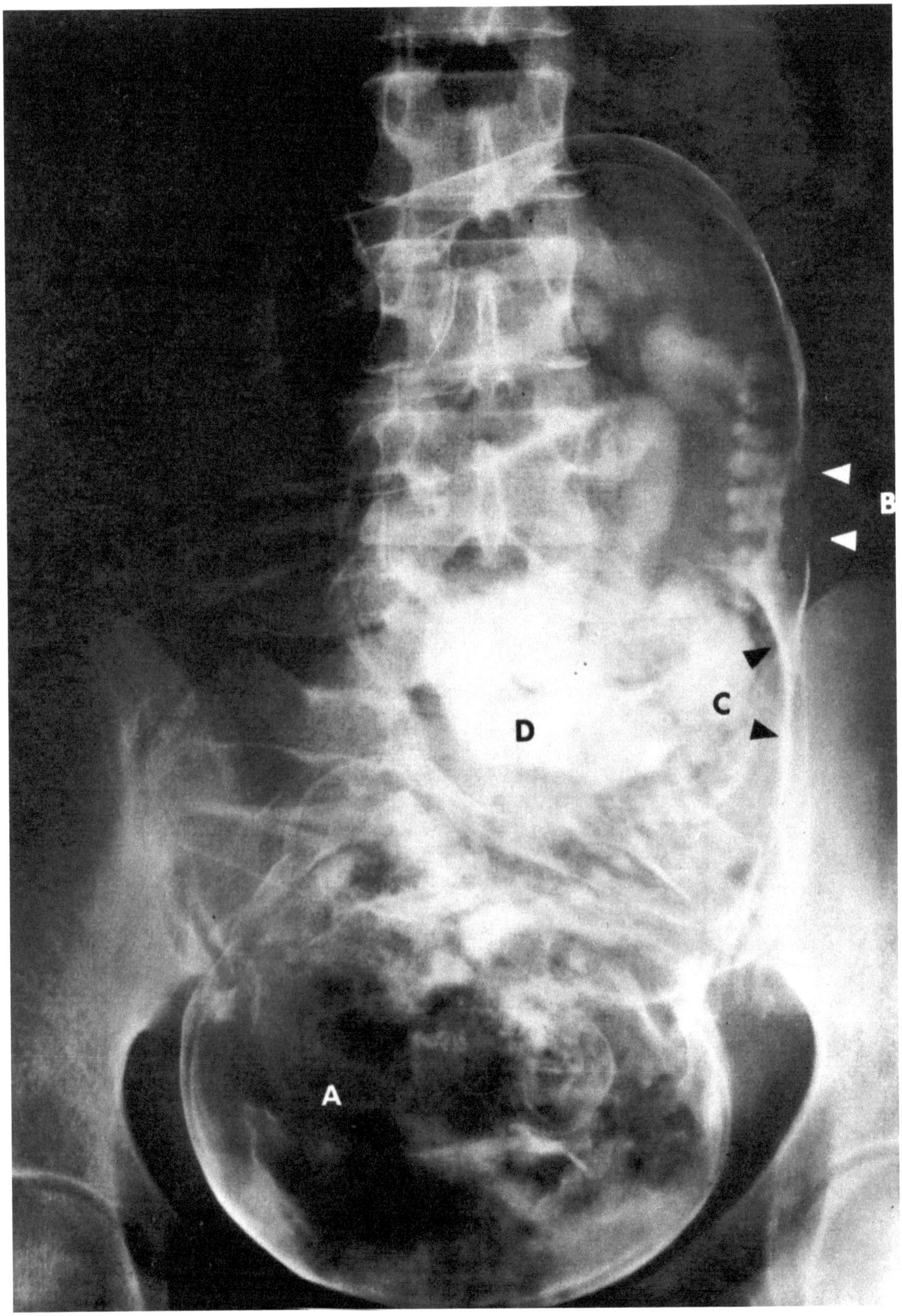

vertebral column difficult for superimpositions.
**Prenatal summary diagnosis:** Hydrocephalus; large neural tube defect with celes at thoracolumbar level; diaphragmatic defect.
**Clinical course:** Termination of pregnancy in 37th week; 2,890 g, 48 cm.
**Radiogram** (Fig. 79): Condition after cranioclasty; confirmation of prenatal diagnosis; additional findings included multiple malformations of vertebral bodies at thoracic and lumbar levels as well as costal abnormalities.
**Post-mortem findings:** Confirmation of prenatal diagnosis; additional findings included mesenterium iliocolicum commune, hypoplasia of right lung, clump kidneys on either side; Potter-like facies. ◁



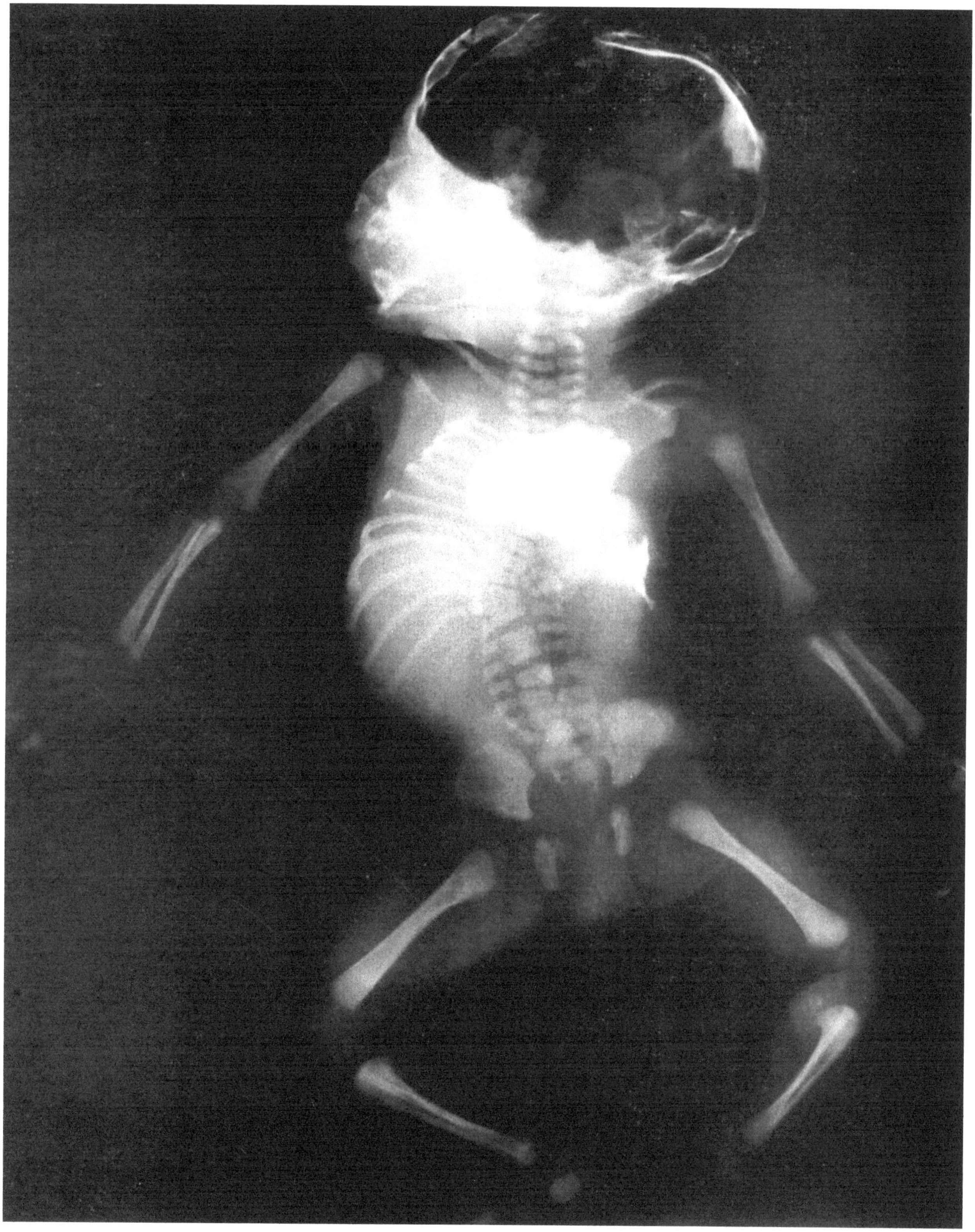

Fig. 79

**Case 45** **Patient R.M./85**, 31 years, second gravidity, one parturition.
**Record:** One clinically intact child.
**Clinical findings:** 33rd week of pregnancy; no contributory findings.
**Ultrasonic findings:** Internal hydrocephalus, maximum thickness of pallium 5 mm; no additional malformation detectable.

**Indication for AFG:** Search for additional malformations.
**AFG findings** (Fig. 80: foetogram 23 hours from injection): Female foetus; breech presentation; projection to thoracic spine shows high-contrast intestinal loops in abdominal region and one intestinal loop filled up with contrast medium (A; arrows); detection of contrast-imaged stomach in ventral position (B); macrocephalia (C); incomplete calcifica-

Fig. 80

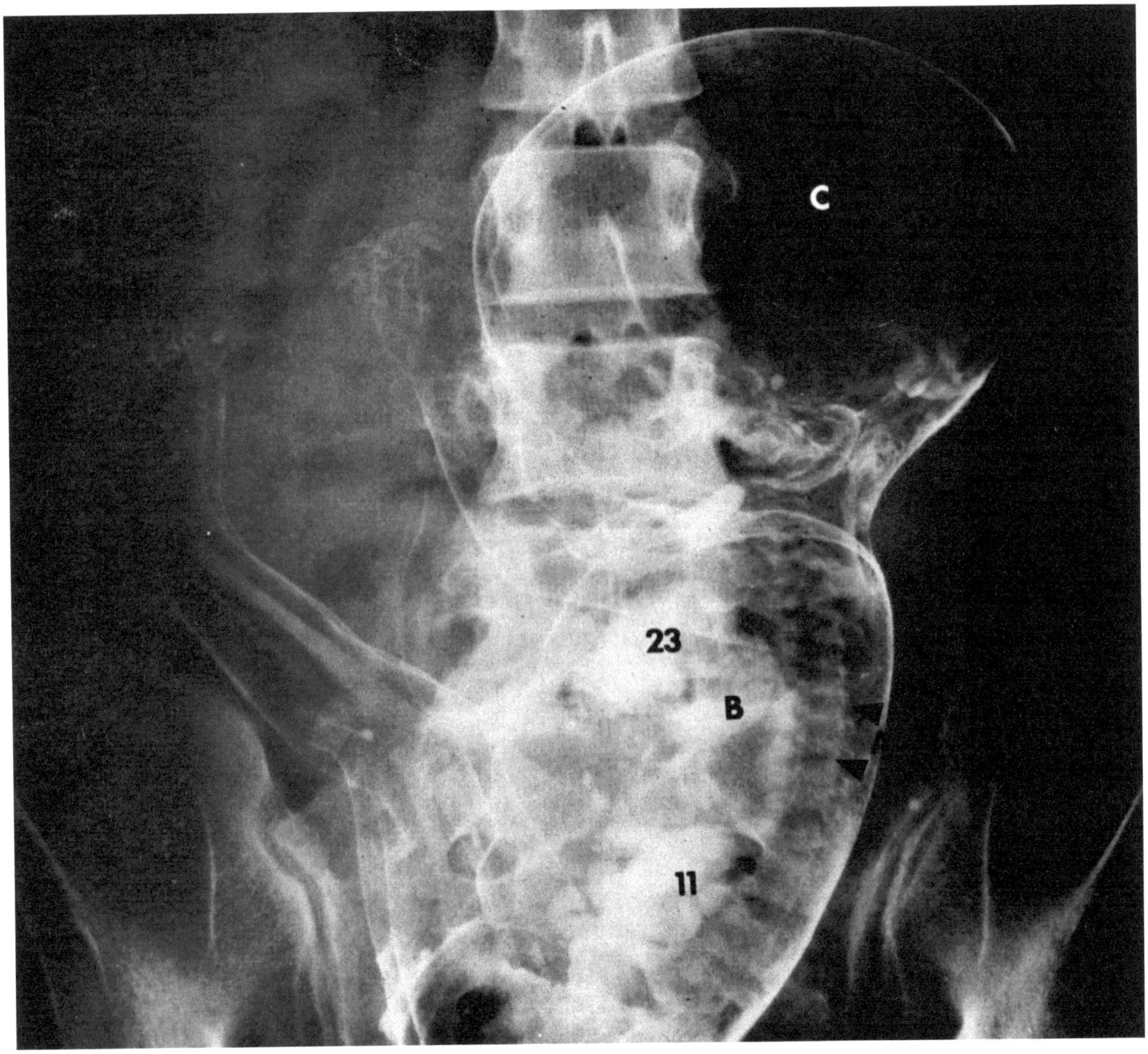

tion of skull cap; free Lipiodol in cervical and thoracic regions.
**Prenatal summary diagnosis:** Internal hydrocephalus; diaphragmatic defect on the left side (left congenital diaphragmatic hernia).
**Clinical course:** Termination of pregnancy in 34th week; intrapartum death; 1,450 g, 38 cm.

Case 45

**Radiogram** (Fig. 81) and **post-mortem findings:** Internal hydrocephalus; large dorsolateral diaphragmatic defect on the left; thoracic displacement of stomach, spleen, pancreas, small intestine, and colon; ventricular septal defect; abnormal mitral valve; complex malformation of urinary drainage system.
**Genetic findings:** Trisomy 18. ◁

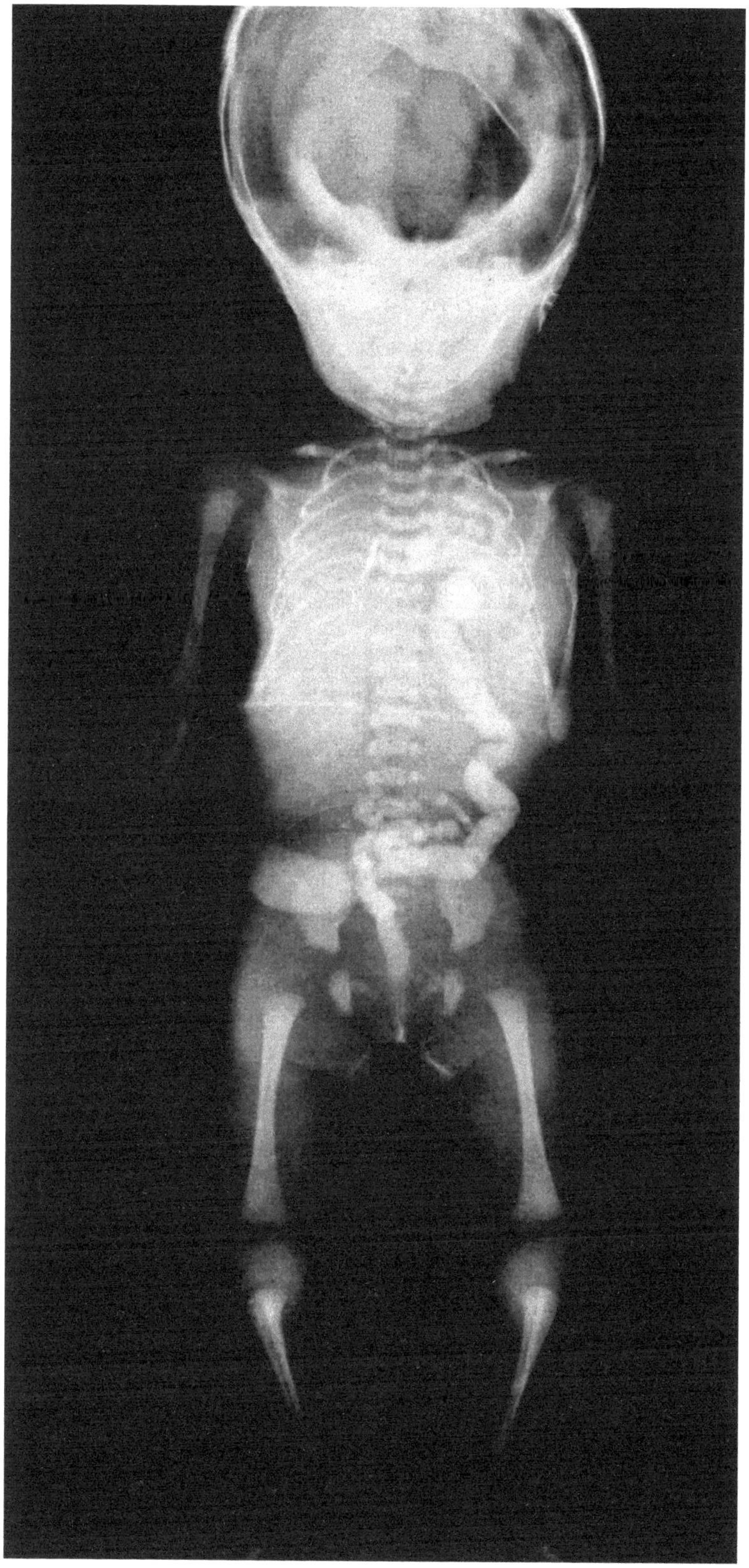

Fig. 81

**Case 46** **Patient E.S./84**, 22 years, first gravidity.
**Clinical findings:** 32nd week of pregnancy; polyhydramnion.
**Ultrasonic findings** (Fig. 82): Twin pregnancy; diamniotic; polyhydramnion in one embryonic cavity; larger of both foetuses in latter cavity; this foetus with pronounced ascites (A) and visualisation of omental bursa (B); struma colli congenita only recorded from second foetus; no malformation.

**Indication for AFG:** Polyhydramnion; search for malformations in either foetus.
**AFG findings** (Fig. 83a: Foetogram 24 hours from injection; Fig. 83b: Foetogram 46 hours from injection): 24-hour foetogram (Fig. 83a) showed condition after puncture of right embryonic cavity; right foetus in foot presentation; left foetus in cephalic presentation; Lipiodol marking of

Fig. 82

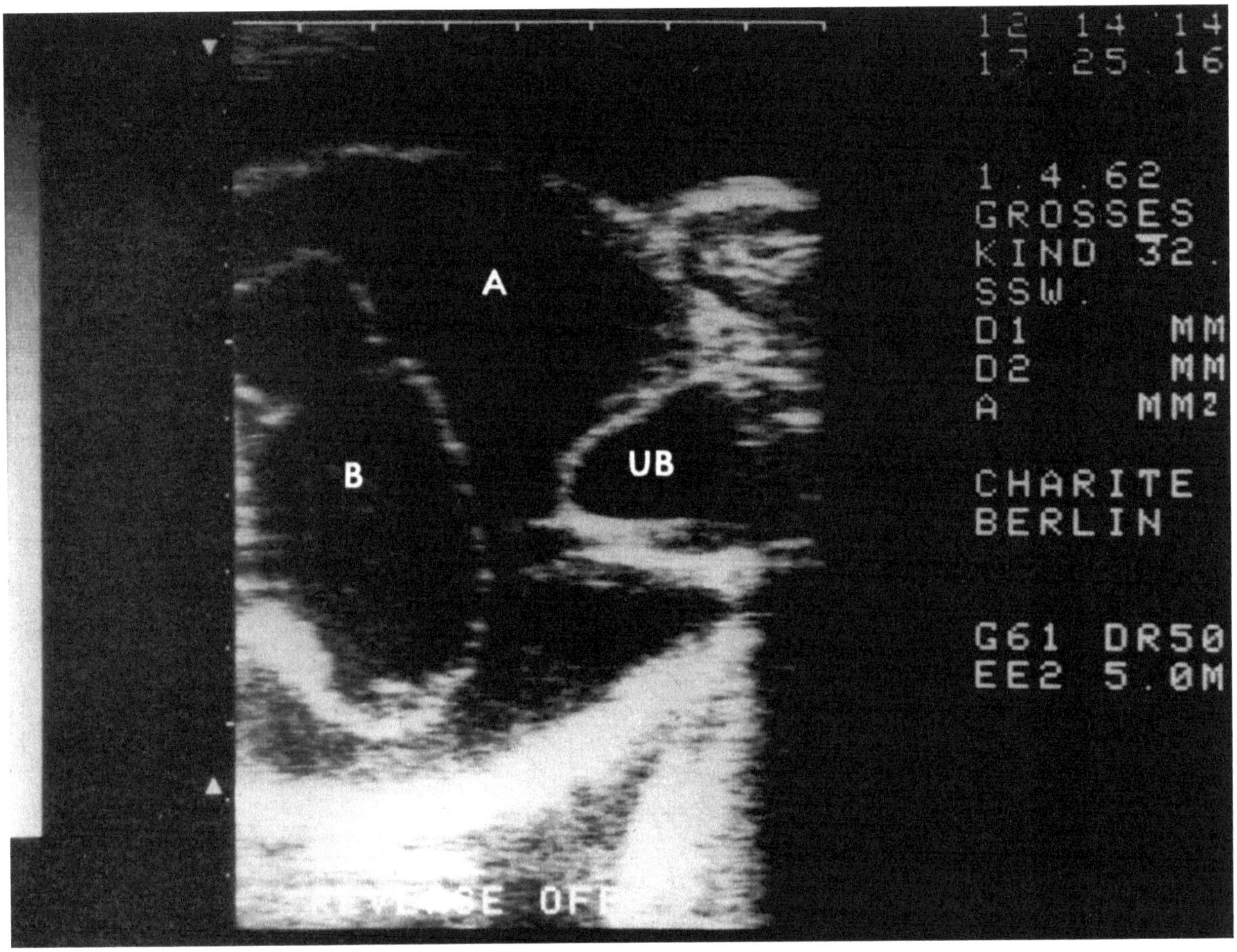

right foetus with delayed gastro-intestinal passage of contrast medium and inhomogeneous contrast of intestines (A; arrows); abdominal protrusion (B; arrow); contrast medium detected in intestine of left foetus (C) without Lipiodol marking of skin surface; hence, water-soluble contrast medium has obviously diffused into left, unpunctured embryonic cavity. 46-hour foetogram (Fig. 83b) showed condition after puncture of either embryonic cavity; large foetus in breech presentation; small foetus in cephalic presentation; both of them male; distension of flanks (B); delayed gastro-intestinal passage of contrast medium, accompanied in large foetus by strongly pronounced calibre variations of lumens of small and large bowels (A); smaller foetus without contributory findings.



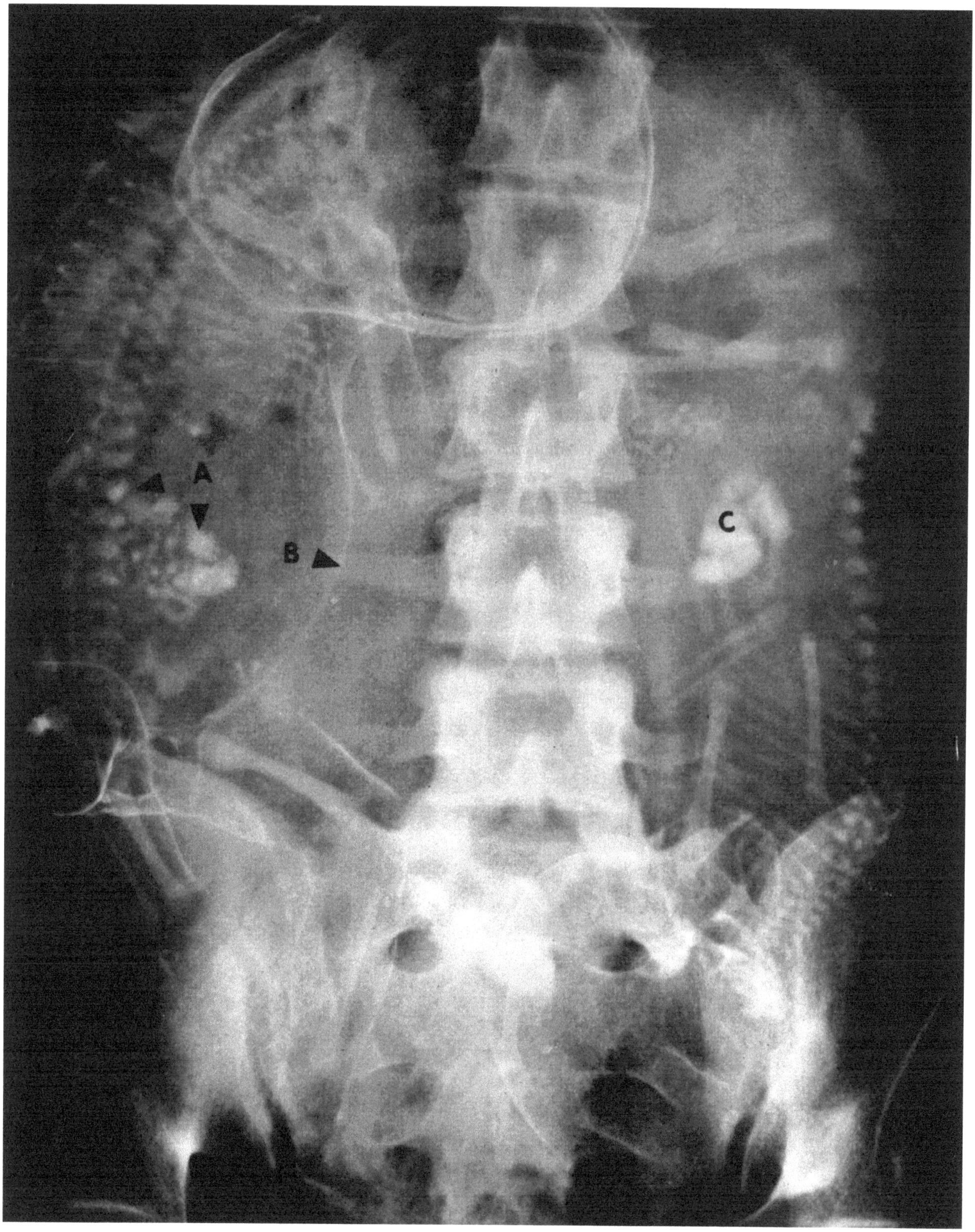


Fig. 83a

Case 46 **Prenatal summary diagnosis:** Peritonitis of right foetus, struma colli congenita of one foetus.

**Clinical course:** Delivery in 33rd week of pregnancy by caesarean section for amniotic infection.

First child: 2,350 g, 46 cm; spontaneous regression of ascites within ten days; clinical suspicion of cerebral haemorrhage was not sonographically secured; development of internal hydrocephalus; valve implantation; possible signs of intrauterine infection but no hard evidence.

Second child: 1,370 g, 40 cm; normal development.

Hypothyreosis of both children in concomitance with struma colli congenita which had been sonographically detected prior to AFG. ◁

Fig. 83 b

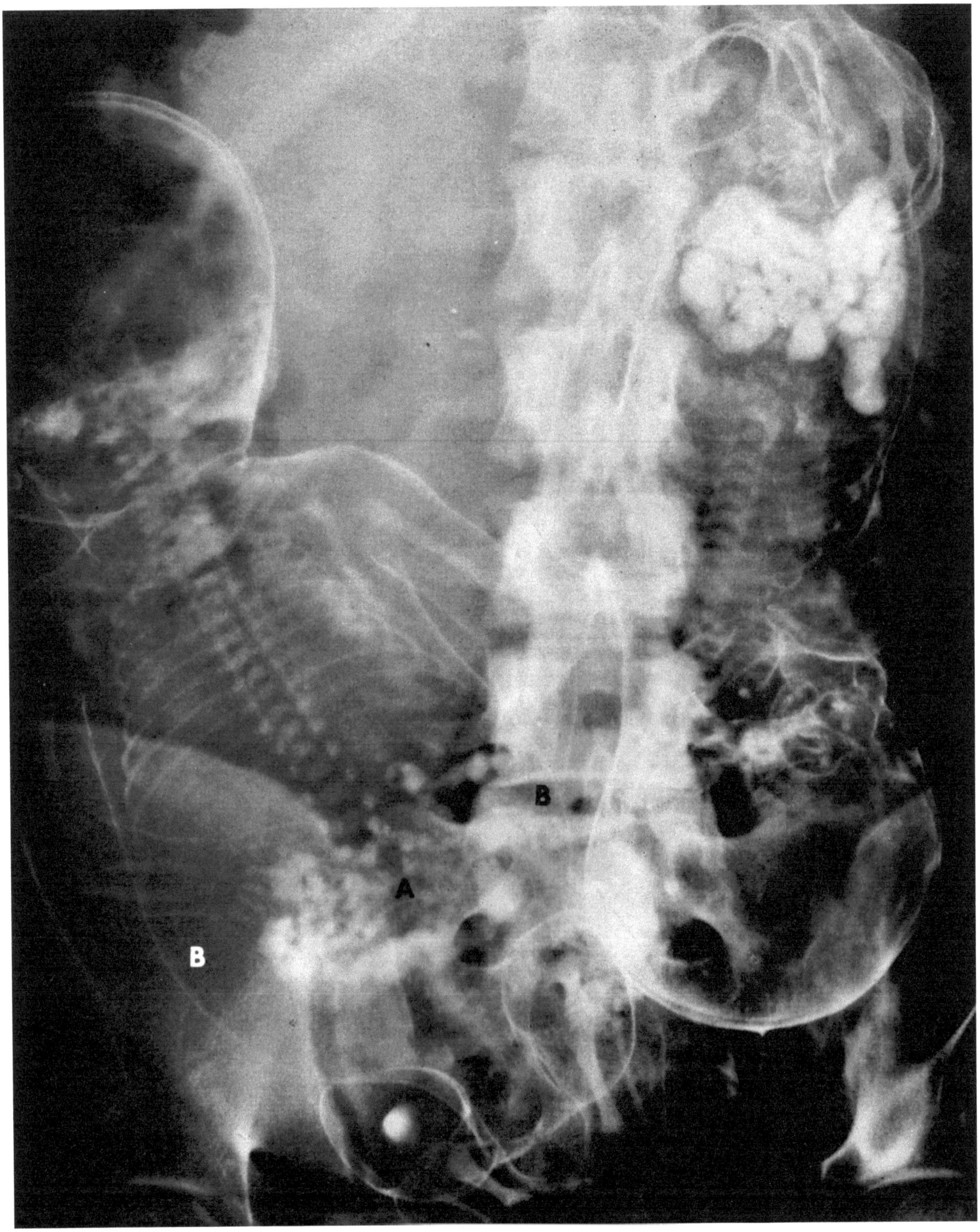

**Case 47**

**Patient S.B./86,** 19 years, first gravidity.
**Clinical findings:** 30th week of pregnancy; no contributory findings.
**Ultrasonic findings:** Twin pregnancy; inconspicuous foetus without detectable malformations; second incomplete foetal trunk without detectability of head, thorax, heart, and upper extremities; incomplete vertebral column; normal development of pelvic girdle and lower extremities.
**Indication for AFG:** Verification of ultrasonic findings; signs indicative of malformations in sonographically inconspicuous foetus.
**AFG findings** (Fig. 84: foetogram 24 hours from injection): Twin pregnancy; Lipiodol marking of both embryonic primordia by one single amniocentesis; only incomplete vertebral column and lower extremities detectable of right embryonic primordium; male foetus on the left apparently displaced by rudimentary embryo; time-adequate gastrointestinal passage of contrast medium, but no visualisation

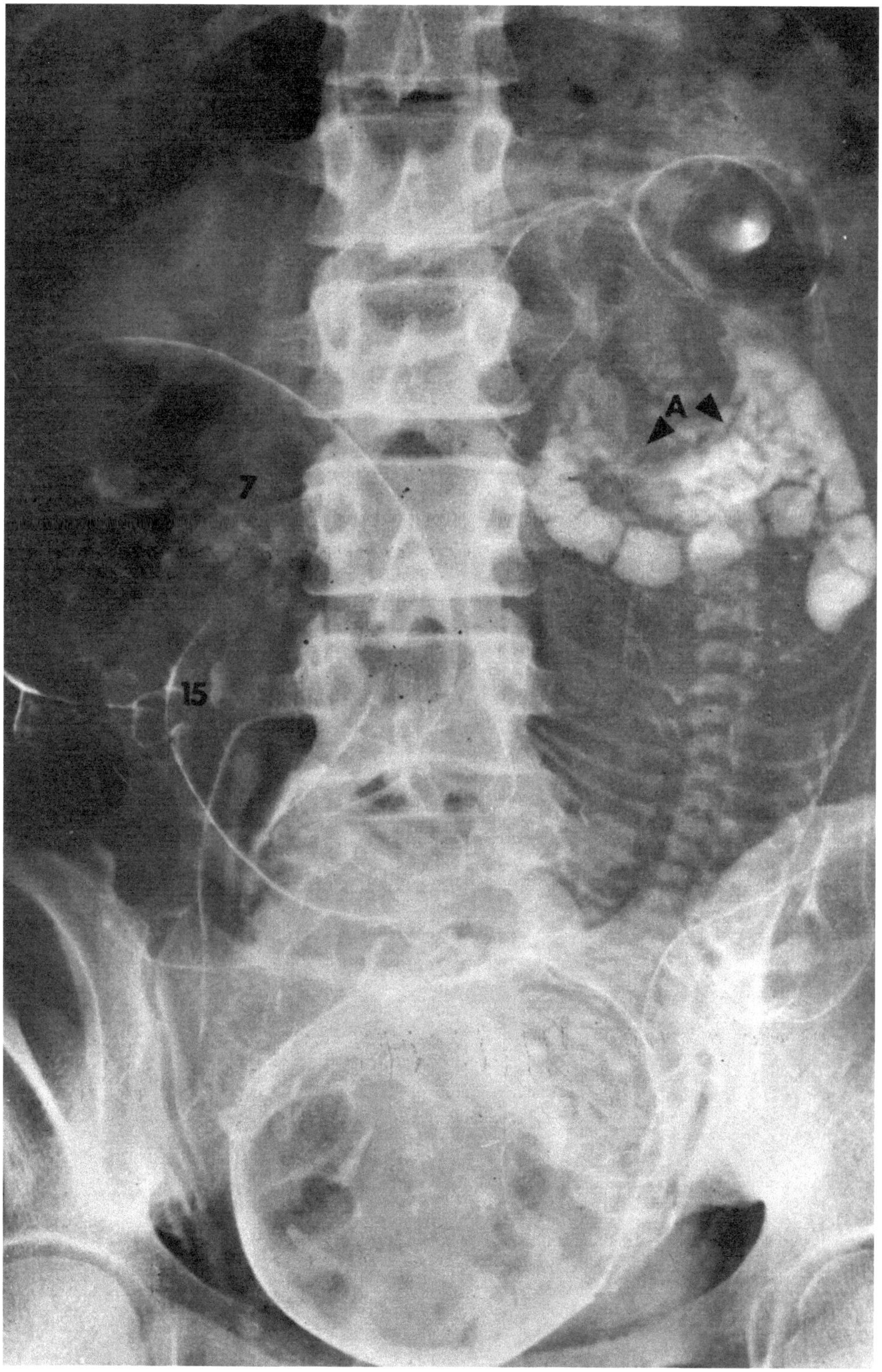


Fig. 84

**Case 47** of rectosigmoid; cranial displacement of small intestine convolution, most probably by completely filled urinary bladder (A; arrows); no detectable maformations.
**Prenatal summary diagnosis:** Twin pregnancy; monamniotic; acardia and acephalus of one embryonic primordium.
**Clinical course:** Spontaneous labour in 32nd week of pregnancy; I. acardia and acephalus; II. child with hydrops, pale, shock symptoms; immediate postnatal ultrasonic investigation revealed slight ascites and perirenal accumulation of fluid on either side; conspicuous echoless structure of kidneys; findings were interpreted as consequence of shock symptoms in response to foeto-foetal transfusion.
**Radiogram** (Fig. 85): Acardius acephalus. Angiography via both umbilical arteries and umbilical veins; no visualisation of heart nor major vessels (aorta, vena cava); vascularisation restricted to segments of undifferentiated trunk. ◁

Fig. 85

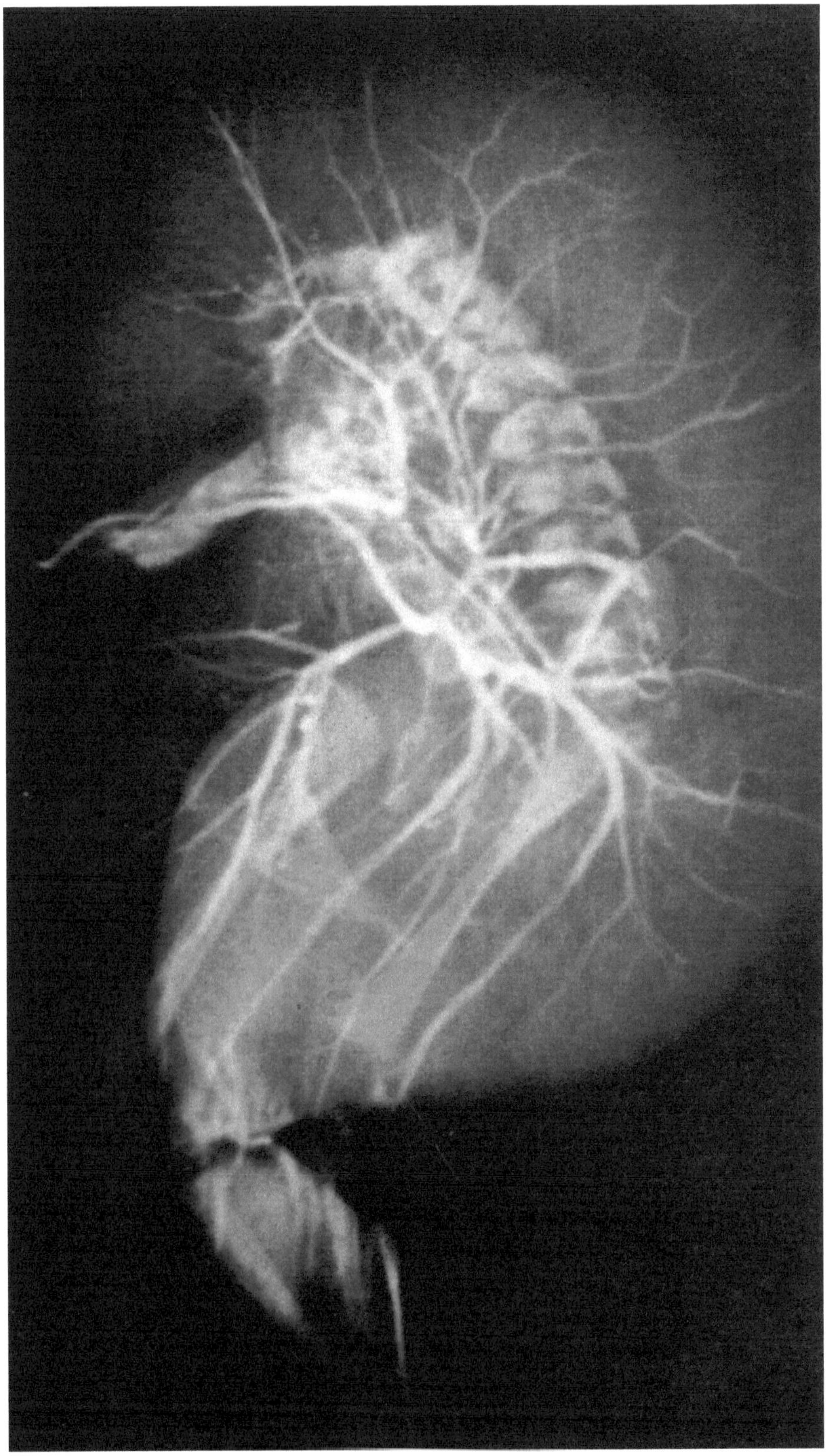

**Case 48**

**Patient R.M./85,** 33 years, fourth gravidity, two parturitions.
**Record:** Two clinically intact children; one interruption.
**Clinical findings:** 16th week of pregnancy; no contributory findings.

**Ultrasonic findings:** Twin pregnancy; amorphous foetal primordium (Fig. 86, arrows); inconspicuous foetus; diamniotic.
**Indication for amniography:** Verification of ultrasonic find-

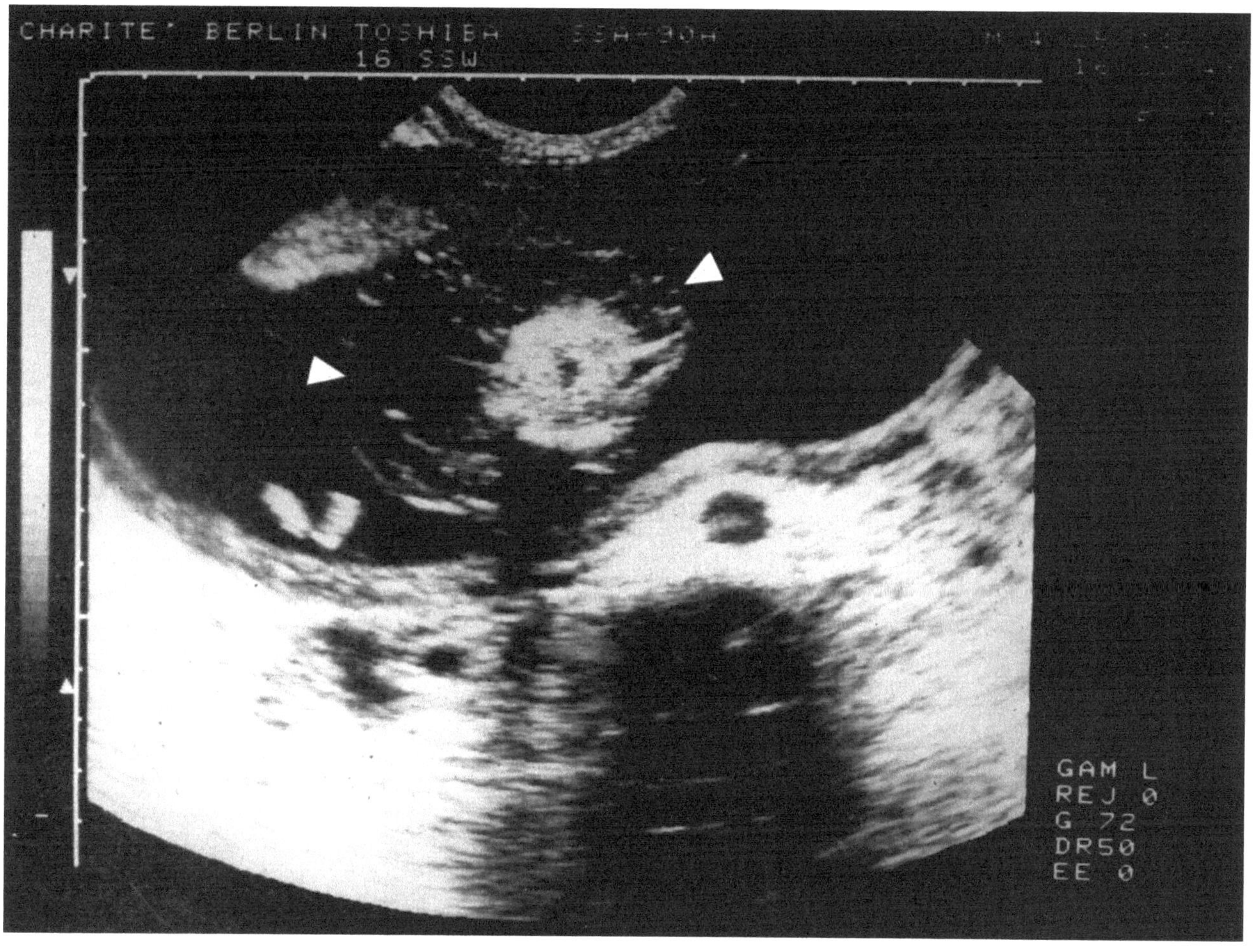


Fig. 86

Case 48 ings; possible detection of malformations in sonographically inconspicuous foetus.

**AFG findings** (Fig. 87: amniography 120 minutes from injection): **Only one amniotic cavity visible**; fluoroscopy shows **sonographically intact foetus** in cephalic presentation as recess in contrast medium; no unambiguous detectability of

g. 87

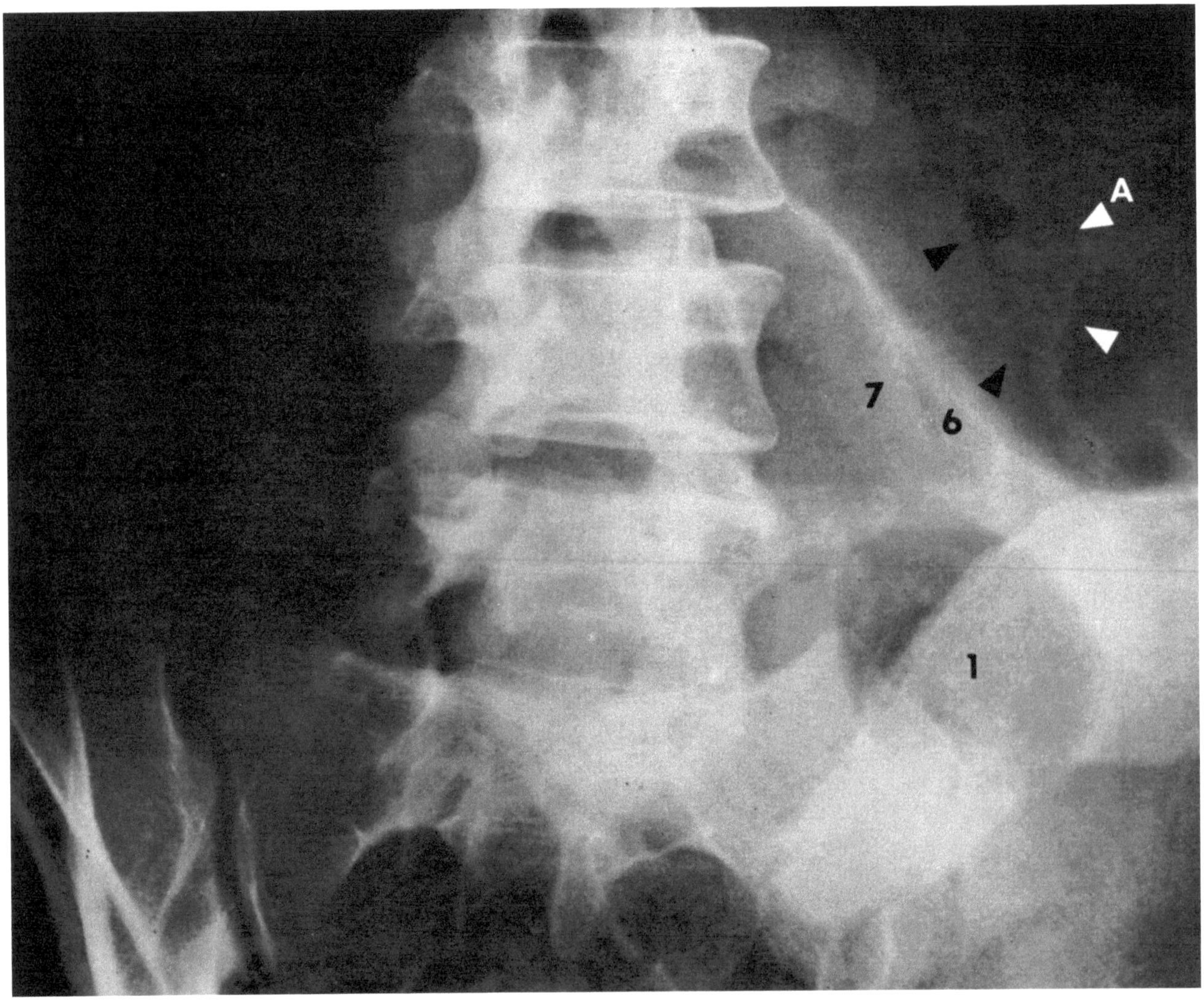

contrast medium in gastrointestinal canal; inconspicuous outer contours; regular configuration of skeleton; skeletal fragments of acephalic acardiacus detectable from non-contrast embryonic cavity (A; arrows).

**Clinical course:** Termination of pregnancy, six hours after amniocentesis.



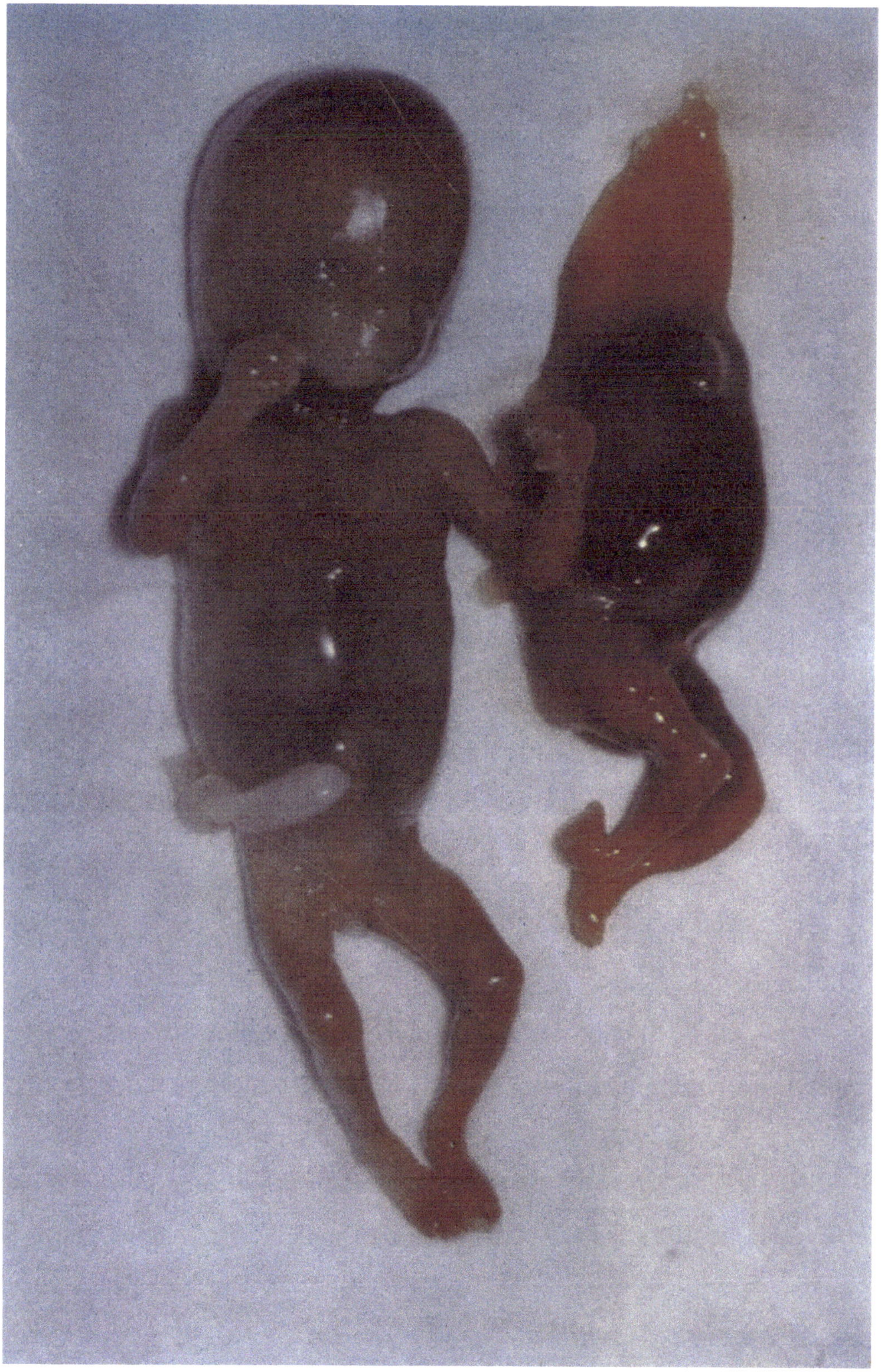

Fig. 88 a

Case 48 **Radiogram** (mammography technique; Fig. 88b):
1. Acardius acephalus, female.
2. No contrast medium detectable in gastro-intestinal tract; no contributory findings from skeleton and soft tissue of second foetus (male); clinical aspect shows Figure 88a.

No section made. ◁

Fig. 88b

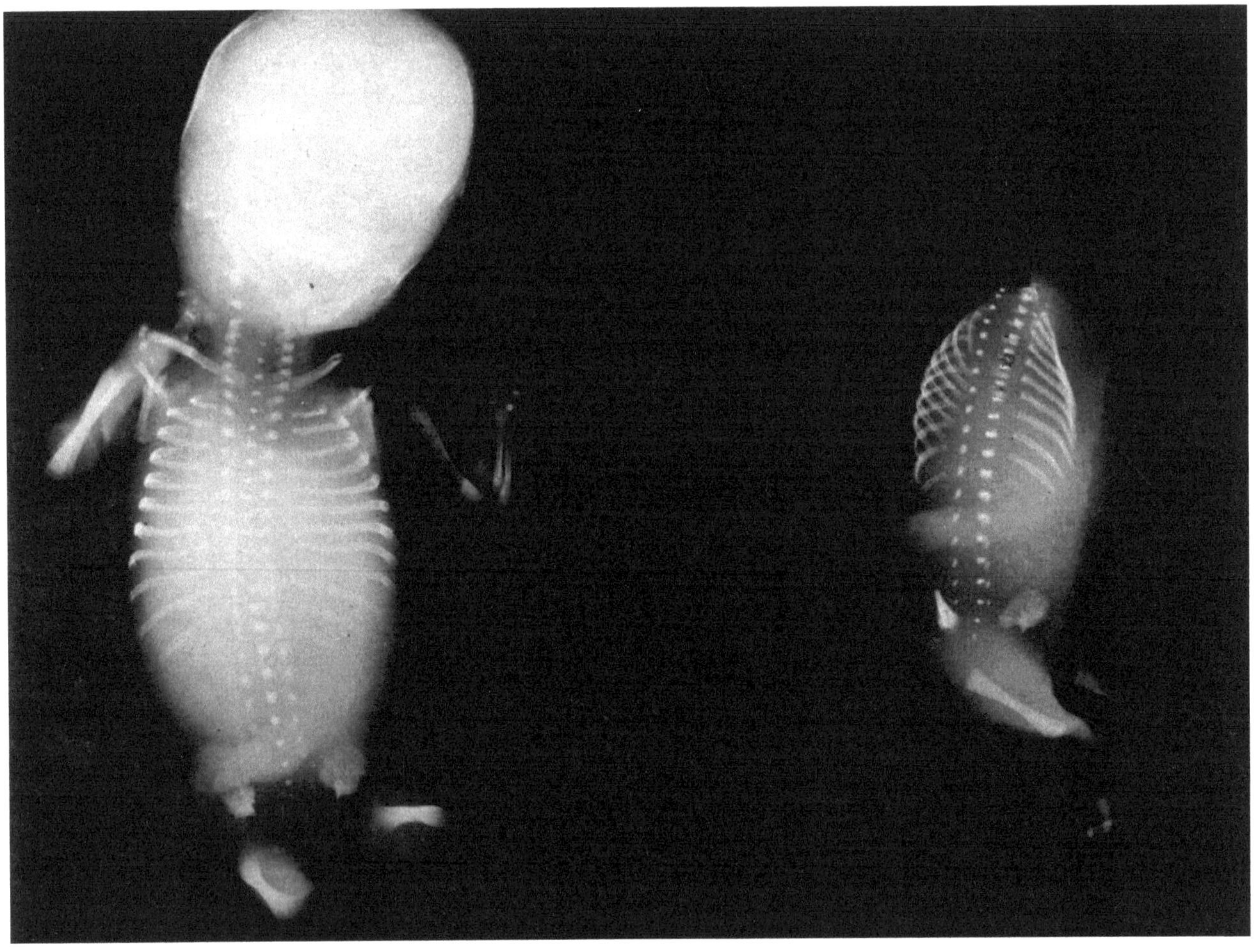

# 11.

## Literature


*Abét, L.; Natho, W.; Richter, J.; Prenzlau, P.:* Die Amniofetographie in der pränatalen Diagnostik fetaler Fehlbildungen und Erkrankungen. DDR-Med.-Report **16** (1987) 515

*Abét, L.; Natho, W.; Bollmann, R.; Prenzlau, P.:* Die Amniofetographie in der hochspezialisierten pränatalen Diagnostik fetaler Fehlbildungen und Erkrankungen. Med. aktuell **14** (1988) 244–247

*Adair, F. L.; Davis, M. E.:* Amniography with skiodan injections. A preliminary report. Amer. J. Obstet. **26** (1933) 881 – Ber. Gynäk. **2b** (1934) 446

*Aducci, J. E.; Olson, R. J.:* Transabdominal amniography and diagnosis of hydatidiform mole. Abdom. Surg. **12** (1970) 43

*Agüero, O.; Zighelboim, I.:* Amniographia en la mola hidatidiform. Rev. Obstet. Ginec. Venez. **29** (1968) 291

*Agüero, O.; Zighelboim, I.:* Fetography and molegraphy. Surg. Gynec. Obst. **130** (1070a) 649

*Agüero, O.; Zighelboim, I.:* Intrauterine diagnosis of fetal diaphragmatic hernia by amniography. Am. J. Obstet. Gynec. **107** (1970b) 971

*Agüero, O.; Zighelboim, I.:* Diagnostic radiology of fetal abnormalities. Int. J. Gynaecol. Obstet. **14** (1976) 314

*Albano, G.:* Amniosgrafia fetografia od orografia? (Qualche osservazione sulla terminologia nella radiodiagnostica da contrasto.) Radiol. med. **21** (1934) 52 – Ber. Gynäk. **26** (1934) 446

*Albano, G.; Gallina, E.:* Amniosgrafia. Tecnica, biologia, resultati. Agostiniana, Roma 1932 – Ber. Gynäk. **25** (1932) 68

*Alex, R.:* Röntgenologische Diagnose eine Thoracophagus während der Schwangerschaft. Zbl. Gynäkol. **74** (1952) 469

*Alumina, R.; Tapia, A.; Capetillo, M.; Hollstein, K.; Sepulveda, A.; Tolia, D.:* Escuriimento de liquido amniotica a amniocentesis. Rev. Chil. Obstet. Ginecol. **46** (1981) 142

*Amy, J. J.; Mandelman, N.:* Fetography: technique and applications. Eur. J. Obstet. Gynecol. Reprod. Biol. (1973) 25

*Ang, A. H.; Chon, W. F.; NG, K. K.:* Amniography in the early diagnosis of hydatiform mole. Brit. J. Radiol. **48** (1975) 979

*Angerstein, W.; Brandt, G. A.; Neumeister, K.:* Die Strahlenbelastung der Bevölkerung der DDR durch röntgendiagnostische Maßnahmen. Moderne Röntgenfotografie Heft **1** (1986) 9

*Arvis, P.; Le Pors, P.; Priou, G.; Fraisse, E.; Grall, J. Y.:* Le blessure de cordon au l'amniocentese tardive. J. Gynecol. Obstet. Biol. Reprod. (Paris) **12** (1983) 501

*Askenazy, M.; Borenstein, R.; Katz, Z.; Segal, M.:* Constriction of the umbilical cord by an amniotic band after mid-trimester amniocentesis. Acta Obstet. Gynecol. Scand. **61** (1982) 89

*Bakharev, V. A.; Karetnikova, N. A.; Moiseeva, E. N.:* Use of fetoamniography in the prenatal diagnosis of fetal congenital developments defects. Akush. Ginekol. – Moskva **3** (1986) 18 (russ.)

*Ballantyne, J. W.:* zitiert nach: *Sheares, B. U.:* Foetal abnormalities that cause difficult labor. J. Obstet. Gynaecol. Br. Emp. **48** (1941) 354

*Balsam, D.; Weiss, R. R.:* Amniography in prenatal diagnosis. Radiology **141** (1981) 379

*Bayer, H.:* Zur Frage der Geburtseinleitung bei Doppelmißbildungen. Zent.bl. Gynäkol. **89** (1967) 28

*Bayer, H.:* Praktische Gesichtspunkte zur Übernahme der Ultraschalldiagnostik in die Routine der Schwangerenbetreuung. Ultraschall **2** (1981) 267

*Becroft, D. M.; Smeeton, W. M.; Stewart, J. H.:* Fetal thyroid hyperplasia, rhesus immunization, and amniography. Arch. Dis. Child. **55** (1980) 213

*Becroft, D. M.; Stewart, J. H.; Smeeton, W. M.:* Rhesus sensitization, amniography, and thyroid hyperplasia. Lancet **II** (1976) 1191

*Bell, M. J.; Ternberg, J. L.:* Antenatal diagnosis of diaphragmatic hernia. Pediatrics **60** (1977) 738–740

*Bernaschek, G.; Dadak, C.; Kratochwil, A.:* Frühzeitige Diagnose fetaler Mißbildungen durch Ultraschall. Geburtsh. u. Frauenheilk. **40** (1980a) 868

*Bernaschek, G.; Kratochwil, A.; Spernol, R.:* Die Ultraschalldiagnose des fetalen Ascites. Geburtsh. u. Frauenheilk. **40** (1980b) 1029

*Berner, H. W.:* Amniography, an accurate way to localize the placenta. Obstet. Gynecol. **29** (1967) 200

*Bishop, P. A.:* The roentgenologic diagnosis of fetal hydrops. Am. J. Roentgenol. **86** (1961a) 415

*Bishop, P. A.:* Roentgenologic diagnosis on soft tissue dystocia. Radiol. Clin. N. Am. **5** (1961b) 8

*Blumberg, M. L.; Wohl, G. T.; Wiltchik, S.:* Placental localization by amniography. Am. J. Roentgenol. **100** (1967) 688

*Blunt, A.:* Conjoined twins: report of a case of thoracophagus. Aust. New Zeal. J. Obstet. Gynaec. **8** (1968) 29

*Bollmann, R.; Schilling, H.; Abét, L.; Zienert, A.; Möckel, A.; Weihrauch, A.:* Ergebnisse invasiver und pharmakosonographischer Untersuchungen in der Schwangerschaft. (I. Mitteilung). Zentralbl. Gynäkol. **110** (1988) 857

*Bollmann, R.; Schilling, H.; Abét, L.; Natho, W.; Zienert, A.; Möckel, A.; Weihrauch, P.:* Ergebnisse invasiver und pharmakosonographischer Untersuchungen in der Schwangerschaft. (II. Mitteilung: Amniofetographie) Zentralbl. Gynäkol. **110** (1988) 864

*Borden, S.; Rider, R. F.; Pollard, J. J.; Hendren, W. H.:* Radiology of conjoined twins. Am. J. Roentgenol. **120** (1974) 424

*Borelli, A. P.:* Amniography: Useful radiographic procedure. NY State J. Med. **67** (1967) 1395

*Boyd, J. J.; Bowman, J. M.; McInnis, A. C.; Kiernan, M. K.:* Fetal diaphragmatic hernia detected at intrauterine transfusion. Can. Med. Assoc. J. **100** (1969) 1105

*Bredow, V.; Schütz, M.; Theel, L.; Seidlitz, G.:* Zur Problematik des nichtimmunologischen fetalen Aszites – Kasuistik. Zentralbl. Gynäkol. **110** (1988) 578

*Bremme, K.; Eneroth, P.; Nilson, B.:* Hormone levels an amniotic fluid and maternal serum in women who undege spontaneous abortion after second trimester amniocentesis. Gynecol. Obstet. Invest. **18** (1984) 78

*Brezina, K.:* Die Röntgendiagnostik in der Geburtshilfe heute (Bedeutung und Strahlenbelastung). Wiener med. Wschr. **123** (1973) 709
*Broome, D. L.; Wilson, M. G.; Weiss, B.; Kellogg, B.:* Needle puncture of fetus: A complication of second-trimester amniocentesis. Am. J. Obstet. Gynecol. **126** (1976) 247
*Brosens, I.; Gordon, H.; Baert, A.:* Prediction of fetal maturity with combined cytological and radiological methods. J. Obstet. Gynaec. Brit. Owlth. **76** (1969) 20
*Bruce, S.; Duffy, J. D.; Wolf, J. E. jr.:* Skin dimpling associated with midtrimester amniocentesis. Pediatr. Dermatol. **2** (1984) 140
*Brusis, E.; Rjosk, H. K.; Kuss, E.:* Wertigkeit der Alpha-1-Fetoprotein-Bestimmung für die Diagnose fetaler Mißbildungen bei Patientinnen mit Hydramnion. Geburtsh. u. Frauenheilk. **40** (1980) 818
*Burke, F. J.:* Placenta praevia – amniography. J. Obstet. Gynacc. Brit. Emp. **42** (1935) 1096
*Burke, F. J.:* Amniography. Ber. Gynäk. **31** (1936) 702
*Cash, M. B.; Kornmesser, J. G.:* Diagnosis of a fetal neck mass by amniography. Radiology **91** (1968) 476
*Caterini, H. R.; Rubino, S. M.; Kaminetzky, H. A.:* Amniography during subsequent pregnancy for evaluating the postcesarean section uterine scar. Obstet. Gynecol. **39** (1972) 717
*Caterini, H. R.; Sama, J.; Iffy, L.; Harrigan, J.; Pelosi, M.:* A revaluation of amniography. Obstet. Gynecol. **47** (1976) 373
*Cerrolaza Asenjo, J.; Gomez de Blas, F.; Caballero Peregrini, P.; Nadal Moncadas, B.:* Valor de la amniografia en la eufermedad hemolitica perinatal. Toko-ginec. pract. pract. **30** (1971) 851
*Cetroni, M.; Azzariti, M.:* Über die Amniographie. Zbl. Gynäkol. **58** (1934) 1132
*Cheng, W. C.:* The value of amniography in early diagnosis of hydatidiform mole. J. Obstet. Gynaec. Brit. Cwlth. **74** (1967) 753
*Chinn, D. H.; Filly, R. A.; Callen, P. A.:* Congenital diaphragmatic hernia diagnosed prenatally by ultrasound. Radiology **148** (1983) 119
*Christensen, J. B.; Hesseldahl, H.; Dorph, S.:* Omfalocele diagnosticeret ved ultralydunders gelse og amniografi. Ugeskr. Laeger. **144** (1982) 3356
*Connon, A. F.:* Antenatal diagnosis of spina bifida. J. Obstet. Gynaecol. Br. Cwlth. **81** (1974) 753
*Cornell, E. L.; Case, J. T.:* Neoskidan in amniography. Amer. J. Obstet. **27** (1934) 894 – Ber. Gynäk. **28** (1935) 199
*Crane, J. P.; Kopta, M. M.:* Genetic amniocentesis: impact of placental position upon risk of pregnancy loss. Am. J. Obstet. Gynecol. **150** (1984) 813
*Creasman, W. T.; Lawrence, R. A.; Thiedes, H. A.:* Fetal complications of amniocentesis. JAMA **204** (1968) 949
*Crosby, W.:* Fetal respiratory distress following fetography. Am. J. Obstet. Gynecol. **121** (1975) 958
*Cruikshank, D. P.; Varner, M. W.; Cruikshank, J. E.; Grant, S. S.; Donnelly, E.:* Midtrimester amniocentesis. An analysis of 932 cases with neonatal follow up. Am. J. Obstet. Gynecol. **139** (1983) 204
*Da Cunha, S. P.; Araujo Bezerra, M. M.; Bailao, L. A.; Yazelle, M. E. H. D.; Franco, J. G.; Martinez, A. E.:* Contribuicào da amniografia no setudo de patologias obstetricas. Obstet. Ginec. lat.-amer. **32** (1974) 93
*Dahl, J.; Witkowski, R.; Prenzlau, P.; Reinhold-Richter, L.; Abét, L.; Nitz, I.:* Kurzrippen-Polydaktylie-Syndrom (Saldino-Noonan) – eine perinatal letale Kombination schwerer Fehlbildungen. Z. Klin. Med. **43** (1988) 493
*Dallaire, L.; Belanger, L.; Smith, C. J.; Kelleher, P. C.:* Origin of amniocenteses-induced rises of alpha-fetoprotein-concentrations in maternal serum. Br. J. Obstet. Gynaecol. **147** (1984) 586
*Daw, E.:* Fetography. Am. J. Obstet. Gynecol. **115** (1973) 718
*Delaplane, D.; Wiringa, K. S.; Shulman, S. T.; Yoger, R.:* Congenital mucocutaneous candidiasis following diagnostic amniocentesis. Am. J. Obstet. Gynecol. **147** (1983) 342
*Dellenbach, P.; Walter, J.; Hartman, J.:* Amniographie, fetographie, amniofetographie. Technique e interet. Rev. Fr. Gynecól. Obstet. **70** (1975) 401
*Denavit, M. F.; Lecointre, C.; Mullet, E.; Menibus, C. de; Bosssier, A.:* Un accident de l'amniofetographie: l'hypothyroidie. Arch. Franc. Ped. **34** (1977) 543
*Duchatel, F.; Delseny, P.; O'Hana, R.; L'Huillier, P.:* Estenose duodenale. Diagnostique echographique et critique de l'amniofetographie. Rev. Franc. Gynécol. Obstét. **74** (1979) 47
*Duenhoelter, J. H.; Santos-Ramos, R.; Rosenfeld, R.:* Prenatal diagnosis of gastrointestinal tract obstruction. Obstet. Gynecol. **47** (1976) 618
*Duenhoelter, H. J.; Santos-Ramos, R.:* Diagnose kongenitaler Mißbildungen vor der Geburt mit Sonographie und Amniofetographie. Arch. Gynäk. **224** (1977) 105
*Dunnihoo, D. R.; Harris, R. E.:* The diagnosis of monoamniotic twinning by amniography. Am. J. Obstet. Gynecol. **96** (1966) 894
*Ehrhardt, K.:* Der trinkende Fetus. Münch. med. Wschr. **42** (1937) 1699
*Elliot, K.:* Candidiasis after diagnostic amniocentesis. Letter. Am. J. Obstet. Gynecol. **149** (1984) 586
*Erbslöh, J.:* Das intrauterine Fetogramm. Arch. Gynäk. **173** (1941/42) 160
*Erbslöh, J.:* Zur Frage der röntgenologischen Darstellung der Körperoberfläche des Feten in utero. Zbl. Gynäk. **66** (1942a) 250
*Erbslöh, J.:* Darstellung der graviden Gebärmutter nach intraamnialer Injektion von Immetal. Zbl. Gynäk. **66** (1942b) 1911
*Erbslöh, J.:* Die Methoden der röntgenologischen Darstellung der schwangeren Gebärmutter mit Hilfe von Kontrastmitteln (Amniographie, Placentographie und Fetographie). Geburtsh. u. Frauenheilk. **4** (1942c) 349
*Erbslöh, J.:* Das intrauterine Fetogramm, ein Beitrag zur geburtshilflichen Röntgendiagnostik. Röntgenpraxis **14** (1942d) 28
*Fagan, C. J.:* Antepartum diagnosis of conjoined twins by ultrasonography. Am. J. Roentgenol. **129** (1977) 921
*Fairweather, D. V. I.; Tacchi, D.; Coxon, A.; Hughes, M. I.; Murray, S.; Walker, W.:* Brit. Med. Journ. **4** (1967) 189

*Fernhoff, P. M.; Marion, J. P.; Priest, J. H.*: Limitations of amniography in the prenatal diagnosis of spina bifida. Am. J. Med. Genet. **7** (1980) 369
*Ferris, E. J.; Shapiro, J. H.; Spira, J.*: Roentgenologic aspects of intrauterine transfusion. JAMA **196** (1966) 635
*Finegan, J. A. K.*: Amniotic fluid and midtrimester amniocentesis: a review. Br. J. Obstet. Gynaecol. **91** (1984) 745
*Finegan, J. A. K.; Quarrington, B. J.; Hughes, H. E.; Rudd, N. L.; Stevens, L. J.; Weksberg, R.; Doran, T. A.*: Midtrimester amniocentesis: Obstetrics outcome and neonatal neurobehavioral status. Am. J. Obstet. Gynecol. **150** (1984) 989
*Fochem, K.*: Einführung in die geburtshilfliche und gynäkologische Röntgendiagnostik. Amniographie und Fetographie. Thieme, Stuttgart 1967, S. 54
*Fracasso, E.*: In proposition della diagnosi radiologica di mola vesciolare. Quad. Red. **18** (1955) 449
*Frigoletto, F. D.; Griscom, N. T.*: Amniography for the detection of fetal myelomeningocele. Obstet. Gynecol. **44** (1974) 286
*Frischkorn, R.*: Hat die Röntgendiagnostik in der Schwangerschaft noch ihre Berechtigung? Geburtsh. u. Frauenheilk. **33** (1973) 125
*Galle, P. C.; Meis, P. J.*: Complications of amniocentesis: a review. J. Reprod. Med. **27** (1982) 149
*Garndt, J.; Hamblin, T. J.; Smith, D. S.; Wellstead, L.*: Plasmaphoresis in the Rh hemolytic disease: The danger of amniocentesis. Int. J. Artif. Organs **6** (1983) 83
*Gautry, J. P.; Vielh, J. P.; Hurraux-Rendu, C.*: Amniocentese enfin de gestation: interet, appreciation du risque. Nouv. Presse Med. **9** (1980) 929
*Gilberg, C.; Rasmussen, P.; Wahlstrom, J.*: Long-term follow-up of children born after amniocentesis. Clin. Genet. **21** (1982) 69
*Glätzner, H.; Halberstadt, E.; Stein, W. W.; Wernicke, K.*: Aussagemöglichkeit der Amniographie. Arch. Gynäk. **224** (1977) 105
*Golbus, M. S.; Stephens, J. D.; Cann, H. M.; Mann, J.; Hensleigh, P. A.*: RH-isoimmunization following genetic amniocentesis. Prenat. Diagn. **2** (1982) 149
*Goldman, J. A.; Peleg, D.*: Massive etraperitoneal bleeding – a rare complication of amniocentesis. Acta Obstet. Gynecol. Scand. **59** (1980) 283
*Granjon, A.*: A propos du diagnostic du sexe pedant la grossesse. Presse Méd. **57** (1948) 688
*Gravenhorst, J. B.*: Intrauterine transfusion, a therapeutic intervention in Erythroblastosis fetalis. Diss. Leyden 1968
*Grech, P.; Spitz, L.*: Fetal complications of amniography. Brit. J. Radiol. **50** (1977) 110
*Grepin, G.; Dela Housse, G.; Decocq, J.*: Incidence de l'amniofoetographie sur la thyroide foetale. J. Gynecol. Obstet. biol. Reprod. 1978, 7/8, S. 1405–1413
*Griscom, N. T.*: Possible radiologic approaches to fetal diagnosis and therapy. Clin. Perinatol. **1** (1974) 435
*Griscom, N. T.*: Radiographic fetal diagnosis. In: Heriditary disorders of the fetus: Diagnosis, prevention and treatment. Edited by: Milemsky, A., Plenum Press, New York 1979a
*Griscom, N. T.; Frigoletto, F. D.; Harris, G. B. G.*: Amniography in second trimester diagnosis of myelomeningocele. Am. J. Roentgenol. **133** (1979b) 1151
*Griscom, N. T.; Harris, G. B. G.; Umansky, I.; Easterday, C. L.; Frigoletto, F. D.*: Internal radiographic anatomy of the intrauterine fetus. Progr. Pediatr. Radiol. **3** (1970) 344
*Haberstroh, W. D.; Hichman, M.; Slate, W. G.*: Fetal bleeding and bradycardia following diagnostic amniocentesis. Del. Med. J. **55** (1983) 211
*Halle, H.; Richter, J.; Prenzlau, P.; Kunz, B.*: Die Amniofetographie in der antenatalen Diagnostik fetaler Mißbildungen. Zbl. Gynäkol. **99** (1977) 37
*Hansmann, M.*: Nachweis und Ausschluß fetaler Entwicklungsstörungen mittels Ultraschall-Screening und gezielter Untersuchung – ein Mehrstufenkonzept. Ultraschall **2** (1981) 206
*Hansmann, M.; Schlächter, H.; Födisch, H. J.; Plotz, E. J.*: Präpartale Diagnose eines Thoracophagus mittels Ultrasonographie. Gynäkologe **12** (1979) 64
*Harrison, M. R.; Adzick, N. S.; Nakayama, D. K.; de Lorimier, A. A.*: Fetal diaphragmatic hernia: Pathophysiology, natural history, and outcome. Clin. Obstet. Gynecol. **29** (1986) 490
*Hasaart, T. H.; Essed, G. G.*: Amniotic fluid embolism after transabdominal amniocentesis. Eur. J. Obstet. Gynecol. Reprod. Biol. **16** (1983) 25
*Hensleigh, P. A.; Cann, H.*: Rh-sensitization after genetic amniocentesis. Letter. Obstet. Gynecol. **58** (1981) 136
*Hesseldahl, H.; Als, O.; Dorph, S.; Kjer, J. J.; Ström, K. V.*: Prenatal diagnosis of omphalocele by ultrasound and amniography. Acta Obstet. Gynecol. Scand. **59** (1980) 83
*Hill, L. M.; Platt, L. D.; Kellogg, B.*: Rh-sensitization after genetic amniocentesis. Obstet. Gynecol. **56** (1980) 459
*Hinselmann, M.*: Die pränatale Diagnostik kindlicher Mißbildungen in der zweiten Schwangerschaftshälfte. Gynäkologe **6** (1973) 189
*Hinst, J.; Stencl, J.*: Komplikácie po transabdominalnej amniocentéze a ich prevencia. Bratisl. lek. listy. **84** (1985) 94
*Hislop, A.; Fairweather, D. V.; Blackwell, R. J.; Howard, S.*: The effect of amniocentesis and drainage of amniotic fluid on lung development in Maccaca fascicularis. Br. J. Obstet. Gynaecol. **91** (1984) 835
*Holzgreve, W.; Hansmann, M.*: Erfahrung mit der "Free Hand Needle"-Technik bei 3215 Amniozentesen im 2. Trimenon zur pränatalen Diagnostik. Gynäkologe **17** (1984a) 77
*Holzgreve, W.; Wagner, H.; Rempen, A.*: Möglichkeiten der pränatalen Beurteilung von normaler und gestörter Neuralrohrentwicklung durch Ultraschall. medwelt **35** (1984b) 1344
*Horger, E. O.; McCarter, L. M.*: Prenatal diagnosis of sacrococcygeal teratoma. Am. J. Obstet. Gynecol. **134** (1979) 228
*Houlton, M. C. C.; Sutton, M.; Aitken, J.*: Antenatal diagnosis of duodenal atresia. J. Obstet. Gynaecol. Br. Commw. **81** (1974) 818
*Hubinont, C.; Pratola, D.; Rothschild, E.; Rodesch, F.; Schwers, J.*: Dicephalus: Unusual case of conjoined twins and its prepartum diagnosis. Am. J. Obstet. Gynecol. **149** (1984) 693

*Jonatha, W.*: Stellenwert von Fetoskopie und Amniographie. – In: Pränatale Diagnostik, 2. Bochumer Symposium/ Herausg.: Engert, J.; Quakernack, K. – Z. Wissenschaftliche Information (MILUPA/Friedrichsdorf) **11** (1985) 31
*Kellner, K. R.; Cruz, A. C.; Gelman, S. R.; Uries, J. K.; Spellacy, W. N.*: Percutaneous fetal ventriculography: a simplified technique to aid in the management of the hydrocephalic fetus. J. Reprod. Med. **24** (1980) 225
*Kelly, D. R.; Grant, E. G.; Zeman, R. K.; Choyke, P. L.; Bolan, J. C.; Warsof, S. L.*: In utero diagnosis of congenital diaphragmatic hernia by CT amniography. J. Comput. Assist. Tomogr. **10** (1986) 500
*Kerr, J. M.; McKay, W. G.*: Amniography. Trans. Edin. Obstet. Soc. **21** (1933a) 75
*Kerr, J. M.; McKay, W. G.*: The diagnosis of placenta praevia with special reference to employment of x-rays for this purpose. Edinburgh M. J. **40** (1933b) 21
*King, T. M.; Wollschlaeger, G. R.*: Amniography in the intrauterine transfusion: Demonstration of an intestinal obstruction in a newborn. South Med. J. **60** (1967) 189
*Kjessler, B.; Hemmingsen, A.; Nilson, B. A.; Johannson, S. G. O.*: Early diagnosis of trophoblastic disease and fetal maldevelopment by determination of alpha-fetoprotein, human choriongonadotropin and amniography. Acta Obstet. Gynecol. Scand. (Suppl.) **69** (1977) 83
*Klein, S. A.; Young, B. K.; Wilson, S. J.; Katz, M.*: Continous fetal monitoring following third-trimester amniocentesis. Obstet. Gynecol. **58** (1981) 444
*Knochel, J. Q.; Lee, T. G.; Melendez, M. G.; Henderson, S. G.*: Fetal anomalies involving the thorax and abdomen. Radiol. Clin. North Am. **20** (1982) 297
*Knox, E.*: The effect of amniography on amniotic fluid L/S ratio. Obstet. Gynecol. **49** (1977) 154
*Kopecki, P.; Jung, H.; Cen, M.*: Zur Technik der intrauterinen Transfusion bei Rhesus-Erkrankungen mittels der Oberflächendarstellung durch Lipiodol-Ultrafluid. Geburtsh. u. Frauenheilk. **29** (1969) 239
*Kopecki, P.; Jung, H.; Lahmann, H.; Lindenfelser, R.*: Klinische Erfahrungen mit der Amniographie bei der pränatalen Transfusion und Untersuchungen zur Frage der Kontrastmittelresorption des Feten. Z. Geburtsh. u. Perinat. **178** (1974) 360
*Kräubig, H.*: Die röntgenologische Darstellung des Kindes in utero durch die Fetographie. Fortschr. Röntgenstr. **86** (1957) 351
*Kurjak, A.*: Ultrasound diagnosis of congenital malformations. In: Handbook of clinical ultrasound. Publ. by Wiley and Sons, New York 1975, S. 189
*Lefebvre, J.; Granjon, A.; Méric, A.*: L'amniographie. J. de. Radiol. Electrol. **29** (1948) 601
*Leitsmann, H.; Schlegel, C.; Ruckhäberle, K. E.*: Erfahrungen zur Amniofetographie in der 2. Hälfte der Schwangerschaft. Zbl. Gynäkol. **102** (1980) 881
*Lele, A. S.; Camardy, P. J.; Hurd, M. E.; O'Leary, J. A.*: Fetomaternal bleeding following diagnostic amniocentesis. Obstet. Gynecol. **60** (1982) 60
*Lenke, R. R.; Ashwood, E. R.; Cyr, D. R.; Gravett, M.; Smith, J. R.; Stenchever, M. A.*: Genetic amniocentesis: Significancy of intraamniotic bleeding and placental location. Obstet. Gynecol. **65** (1985) 798
*Lennon, G. G.*: Intrauterine foetal visualization. J. Obstet. Gynaecol. Br. Cwlth. **74** (1967) 227
*Leschot, N. J.; Verjaal, M.; Treffers, P. E.*: Risks of midtrimester amniocentesis: Assesment in 3000 pregnancies. Br. J. Obstet. Gynaecol. **92** (1985) 804
*Liley, A. W.*: Intrauterine transfusion of foetus in haemolytic disease. Brit. Med. J. **2** (1963) 1107
*Lindinger, A.; Huhn, W.*: Hypothyreote Struma nach Amniofetographie. Z. Geburtsh. u. Perinat. **183** (1979) 461
*Mandelbaum, B.*: Increased fetal scalp thickness: A new sign of fetal death. Am. J. Obstet. Gynec. **114** (1972) 809
*McLain, C. R. jr.*: Amniography studies of the gastrointestinal motility of the human fetus. Am. J. Obstet. Gynec. **86** (1963) 1079
*McLain, C. R.*: Amniography, a versatile diagnostic procedure in obstetrics. Obstet. Gynecol. **23** (1964) 45
*McLain, C. R.*: Amniography for diagnosis and management of fetal death in utero. Obstet. Gynecol. **26** (1965) 233
*McLain, C. R.; Russel, P. T.*: Amniography studies of chronic distress in hypertensive disorders of pregnancy. Am. J. Obstet. Gynecol. **107** (1970) 673
*Melin, J. R.*: Intrapartum diagnosis of conjoined twins. Obstet. Gynecol. **29** (1967) 50
*Menees, T. O.; Miller, J. D.; Holly, J. E.*: Amniography. Am. J. Roentgenol. **24** (1930) 363
*Mennuti, M. T.*: Neural tube defects. Obstet. Gynecol. **52** (1978) 510
*Mennuti, M. T.; Moranz, J. G.; Schwarz, R. H.; Mellman, W. J.*: Amniography for the early detection of neural tube defects. Obstet. Gynecol. **49** (1977) 25
*Mennuti, M. T.; Brummonf, W.; Cromebleholme, W. R.; Schwarz, R. N.; Arvan, D. A.*: Fetal-maternal bleeding associated with genetic amniocentesis. Obstet. Gynecol. **55** (1980) 48
*Mennuti, M. T.; Di Gaetano, A.; McDonnell, A.; Cohen, A. W.; Listen, R. M.*: Fetal-maternal bleeding associated with genetic amniocentesis real-time versus static ultrasound. Obstet. Gynecol. **62** (1982) 26
*Merin, S.; Beyth, Y.*: Uniocular congenital blindness as a complication of midtrimester amniocentesis. Am. J. Ophthalmol. **89** (1980) 299
*Meschan, I.; Nelson, L. H.; Watson, N. E.; Ott, D. J.*: Geburtshilfe und Gynäkologie. In: *Meschan, I.*: Diagnostik mit bildgebenden Verfahren. Band I/1: Abdomen, Teil 1. Ferdinand Enke Verlag, Stuttgart, 1988, S. 312–389
*Messana, V.; Rubino, S. M.; Sorrentino, A.*: La fetografia. Rad. Prat. **20** (1970) 37
*Messana, V.; Rubino, S. M.*: An application of fetography. JAMA **228** (1974) 1639
*Messana, V.; Rubino, S. M.*: La fetografia per la diagnosi di post-maturità fetale. Min. Gin. **27** (1975) 858
*Miething, R.*: Transitorische Hypothyreose bei Früh- und Neugeborenen nach Amniofetographie während der Schwangerschaft. Klin. Pädiatr. **193** (1981) 372
*Mikusova, M.; Kodl, D.; Snobr, J.*: Odhad d avky v plodu. Cesk. Radiol. **36** (1982) 326

*Möbius, W.*: Geburtshilfliche Strahlen- und Röntgendiagnostik. Akademie-Verlag, Berlin 1967, S. 42–47
*Moessinger, A. C.; Blanc, W. A.; Byrne, J.; Andrews, D.; Warburton, D.: Blom, A.*: Amniotic band syndrom associated with amniocentesis. Am. J. Obstet. Gynecol. **141** (1981) 588
*Moessinger, A. C.; Bassi, G. A.; Ballantyne, G.; Collins, M. H.; James, L. S.; Blanc, W. A.*: Experimental production of pulmonary dysplasia following amniocentesis and oligohydramnios. Early Hum. Dev. **8** (1983) 343
*Mohr, J.*: Fetal genetic diagnosis: development of techniques for early sampling of fetal cells. Acta Pathol. Microbiol. Scand. **73** (1968) 37–41
*Müller-Holve, W.; Garbe, U.; Kohlmann, H.; Martin, K.*: Ultraschall-Basis-Untersuchung (U.B.U.) in der Schwangerschaft. Geburtsh. u. Frauenheilk. **41** (1981) 607
*Murray, J. C.; Karp, L. E.; Williamson, R. A.; Cheng, E. Y.; Luthy, D. A.*: Rh isoimmunization related to amniocentesis. Am. J. Med. Genet. **16** (1983) 527
*Muti, W.; Wanjun, L.; Hong, F.; Yueying, W.; Fengxian, H.*: Neonatal screening for congenital hypothyroidism by using RIA determination of TSH in dried blood spot. Acta Univ. med. Tongji **15** (1986) 81
*Natho, W.*: Indikationen zur Amniofetographie in der pränatalen Diagnostik. Dissertation A, Humboldt-Universität zu Berlin, 1988, 123 S.
*Natho, W.; Abét, L.; Bollmann, R.; Kursawe, R.; Giest, H.; Körner, H.*: Pränatale Diagnose einer Duodenalstenose – Ein Fallbericht. Radiologia diagn. **29** (1988) 71
*Natho, W.; Abét, L.; Bollmann, R.; Prenzlau, P.; Halle, H.; Richter, J.*: Röntgendiagnostik in der Schwangerschaft heute? Die Amniofetographie in der pränatalen Diagnostik. Zeitschr. Klin. Med. **45** (1990) 573
*Natho, W.; Abét, L.; Bollmann, R.; Prenzlau, P.*: Indikationen zur Amniofetographie in der pränatalen Diagnostik fetaler Fehlbildungen und Erkrankungen. Radiol. diagn. **30** (1989) 271
National Council on Radiation Protection and Measurement (NCRP): Medical radiation exposure of pregnant and potentially pregnant woman. Washington D.C., 1977. (NRCP report No. 54, p. 11)
*Neering Tessaro, A., Chasler, C. N.*: Amniography as an aid in intrauterine transfusion. Am. J. Roentgenol. **103** (1968) 195
*Neldam, S.; Pederson, J. F.*: Fetal heart rate response to amniocentesis in early pregnancy. J. Perinat. Med. **8** (1980) 209
*Nolan, G. H.; Schmickel, R. D.; Chantaratherakitti, P.; Knickerbocker, C.; Hamman, J.; Louwsma, G.*: The effect of ultrasonography on midtrimester genetic amniocentesis complications. Am. J. Obstet. Gynecol. **140** (1981) 531
*Noonan, C. D.*: Antenatal diagnosis of fetal abnormalities. In: Symposium on obstetric and gynecologic radiology. Ed. by *Schreiber, M. H.*, The radiologic clinics of North America, W.B. Saunders Company, Philadelphia – London – Toronto, April 1974, Vol. XII, No. 1, p. 13
*Neumeister, N.*: Genetische und somatische Risiken in der Röntgendiagnostik. Radiol. diagn. **23** (1982) 408
*Ogden, J. A.; Wade, M. E.; Davis, C. D.*: Radiology **93** (1969) 1315
*Ogita, S.; Hasegawa, H.; Matsumoto, M.; Kamei, T.; Shimamoto, T.; Ohnishi, M.; Sugawa, T.*: Prenatal diagnosis of E trisomy syndrome by fetography. Obstet. Gynecol. **43** (1974) 887
*Ogita, S.; Kamei, T.; Matsumoto, M.; Shimamoto, T.; Shimura, K.*: Prenatal diagnosis of osteogenesis imperfecta congenita by means of fetography. Eur. J. Pediatr. **123** (1976) 179
*Ogita, S.; Kamei, T.; Sugawa, T.*: Estimation of fetal weight by fetography. Am. J. Obstet. Gynecol. **127** (1977) 37
*Oide, S.; Yamaguchi, H.; Niizu, N.; Takahashi, S.; Takashima, K.*: Transient neonatal hypothyroidism probably due to contrast media used in fetal radiography. Hornman T. Rinsho. **31** (1983) 76
*Opri, F.; Kirchner, H.*: Diagnostik fetaler Mißbildungen – eine seltene Komplikation bei der Amniographie. Zbl. Gynäkol. **100** (1978) 1044
*Opri, F.; Kirchner, H.*: Die Stellung der Amniozentese in der pränatalen Diagnostik. Amniozentese und Amniografie im Rahmen der pränatalen Diagnostik. Zbl. Gynäkol. **102** (1980) 71
*Palle, C.; Andersen, J. W.; Tabor, A.; Lauritsen, J. G.; Sang, J.; Philip, J.*: Increased risk of abortion after genetic amniocentesis in twin pregnancies. Prenat. Diagn. **3** (1983) 83
*Panayobon, P. P.; Vrettos, A. S.; Koliopoúlos, C.*: Amniofetography in obstetrics: diagnostic procedure. Int. Surg. **57** (1972) 137
*Pauwen, J. G.; Lammers, B.*: Über die röntgenologische Darstellung der Frucht im Mutterleib (Fetographie) beim akuten Hydramnion. Z. Geburtsh. Gynäk. **129** (1948) 268
*Persand, F. V. N.*: Problems of birth defects. – MTP Press: Lancaster, England
*Porreco, R. P.; Young, P. E.; Resnik, L.; Cousins, L.; Jones, O. W.; Richards, T.; Kernahan, C.; Matson, M.*: Reproductive outcome following amniocentesis for genetic indications. Am. J. Obstet. Gynecol. **143** (1982) 653
*Portes, L.; Lefebvre, J.; Granjon, A.*: L'amniografie. Gynéc. et Obst. **47** (1948) 378
*Portman, M. A.; Brouiletee, R. T.*: Fatal intracranial hemorrhage complicationg amniocentesis. Am. J. Obstet. Gynecol. **144** (1982) 731
*Prenzlau, P.; Abét, L.*: Sonographische Darstellung intrafetaler Zysten und deren Differentialdiagnose. Zbl. Gynäkol. **105** (1983) 982
*Prenzlau, P.; Witt, J.; Götze, W.*: Verletzung des fetalen Thorax nach Amniozentese. Z. Klin. Med. **41** (1986) 2223
*Queenan, J. T.*: Amniocentesis and transamniotic fetal transfusion for Rh-diseases. Clin. Obstet. Gynec. **9** (1966) 491
*Queenan, J. T.; von Gal, H. V.; Kurarych, S. F.*: Amniography for clinical evaluation of erythroblastosis fetalis. Am. J. Obstet. Gynecol. **102** (1968) 264
*Queenan, J. T.; Gadow, E. C.*: Amniography for detection of congenital malformation. Obstet. Gynecol. **35** (1970) 648
*Raimer, S. S.; Raimer, B. G.*: Needle puncture scars from midtrimester amniocentesis. Arch. Dermatol. **120** (1984) 1360
*Ranke, M.; Nothjunge, J.; Mentzel, H.*: Kongenitale Struma bei einem Frühgeborenen nach Amniographie. Monatsschr. Kinderheilkd. **125** (1977) 941

*Raphael, M. J.; Gordon, H.; Schiff, D.*: Radiological aspects of intra-uterine blood transfusion. Br. J. Radiol. **40** (1967) 520
*Ravina, J.; Hazout, A.; Touratier, P.; Jamain, B.*: L'amniofetographie. Nouv. Press. Med. **5** (1976) 787
*Reifferscheid, W.; Schliemann, R.*: Röntgenographischer Nachweis der intrauterinen Atembewegungen des Fetus. Zent. Bl. Gynäk. **63** (1939) 146 und Zent. Bl. Gynäk. **64** (1940) 75
*Roberts, N. S.; Dunn, L. K.; Weiner, S.; Godmilow, L.; Miller, R.*: Midtrimester amniocentesis. J. Reprod. Med. **28** (1983) 167
*Rodesch, F.; Camus, M.; Ermans, A. M.; Dodion, J.; Delange, F.*: Adverse effect of amniofetography on fetal thyroid function. Am. J. Obstet. Gynecol. **126** (1976) 723
*Ron, M.; Cohen, T.; Yaffe, H.; Beyth, Y.*: The clinical significance of blood-contaminated midtrimester amniocentesis. Acta Obstet. Gynecol. Scand. **61** (1982) 43
*Rubino, S. M.*: The diagnosis of an intact hydatiform mole with coexistent fetus by amniography. Obstet. Gynecol. **46** (1975) 364
*Rubino, S. M.; Messana, V.*: L'utilita dell'amniografia uella practica ostetrica. Att. Ost. Gin. **15** (1969) 465
*Rubino, S. M.; Messana, V.; Rossi, T.*: L'opacizzazione delle vie urinarie come segno indiretto per la diagnosi amniografica di mola vescicolare. Rad. Prat. **20** (1970) 45
*Rubino, S. M.; Messana, V.*: Amniografia et amniocentesi: due tecniche diagnostiche complementari. Pat. Clin. Ostet. Gin. **2** (1974a) 132
*Rubino, S. M.; Messana, V.*: Amniografia: nouve possibilita diagnostiche di una "vecchia" tecniche. Pat. Clin. Ostet. Gin. **2** (1974b) 177
*Rubino, S. M.; Messana, V.; Fiorino, S.*: Amniografia e fetografia: due tecniche diagnostiche spesso complementari. Ann. Ost. Gin. Med. Perin. **97** (1976) 374
*Russell, J. G. B.*: Radiology in the diagnosis of fetal abnormalities. J. Obst. Gynaec. Brit. Comm. **76** (1969) 345
*Sadovsky, E.; Eyal, F. G.; Perlman, M.; Beyth, Y.*: Decreased fetal activity and fetal heart rate changes after amniocentesis complicated by fetal hemorrhage. Int. J. Gynaecol. Obstet. **19** (1981) 395
*Salvador Monte, R.; Muxi Olives, A.; Perez Soler, J.; Duran de Hoyos, A.*: La amniografia en al diagnostico de la fetopathia diabetica. Radiologia – Madrid **15** (1973) 201
*Salzman, L.; Kuligowska, E.; Semine, E.*: Pseudoomphalocele: Pitfal in fetal sonography. Am. J. Roentgenol. **146** (1986) 1283
*Sand, H.; Bock, J. E.*: Prenatal diagnosis of soft-tissue malformations by ultrasound and X-ray. Acta Obstet. Gynecol. Scand. **55** (1976) 191
*Santarelli, J.; Duval, C.; Baudelot, J.*: CENT transfusions de sang an foetus. Rev. Franc. Gynéc. **67** (1972) 451
*Sant-Cassia, L. J.; MacPherson, M. B. A.; Tyack, A. J.*: Midtrimester amniocentesis: is it safe? A single centre controlled prospective study of 517 sonsecutive amniocentesis. Br. J. Obstet. Gynecol. **91** (1984) 736
*Savignac, E. M.*: Roentgen amniography: a valuable and safe aid to obstetrical diagnosis. Radiology **60** (1953) 545
*Savignac, E. M.*: The prenatal roentgen diagnosis of fetal hydrops. Am. J. Roentgen. **80** (1958) 673
*Scheuermann, R.*: Amniographie als Methode zur pränatalen Diagnose angeborener Fehlbildungen. In: *Murken, J.-D.; Stengel-Rutkowski, S.* (Herausg.): Pränatale Diagnostik. Stuttgart 1978, S. 135–147
*Schinzel, A.*: Porencephalic cysts as a result of placental damage at amniocentesis? Arch. Dis. Childh. **56** (1981) 405
*Schlensker, K. H.; Citoler, P.; Bolte, A.*: Schwangerschaftsausgang nach Amniozentese. Zur pränatalen Diagnostik genetisch bedingter Defekte. Geburtsh. u. Frauenheilk. **44** (1984) 137
*Schmidt, W.; Gabelmann, J.; Boss, R.; Garoff, L.; Kubli, K.*: Feto-maternale Transfusionen nach Amniocentese in der Frühschwangerschaft – eine Auswertung von 1000 Fällen. Z. Geburtsh. u. Perinat. **184** (1980) 359
*Schreiner, W. E.; Maroni, E.*: Morbus haemolyticus neonatorum. Praenatale Diagnose, Prognose und intrauterine Transfusion an dem schwer erkrankten Fetus. Med. Klin. **64** (1969) 78
*Schwarz, R.; Kyank, H.*: Amniographische Diagnose der Blasenmole. Zent. Bl. Gynäkol. **95** (1973) 145
*Schwarzlos, G.; Stark, K.-H.; During, R.; Hille, M.; Müller, S.; Plesse, R.; Scheunemann, P.; Wilken, H.*: Erfahrungsbericht über 20 Jahre der Anwendung der intrauterinen fetalen Transfusion bei schwerem Rh-bedingten Morbus haemolyticus fetalis. Zent. bl. Gynäkol. **110** (1988) 18
*Sepulveda, W.; Quiroz, V.; Fernandez, R.*: Traumatismo desvasos fetales durante la amniocentesis. Rev. Child. Obstet. Ginecol. **49** (1984) 99
*Shapiro, L. R.; Singer, N.; Mannor, S. M.*: Immediate and unexplained fetal death during midtrimester amniocentesis. Prenat. Diagn. **3** (1983) 151
*Simpson, J. L.; Socol, M. L.; Aladjem, S.; Elias, S.*: Normal fetal growth despite persistent amniotic fluid leckage after tic amniocentesis. Prenat. Diagn. **1** (1981) 277
*Skovbo, P.; Smith-Jensen, S.*: Ultrasonic scanning and fetography at polyhydramnios. Acta Obstet. Gynecol. Scand. **60** (1981) 51
*Spinapolise, R. X.; Wallace, D.; Kennedy, P.*: Fetal distress secondary to fetal vessels perforation after amniocenteses. A case report. J. Reprod. Med. **28** (1983) 551
*Steele, M. W.; Breg, W. R. jr.*: Chromosome analysis of human amniotic fluid cells. Lancet **1** (1966) 383
*Stock, J. R.*: Fetal death secondary to needle laceration during 2nd trimester amniocentesis: a case report. Prenat. Diagn. **2** (1982) 133
*Storm, W.*: Transitorische Hypothyreose des Neugeborenen nach Amniofetographie mit jodhaltigem Kontrastmittel. Geburtsh. u. Frauenheilk. **46** (1986) 185
*Stubbe, P.; Heidemann, P.; Schurnbrand, P.; Ulbrich, R.*: Transient congenital hypothyroidism after amniofetography. Eur. J. Pediatr. **135** (1980) 97
*Sutter, J.; Arab, H.; Manning, F. A.*: Monamniotic twinning: Antenatal diagnosis and management. Am. J. Obstet. Gynecol. **155** (1986) 836
*Suzumori, K.; Yoshiaki, Y.*: Diagnosis of human fetal abnormalities by fetography. Teratology **12** (1975) 303
*Szendi, B.*: Weitere Aufklärung der Morphologie und Biologie des schwangeren Uterus und des Fetallebens mittels Röntgenuntersuchungen (Embryographie). Arch. Gynäk. **170** (1940) 429

*Tabsh, K. M.; Lebherz, T. B.; Grandall, B. F.:* Risk of prophylactic anti-D-immunglobulin after second trimester amniocentesis. A. J. Obstet. Gynecol. **149** (1984) 225

*Talledo, E. O.:* Further experience with amniography in fetal death in utero. South Med. J. **61** (1968) 101

*Tetti, A.; Barbanti, A.:* Possibilitá diagnostiche dell'amniosgrafia. Radiol. med. (Torino) **44** (1958) 929 – Ber. Gynäk. **68** (1959) 154

*Therkelson, A. J.; Rehder, H.:* Intestinal atresia caused by second trimester Amniocentesis. Case report. Br. J. Obstet. Gynaecol. **88** (1981) 559

*Thomsen, S. G.; Isager-Sally, L.; Lange, A. P.; Saurbrey, N.; Grouvall, S.; Schiller, V.:* Elevated maternal serum alphafetoprotein caused by midtrimester amniocentesis: a prognostic factor. Obstet. Gynecol. **62** (1983) 297

*Torres, H. A.; Pelegrina, I. A.:* Transabdominal intrauterine contrast medium injection. An aid in the early diagnosis of hydatidiform mole. Am. J. Obstet. Gynecol. **94** (1966) 936

*Utiger, R. D.:* The diverse effects of jodide on thyroid function. N. Engl. J. Med. **287** (1972) 562

*Utzuki, A.; Hashidzume, H.:* Über die röntgenologische Darstellung der Körperoberfläche des Feten in utero mit besonderer Berücksichtigung von Mißbildungen und von Totenzeichen. Zbl. Gynäkol. **65** (1941) 194

*Uzeta, H.:* Rev. Cir. (Mexico) **3** (1935) 309

*Vago, T.; Charkin, J.:* Extramembranous pregnancy: An unusual complication of amniocentesis. Am. J. Obstet. Gynecol. **137** (1980) 511

*Verjaal, M.; Leschot, N. J.; Treffers, P. E.:* Risk of amniocentesis and laboratory findings in a series of 1500 prenatal diagnosis. Prenat. Diagn. **1** (1981) 173

*Vincenzoni, M.; Bellati, U.; Morici, A.; Baldelli, S.:* Vantaggi dell'amniografia con mezzo di contrasto liposolubile. Ann. Radiol. diagn. (Bologna) **45** (1975) 343

*Waldi, N. J.; Terzian, E.; Vickers, P. A.; Weatherhall, J. A.:* Congenital talipes and hip malformation in relation to amniocentesis: a case-control study. Lancet **2** (8344) (1983) 246

*Weise, W.; Gabriel, D.:* Pränatale Diagnostik genetischer Defekte mittels Chromosomenanalyse, Alpha-Fetoproteinbestimmung, Amniofetographie und Fetoskopie. Dtsch. Ges.-wesen **38** (1983) 2034

*Weise, W.; Gabriel, D.:* Erfahrungsbericht über 8 Jahre pränatale Diagnostik genetischer Defekte. Zent. Bl. Gynäkol. **106** (1984) 216

*Weise, W.; Quent, P.:* Infertilitätsrisiko nach Feto- und Amniographie. Zbl. Gynäkol. **101** (1979) 1239

*Weiss, R. R.; Macri, J. N.; Balsam, D.:* Amniography in the prenatal diagnosis of neural tube defects. Obstet. Gynecol. **51** (1978a) 299

*Weiss, R. R.; Balsam, D.; Macri, J. N.:* Neural tube defects. Obstet. Gynecol. **52** (1978b) 510

*Wiesenhaan, P. F.:* Fetography. Am. J. Obstet. Gynecol. **113** (1972) 819

*Witkowski, R.; Bollmann, R.; Natho, W.; Abét, L.; Zieger, U.; Weber, K.; Losanova, T.; Schaldach, K. P.; Ukrow, S.; Schilling, H.; Zienert, A.; Kohl, G.:* Homozygote Translokation der Chromosomen 13 und 14 bei einem Feten mit partiellem gefäßbedingten Riesenwuchs und weiteren Fehlbildungen. Z. Klin. Med. **43** (1988) 549

*Wurster, K. G.; Roemer, V. M.; Decker, K.; Hirsch, H. A.:* Amnioninfektionssyndrom nach Amniozentese. Ein kasuistischer Beitrag. Geburtsh. u. Frauenheilk. **42** (1982) 676

*Ye, L.:* Amniography in the diagnosis of hydatiform mole (a report of 7 cases). Chúng Hua Fang She Hsueh Tsa Chih **15** (1981) 298

*Yeast, J. D.; Garite, T. J.; Darchester, W.:* The risks of amniocentesis in the management of premature rupture of the membranes. Am. J. Obstet. Gynecol. **149** (1984) 505

*Youroukos, S.; Papadelis, F.; Matsaniotis, N.:* Porencephalic cysts after amniocentesis. Arch. Dis. Childh. **55** (1980) 814

*Zakut, H.; Lotan, M.; Achiron, R.:* Umbilical cord damage and placental abruption during amniocentesis. Acta Obstet. Gynecol. Scand. **63** (1984) 279

*Zanke, S.:* Amniofetographie. In: Aktuelle Probleme der Geburtsmedizin. Ed. by: Krause, W., VEB Georg Thieme, Leipzig 1983, p. 60

*Zaron, D. N.; Imlolean, Y.; Zaron, G. S.:* The radiographic diagnosis of molar pregnancy. Report on three patients. Obstet. Gynecol. **35** (1970) 89

*Zhu, X. G.:* Report on 12 cases of amniofetography and fetography. Chúng Hua Fu Chan Ko Tsa Chih **16** (1981) 26

# 12.

## Subject Index

**Key of numerals denoting normal findings**

1. Head
2. Face
3. Ear
4. Nape
5. Hair
6. Shoulder
7. Vertebral column
8. Abdomen
9. Stomach
10. Small intestine
11. Colon
12. Rectum
13. Scrotum

13a. Penis

14. Labia
15. Insertion of umbilical cord
16. Umbilical cord
17. Upper arm
18. Forearm
19. Hand
20. Thigh
21. Lower leg
22. Foot
23. Intra-amniotic free lipiodol
24. Iliac bone
25. Ribs
26. Renal pelvis of mother
27. Urinary bladder of mother

Bei Fragen zur Produktsicherheit wenden Sie sich bitte an:
If you have any questions regarding product safety,
please contact:

Walter de Gruyter GmbH
Genthiner Straße 13
10785 Berlin
productsafety@degruyterbrill.com